Human frontiers, environments and disease

This compelling account charts the relentless trajectory of humankind and its changing survival patterns across time and landscape, from when our ancestors roamed the African savannah to today's populous, industrialised, globalising world. This expansion of human frontiers – geographic, climatic, cultural and technological – has entailed many setbacks from disease, famine and depleted resources. The changes in human ecology due to agrarianism, industrialisation, fertility control, social modernisation, urbanisation and modern lifestyles have profoundly affected patterns of health and disease. Today, while life expectancies rise, Earth's ecosystems are being disrupted by the combined weight of population size and intensive consumption. The resultant climate change, stratospheric ozone depletion, loss of biodiversity and other environmental changes pose risks to human health, perhaps survival. Recognising how population health, long term, depends on environmental conditions, can we achieve a transition to sustainability?

Whilst the canvas that Tony McMichael covers is vast, the detail he brings to bear on this immense subject is both illuminating and dramatic. This account succeeds on many levels: as a chronicle of human colonisation and environmental impact; as a description of how recent technological changes have induced mismatches between our biological needs and our ways of living; and as an analysis of our rapidly changing demographic and social profile and its environmental and health consequences. As Tony McMichael argues in the Preface, 'Humankind is now treading heavily upon the Earth. We have greatly increased the size of our "ecological footprint". As we perturb Earth's life-support systems, so we endanger the prospects for human population health and survival. The trail cannot continue much longer with footprints like these.'

Tony (A.J.) McMichael is Professor of Epidemiology, London School of Hygiene and Tropical Medicine. He has held positions in Australia, USA and UK, and has taught widely in Asia, Africa and Europe. He has advised WHO, UNEP, the World Bank and Intergovernmental Panel on Climate Change on dietary, environmental and climatic influences on health. He has enthusiasms for palaeoanthropology and social history. His previous book published by Cambridge University Press in 1993 was *Planetary Overload* (ISBN 0 521 55871 9), a widely acclaimed and influential account of global environmental change and health of the human species.

Human frontiers,

environments
and disease

Past patterns, uncertain futures

Tony McMichael

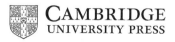

CAMBRIDGE
UNIVERSITY PRESS

CAMBRIDGE UNIVERSITY PRESS
Cambridge, New York, Melbourne, Madrid, Cape Town, Singapore,
São Paulo, Delhi, Dubai, Tokyo, Mexico City

Cambridge University Press
The Edinburgh Building, Cambridge CB2 8RU, UK

Published in the United States of America by Cambridge University Press, New York

www.cambridge.org
Information on this title: www.cambridge.org/9780521803113

First published 2001
Reprinted 2003

A catalogue record for this publication is available from the British Library

ISBN 978-0-521-80311-3 Hardback
ISBN 978-0-521-00494-7 Paperback

Some comments on *Human frontiers, environments and disease*

'This impressive book by an eminent public health scientist explores our most important relationship: our interaction with the environment. It is essential reading for all concerned with assuring future human health – and our very survival.'

   Robert Beaglehole *Professor of Community Health, University of Auckland*

'This book achieves an unusual and important synthesis of the large-scale evolutionary, social and environmental influences on human health and survival. This ecological perspective, highlighting the history of disease and wellness, the state of our epidemiological environment, and the general impacts of recent cultural trends on well-being, is essential if we are to achieve a sustainable future.'

   Paul R. Ehrlich *Bing Professor of Population Studies, Stanford University, and author of 'Human Natures'*

'*Human Frontiers, Environments and Disease* is an innovative and constructive analysis of a problem fundamental to mankind, past, present and future. No one concerned with the bio-medical prospects of the human race could fail to find Professor McMichael's accomplished account thought-provoking and eye-opening.'

   Roy Porter *The Wellcome Trust Centre for the History of Medicine at University College London*

'This is a splendidly written book – a revelation about human health over the millennia. From yellow fever to hypertension it underscores the larger framework of environment-health links. We will be better able to handle the future if more people read this insightful book.'

   Thomas E. Lovejoy *Smithsonian Institution, Washington, DC*

'Today, worldwide, most people live longer and are better fed than ever before. These benefits, however, have environmental and other costs. Tony McMichael's book gives a well organised and wide ranging account of this human story and of its ecological underpinnings. The book concludes with a clear-eyed analysis of current threats to sustainability.'

   Sir Robert May *President, The Royal Society*

To Judith

for lives shared

Contents

Sources for illustrations

Preface

Human life expectancy, in the space of a mere century or so, has become much longer than ever before. This primarily reflects the improved social and physical conditions of living, along with the strengthening of civil institutions; circumstances which, in particular, have greatly diminished childhood deaths from infection and malnutrition. We have thus partially reined in two of the four biblical Horsemen of the Apocalypse: *Famine* and *Pestilence* on their black and pale horses, respectively.[1] Meanwhile, the other two Horsemen, *War* and *Conquest*, still roam menacingly on their red and white steeds.

Warfare continues. The recent conflicts in Kosovo, Chechnya and Sierra Leone testify to the destructiveness of modern firepower and the attendant toll in civilian casualties. Conquest persists, albeit mostly in modern commercial guise, reflecting aspects of economic globalisation and deregulated trade. The ascendancy of free markets, while conferring some health gains via material improvements and the restoration of dietary diversity, adversely affects the health of many vulnerable populations. Our modern economic system has widened the rich–poor gap and, in many settings, has weakened social institutions, eroded environmental conditions, fostered exploitative labour practices and displaced peasant farmers onto more marginal land. Meanwhile, in the world's expanding cities, commercial pressures promote cigarette smoking, automobile dependency and the consumption of energy-dense processed foods.

The profile of human health remains mixed.[2] The health of the wealthy and fortunate continues to exceed that of the poor and disadvantaged, both between and within countries. New diseases emerge alongside the old as societies change, as urbanisation proceeds, and as life expectancy rises. Further, we face various unfamiliar large-scale risks to health.[3] Changes in human demography and mobility, and heightened environmental disruption, have contributed to increases in both new and resurgent infectious diseases. Meanwhile, nature's food-producing resources and fresh-water supplies, now under great pressure, must somehow suffice for a world population that has rising material expectations and is likely to increase from 6 billion to 9 billion by 2050. More generally, the increasing impact of human economic activity on Earth's atmosphere, oceans, topsoil and biodiversity is weakening the planet's life-support systems, changing the climate, and thereby casting a long shadow over humankind's future prospects.

Even so, our health indices are generally improving. Infant mortality has fallen markedly in most populations in response to gains in nutrition, female literacy, family planning, sanitation and vaccination. Modern medicine is increasingly able to defer death, if not always to maintain or restore good health. Epidemiologists continue to whittle away at identifying the factors that contribute to the causation of each specific disease, thereby facilitating its prevention. Meanwhile, on the horizon looms the prospect of disease prevention or alleviation by genetic engineering.

How can we explain this seeming paradox of extended life expectancy in an increasingly environmentally stressed world? Optimists might argue that our improved social institutions and technological capacities can more than compensate for this 'external' environmental decline. Meanwhile, ecologically attuned scientists suspect that we have achieved better population health substantially via material advances that have eroded natural environmental capital – that, in Tim Flannery's words, we have been 'future eaters'.[4] In all other species, sustained population health depends on the continuation of natural processes that yield energy, nutrients and fresh water. This life-supporting 'dividend' from nature is consumed on a recurrent basis, leaving nature's capital stock essentially intact. Human populations, however, have become increasingly dependent upon consuming that natural capital, a process that has now culminated in unprecedented global environmental changes. Those changes pose risks to the health of future generations.

We can understand the significance of these emerging large-scale influences on human health best within an ecological framework. Such a framework elucidates the evolutionary, historical and cultural dimensions of the patterns of human health, disease and survival. We forfeit much understanding of the determinants of health and disease *unless* we can stand back and consider how the changing conditions of life, the collective experiences of whole populations over time, shape the larger patterns of health and survival. This means extending beyond the recent focus of epidemiologists on an individual-based 'biographical' account of disease risk – that is, a risk that is the product of itemised personal behaviours, exposures and biomedical characteristics. Rather, we should apply a more integrative approach of a kind that, during the twentieth century, was largely overshadowed by the reductionist ideas inherent in the classic germ theory and the ensuing biomedical model; an approach which must now engage with the often naive determinism of 'post-genome' molecular genetics.

THERE ARE THREE distinctive, yet inter-related, features in this long history of the changing patterns of human ecology and disease. They are: (i) the encountering by human societies, over time, of many new environmental hazards; (ii) the recurring tensions between changes in living conditions and the needs and capacities of human biology; and (iii) in recent times, the impacts upon patterns of health and disease of population ageing and urban living. These important transitions each deserve a few more introductory words. They encapsulate the unusual, evolving experiences of health and disease in a uniquely dominant, environmentally invasive, species.

First, human populations have colonised, adapted to and ultimately changed many of the world's regional environments. As our *Homo sapiens* forebears dispersed out of Africa from around 80,000 years ago, they encountered unfamiliar types of infections, foods and physical hazards. The particularities of those environments induced cultural and, in some cases, genetic adaptations. Social and technological adaptation has been the real key to global colonisation, enabling humans to increase the 'carrying capacity' of local environments. These changes in human ecology and living conditions also changed the spectrum of diseases. Agriculture and settled living, originating a brief 10,000 years ago, increased the local food yield. As staples came to predominate, agrarianism reduced the range of dietary nutrients and incurred risks of occasional famines. Settled human living, in close proximity with livestock, created unprecedented new ecological opportunities for microbes to adapt to and colonise humans. Hence the emergence of measles, smallpox, tuberculosis and so on. Subsequently, military, commercial and colonial contacts amplified the spread of these infectious diseases. Much later, industrialisation brought new material wealth, various localised environmental hazards, occupational diseases, and the health impacts of modern transport systems. The subsequent generalisation of more 'affluent' ways of living within developed countries consolidated the health gains that had followed the retreat of infectious epidemics – but at the price of acquiring various chronic noncommunicable diseases of late adulthood, particularly those associated with dietary imbalances, physical inactivity and tobacco. Heart disease, peaking in late twentieth century, became the hallmark of modern Western societies, even as infectious disease continued to account for almost half the deaths in the world's poorest populations.

Second, the increasing rapidity and intensity of technological change, urbanisation, material consumption and migration in recent centuries has heightened various mismatches between the biological attributes of humans and their living environment. Some of these mismatches influence the occurrence of particular diseases. For example, the advent of abundant energy-dense foods in increasingly physically inactive urban populations, and the resultant obesity, is causing a worldwide surge in diabetes. The sickle-cell trait in African Americans no longer confers benefit in the absence of malaria, but it does cause pain and suffering. Skin cancer rates are greatly elevated in fair-skinned people of northern European ancestry living now at more sun-exposed latitudes in Australia, New Zealand and the southern USA.

Third, the human demographic profile is now changing dramatically as numbers increase, as urbanisation gathers pace, and as life expectancy extends well beyond our reproductive years. We will thus incur considerably more chronic disability and disease than occurs in other animal species, most of whose members do not survive beyond middle adulthood. We face a social future in which a much greater proportion of the population is elderly, and in which patterns of community and family support differ markedly from historical traditions.

On the horizon, meanwhile, are two other momentous developments. Each has far-reaching consequences for human population health. At the micro-scale we are revealing, intentionally, nature's molecular secrets; we are learning about our genetic code and beginning to rearrange genetic structures. At the macro-scale, as mentioned above, we are unintentionally overloading Earth's life-supporting systems. We have already modified the social, material and environmental foundations of human health over the past two centuries, much of it for the good. Today, as human intervention in the global environment and its life processes intensifies, we need better understanding of the potential consequences of these ecological disruptions for health and disease. These insights should then guide our search for sustainable ways of living.

IN THIS BOOK I explore the story of how changes in human biology, culture and the surrounding environment have influenced patterns of health and disease over many millennia. I offer a narrative account of the evolution of human biology, society, environmental impact and ways of living and how those have affected patterns of health. The *message* is that the health of populations is primarily a product of ecological circumstance: a product of the interaction of human societies with the wider environment, its various ecosystems and other life-support processes. Within the larger scheme of things, human health and survival depends on our maintaining a functional ecosphere that can continue to support human biological and social needs.

A *metaphor* that illuminates the ecological dimension of human population health is that of our species' 'footprints': our footprints along the trail of bio-history. Four types of footprints lead from our distant past into today's world, and then on into an uncertain future.

First, we have a wonderful reminder of the evolutionary trajectory of our hominid ancestors in the mud-preserved Laetoli footprints. These were the footprints, from 3.5 million years ago, of a little band of three upright-walking australopithecines in the African savannah of Laetoli Gorge, Tanzania. The height of these australopithecines was two-thirds that of modern humans; their brain capacity was one-third of ours. Their toes were still a little curved; they were predominantly vegetarians; their communications probably lacked syntax; and adult sexual pair-bonding may have been tentative and temporary. But here, in these footprints, were pointers to the eventual physical, cognitive and emotional attributes of the hominines, the successors to the australopithecines. These, in retrospect, were footprints wandering into the human future.

Second, as these early hominids responded to local environmental changes and the pressures of competition for food within their African environment, so their biology evolved. The brain enlarged; the anatomy of the gut changed; the metabolic handling of altered diets adapted; and skin, hair, stature and blood-vessel tone were all modulated in response to climatic shifts. Similar genetic adaptation occurred in response to regional diets and, later, the adoption of agrarianism. Successful biological adaptations were preserved in genes, to be passed to future generations. Today, various of those genetic adaptations affect our susceptibility to certain diseases, especially in situations of markedly altered ways of living. Those genetic adaptations are molecular footprints that reach from our past into the present and future.

Third, the capacity for cumulative culture enabled humans to leave their primordial evolutionary patch. From around 80,000 years ago, the modern human species, *Homo sapiens*, spread from Africa to West Asia, then South-Central Asia, Australia, East Asia, Europe, North America and so on. The footprints of this global diaspora remain in many forms: stone tools, fire-hearths and permanently modified local environments. Those are our species' palaeoanthropological footprints across the landscape of time and place.

And what of that future? Humankind is now treading very heavily upon the Earth. We have greatly increased the size of our 'ecological footprint'.[5] We used ten times more energy in the twentieth century than our ancestors used in the previous thousand years.[6] As we perturb Earth's life-support systems, such as the climate system and the stocks of biodiversity, so we endanger the prospects for human population health and survival. The trail cannot continue much longer with footprints like these. Yet we cannot reverse, and need not apologise for, human dominance over other species and the environment at large. Humans, after all, are a part of nature. We are a species that, by evolutionary happenstance, has the unique capacity to transform and control the natural world. But we must find a way of living within the limits of this essentially closed biophysical system, Planet Earth. To this end we must now redirect our wonderfully inventive and versatile brains – to date, the most distinctive product of hominoid evolution. Otherwise the hominid chapter in life's grand evolutionary narrative may end unhappily.

MEANWHILE, and on a happier note, I must acknowledge the many and diverse persons who have directly and indirectly assisted me in writing this book. Various colleagues at the London School of Hygiene and Tropical Medicine have been a rich source of ideas and critical comment. These include in particular Dave Leon, Simon Strickland, Astrid Fletcher, David Bradley, Paul McKeigue, John Cleland, Prakash Shetty, Sari Kovats, Andrew Haines, Virginia Berridge, Andy Hall, Emily Grundy, Pat Doyle, Lucy Pembrey, Chris Curtis and Paul Fine. Other colleagues from outside the School whose ideas and suggestions I have appreciated include John Powles, Kirk Smith, Bill Rees, George Davey Smith, Nancy Krieger, Alistair Woodward, Tord Kjellstrom, Jack Caldwell, Robert Beaglehole, Kris Ebi, Philip McMichael, Neil Pearce, Peter Newman, Ruth Bonita, David Waltner-Toews, Leslie Aiello, Laura Westra, Norman Myers, Paul Ehrlich, David Rapport, Paul Epstein, Steve Kunitz, Paolo Vineis, Jonathan Patz, Pim Martens, Maurice King, Tim White and Colin Butler. My thanks to Phillip Raponi for typing the rather arduous final round of revisions, and to Peter Silver my editor at Cambridge University Press – both for his encouragement and for his understanding that a busy academic life does not permit books to be written by the agreed date, or even soon thereafter. My wife, Judith, immersed in her own writing commitments, has known that it meant much to me to finish this book. We will find more weekend time in future to tread lightly on the countryside.

Disease patterns in human biohistory

We are living through an unprecedented transformation in the pattern of human health, disease and death. There have been many great episodes of pestilence and famine in local populations over the ages, but there has been nothing as global and rapid as the change in the profile of human disease and longevity over the past century or so. For hundreds of thousands of years as hunter-gatherers, and subsequently in agrarian societies, our predecessors had an average life expectancy of approximately 25–30 years. Most of them died from infectious disease, and many died of malnutrition, starvation or physical trauma. A large proportion died in early childhood. Today, for the world as a whole, average life expectancy is approaching the biblical 'three score years and ten', and in some rich countries it has reached 80 years.

Two immediate questions arise. What has caused this radical shift in health profile? Can future health gains be shared more evenly around the world? During the 1990s, the combined burden of premature death and chronic or disabling disease was about four times greater, per 1,000 persons, in sub-Saharan Africa than in the Western world.[1] An even more important question looms in a world that is undergoing rapid social and environmental change: can those gains in population health be sustained? To answer the second and third questions we will need to answer the first question.

Over the past two centuries human ecology has been transformed, albeit very unevenly between rich and poor regions. Little more than a century ago, in Manchester, England, half of all young children died before age five. Subsequently, in much of the world, food supplies, housing, water quality and sanitation have improved; ideas of personal and domestic hygiene and of family planning have spread; and workplaces have become safer. Literacy has increased and social modernisation has occurred. Various public health and medical interventions have arisen: anaesthesia and antiseptic surgery in the second half of the nineteenth century, followed by vaccination, contraception, antibiotics, pesticides and oral rehydration therapy for diarrhoeal disease. Death rates in early childhood, particularly from infectious diseases, have declined markedly, first in Western countries from around mid-nineteenth century and then in low-income countries from the 1920s onwards. Maternal deaths in childbirth have declined. Deaths from adult infectious disease, particularly from tuberculosis, have receded.

As more people survive to older age, and as patterns of living, consuming and environmental exposures change, so noncommunicable diseases such as coronary heart disease, diabetes and cancer have come to dominate. Low-income countries are following in the footsteps of the rich countries (Figure 1.1). An epidemic of obesity now looms in rich countries and in urban middle-class populations elsewhere – even as a similar proportion of the world population continues to be underfed and hungry. The world's three leading causes of disease burden (comprising premature death and disabling disease) in the early 1990s, as assessed by the World Health Organization in 1996, were pneumonia, diarrhoeal disease and perinatal disorders.[1] The three conditions projected to take their place by 2020 were coronary heart disease, mental depression and road traffic accidents. Even so, the human immune-deficiency disease, HIV/AIDS, had moved rapidly into second position by 1999, after pneumonia.

Most of this transformation in population health has resulted from broad social changes, from radical shifts in human ecology. Even so, most health-related research continues to focus on specific behavioural, clinical and technological interventions. That, of course, is the style of mainstream science, which deals with discrete, measurable and manipulable units. It also reflects the difficulty we have in seeing the larger picture, in recognising that a population's profile of health and disease is essentially an expression of its social and physical environments. That is, it is an 'ecological' characteristic that reflects the population's collective experiences and way of life. In early 2000, Britain's Labour government announced a national initiative for the *prevention* of heart disease deaths. Along with a familiar 'quit smoking' campaign came an ill-conceived strategy that gave precedence to quicker treatment of heart attack cases (including placing life-saving defibrillators in public venues), training more heart surgeons and more effective prescribing of drugs. Little attention was given to modifying the nation's heart-unfriendly diet, or to changing transport systems and physical activity patterns in order to counter the rise in obesity and its associated metabolic disorders and high blood pressure. The 'Mediterranean diet' keeps heart disease rates low in Greece and Italy. The greater reliance on public transport, cycling and walking has slowed the rise of obesity in the Netherlands. British surgeons at the ready will achieve little in the way of actual prevention (but may, of course, win votes).

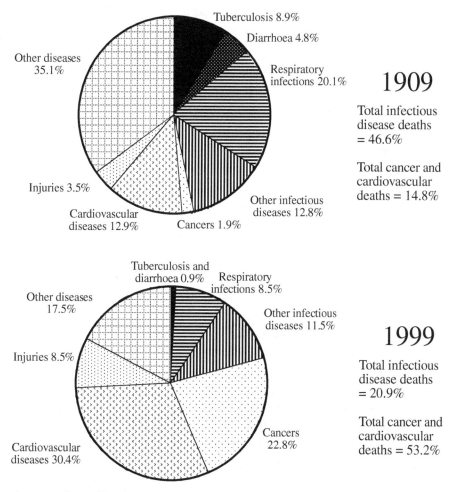

Figure 1.1   Change in the profile of causes of death in Chile between 1909 and 1999. Note the marked reduction in deaths from infectious diseases, and the rise in noncommunicable diseases, especially cardiovascular disease.

Our awareness of these larger influences on health and disease, reflecting the population's relationships with both the natural world and other populations and its own history and internal social structures, ought to have increased in recent years. Various recent developments have underscored this ecological dimension – including, for example, evidence of the health hazards of intensified food production, of the adverse impacts of increased climatic instability attributable to global warming, and of the many social and environmental influences on the emergence and spread of infectious diseases.

A grim reminder of the power of social change to alter patterns of population health comes from HIV/AIDS. Both the origins and the spread of this infectious disease, first identified in the early 1980s, reflect aspects of human ecology. These include: the initial contact with chimpanzee or monkey sources of a human-compatible strain of the ancestral simian virus, the amplified local spread in humans via rural–urban migration in Africa, long-distance dissemination via movements of tourists and military mercenaries, patterns of sexuality and intravenous drug use, and (especially in Africa) the roles of poverty, political denial and the subordination of women. HIV/AIDS may well become numerically the greatest epidemic scourge in human history. Currently there are 40 million infected persons; two-thirds of them are in Africa.

MEANWHILE, NEW large-scale influences on population health are emerging. The future patterns of disease will be much affected by the rapid increase in the proportion of older people, the worldwide process of urbanisation, gains (unequally shared) in affluence and its associated patterns of consumption, and new genetic technologies. The advent of unprecedented global environmental changes, especially human-induced climate change, stratospheric ozone depletion, biodiversity loss and the depletion of fertile soils and fresh water supplies, will have a range of adverse effects on human health. The prospects for human health are being further affected by the processes of globalisation, especially the liberalisation of production, trade and investment with its often inadvertent collateral damage to economic equity, social wellbeing, labour standards, environmental resources and human health.

Patterns of health and disease in the twenty-first century will differ greatly from those of previous centuries. In Western societies, deaths from infectious disease dominated in 1900 and those from heart disease and cancer dominated in 2000. What will dominate in 2100? We are entering a new phase of human ecology as we restructure our relationships with the natural world, convert the global village into a global supermarket, and accelerate the through-traffic of materials, money, people, microbes, information and ideas. The 1.5 billion humans of 1900 will have become 8–9 billion by 2050. We may yet face adversity and crisis as a result of unconstrained climate change and deterioration in the vitality of the planet. There is great uncertainty about these unfamiliar 'futures' – and, as yet, little experience in seeking effective international solutions.

Over the next few decades, life expectancies will probably continue their historically unprecedented rise, especially in low-income countries. However,

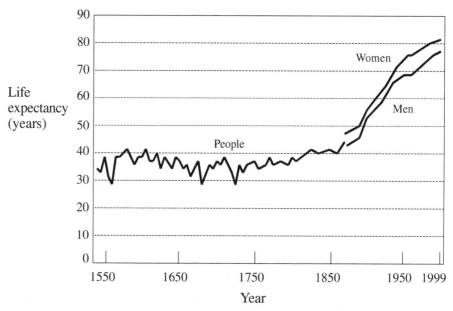

Figure 1.2 Gains in life expectancy in England and Wales over the past two centuries. Social, economic and climatic conditions deteriorated during the seventeenth century. From around 1750 there was a gradual rise in average life expectancy, accelerating after 1850. Much of that rise reflected the decline in infant and child deaths.

if the HIV/AIDS pandemic intensifies, then life expectancies will decline in afflicted countries as they have already done in many sub-Saharan African countries. Globally, the proportion of deaths from infectious diseases will halve from around one-third to one-sixth of total deaths, whereas the proportion due to coronary heart diseases, stroke, cancer and other noncommunicable adult diseases will rise from around one-half to three-quarters.[1] The proportion of deaths from injuries, too, will increase. Malnutrition and unsafe drinking water in the less-developed countries, along with indoor air pollution from cooking and heating in poor households, will remain major killers – even as cigarette smoking, alcohol consumption and dietary excesses cause increasing rates of adult disease and premature death. The burgeoning global tobacco epidemic killed at least 4 million people in 2000. By 2020 it will be killing 10 million per year – that is, about one in every three adult deaths.[1] Diabetes, currently afflicting around 4% of the world's adults, is becoming more prevalent as urban populations everywhere get older and fatter. The widespread decline in traditional family and social supports may contribute to mental depression becoming a major source of chronic health impairment within several decades.

In this changeable world surprising shifts in disease patterns may become more frequent. Life expectancy plummeted in Russia in the early 1990s as social structures and controls dissolved following the collapse of communism. Elsewhere during the 1990s, adult life expectancy fell by at least two years in around 10 other (non-African) countries, including Haiti, Ukraine, Moldova, North Korea and several countries of Central Asia. The newly named variant Creutzfeld-Jakob disease (human 'mad cow disease') appeared unexpectedly in Britain in the mid-1990s, and its future course remains ominously uncertain. For much of the past half-century we imagined that humankind's ancient foe, infectious disease, was in terminal retreat: antibiotics, pesticides, vaccinations, modern sanitation and environmental controls seemed like a winning hand. But then HIV/AIDS emerged and, by the year 2000, was killing over 2 million people annually. Cholera has extended its dominion over the past quarter-century, having embarked on its longest-ever pandemic. Tuberculosis, assisted by HIV, has rebounded. During that same period, the mosquito-borne diseases, malaria and dengue fever, have become resurgent.

So, it is appropriate to stand back from the details and ask big questions about the determinants of population health – and about the sustainability of human health across future generations. The great theme permeating that long-running story is the intimate relationship between environmental circumstances, social conditions, human biology and the occurrence of disease. It is an *ecological* story that reflects the shaping of both human biology and society by environment. It reflects the dependence of human population health upon stocks of natural resources, the functioning of ecosystems, and cohesive social relations.

Disease in history: seeking patterns

The historical record contains many spectacular one-off disease events. One thinks of the great killing epidemics of classical Athens and of Justinian Constantinople; the fourteenth-century Black Death; the Irish potato famine in the 1840s; and the 'Spanish influenza' pandemic that killed around 25 million people in 1918–19. The history of human disease is replete with anecdote and intrigue. Perhaps the Fall of Rome was hastened by lead-induced dementia in the ruling class who stored their wine in lead-lined vessels. The porphyria and resultant intermittent madness of Britain's King George III in the late eighteenth century helped precipitate the fiscal feud that caused the American War of Independence. Smallpox in the seventeenth and eighteenth centuries killed emperors in Japan and Burma and kings and queens in Europe. Beethoven's deafness may have been caused by a markedly raised blood lead concentration (as evidenced in preserved samples of his hair). The Battle of Waterloo may have turned upon Napoleon's haemorrhoids and his resultant sleeplessness.

But those are merely history's eye-catching headlines. The story runs much deeper. It is embedded in the long biological and social evolution of humans and their australopithecine ancestors over the past 5 million years. It is a story of genetic adaptations acquired by globally dispersing hunter-gatherer populations when confronted by unfamiliar local environments. Some of those genetically based traits affect the health of today's populations even though they may now live in environments free of the original hazard. Sickle-cell anaemia in African Americans who are no longer threatened by malaria, and skin cancer in fair-skinned Australians who no longer live under clouded northern European skies are two simple examples. The story is also embedded in human cultural evolution, particularly over the past 10,000 years since agriculture emerged, entailing changes in diet, patterns of infectious diseases, urban living, workplace hazards, and social inequalities. As the scale of human intervention in the natural environment has increased, depleting resources and disrupting ecosystems, so the plot has thickened further.

The scale of real interest, then, is not that of personal haemorrhoids or porphyria. Rather, it lies in the ebb and flow of diseases in whole populations. These are the deeper currents that signify changes in the ecological circumstances of human populations, and which have often affected the course of history. Consider how the warming and climatic instability that followed the end of the last ice age, around 15,000 years ago, induced landscape changes, species dispersals and regional food scarcity that eventually pressed many human groups into growing their own food and herding animals. Consider how the subsequent crowded early villages and towns acted as incubators for novel infectious diseases able to enter human populations from cohabiting animal sources. During the first millennium AD, the repeated ravaging of the Roman Empire and the vast Chinese Han Empire by imported epidemic diseases affected the political map of Eurasia. Later, following the devastating Black Death in Europe, the loss of faith in church and politics contributed to a new social fluidity, scepticism and individualism that potentiated the

Renaissance in Europe and the rise of post-Aristotelian empirical science. With Europe becoming expansionary in trade and conquest, the unwitting reinforcement of adventurous bands of Spanish conquistadors by deadly legions of measles, influenza and smallpox viruses facilitated the conquest of the vast and opulent civilisations of Central and South America. And so the story continues. During the past century, the profile of disease has changed radically, first in Western countries and now in the rest of the world.

We are transient participants in this great, unfinished adventure. Hominids have processed from humble australopithecine origins on the margins of the African savannah several million years ago to today's world, in which modern humans stand, mightily, centre-stage. Central to this unfinished story is the ever-changeable pattern of human health and disease, reflecting the shifts in human ecology and the extent to which our way of life is materially provident, socially equitable and ecologically sustainable. Historical anecdotes make fascinating reading, of course, but it is the larger story at the population level that will assist us to find a sustainable path to the future.

OUR PERCEPTIONS of the causes of disease have evolved rapidly over the past century. Earlier longstanding ideas of divine wrath, astrological conjunctions and non-specific miasmas were replaced in the late nineteenth century by the idea of specific casual agents. That idea arose particularly from the influential germ theory as propounded by Louis Pasteur and Robert Koch. It was reinforced by the elucidation of vitamin deficiency disorders and the identification of particular disease-inducing exposures in the workplace. As the science of genetics evolved; as neo-Darwinism arose in the early twentieth century from the blending of Darwin's theory of evolution with Mendel's theory of inheritance; and as Erwin Schrodinger and others plumbed the mysteries of the nature and origins of life itself, so by mid-twentieth century deeper questions were being asked about human biology and disease. These included questions about the biological ancestry of the human species, about human susceptibility or resistance to agents of disease, and about the social and environmental modulation of disease occurrence.

By the 1960s it became clear that high-income, urbanising populations in the West and Japan had substantially exchanged the ancient burden of infectious diseases for a new set of noncommunicable diseases of later adulthood. The overly simplistic assumption emerged that health and disease were mainly determined by personal behaviours and local environments.[2] With infectious disease seemingly under control and with modern energy-intensive agriculture yielding larger harvests, any sense of dependence on the wider environment had receded. Western epidemiologists led the way in demonstrating the health hazards to individuals of cigarette smoking, of excessive alcohol consumption, of diminished physical activity, and of acquiring high levels of blood pressure and blood cholesterol. Even so, there were other stirrings: there was new talk of 'human ecology', a growing awareness of the insidious hazards to species and ecosystems from DDT and other human-made organic chemicals,[3] accruing evidence of adverse respiratory effects from exposure to a range of urban air pollutants, and, in the 1970s, discussion about the 'limits to growth'.[4] During the 1980s, concerns over human-induced stratospheric ozone depletion and impending global climate change grew stronger. By century's end we could see more clearly that the sheer weight of the human enterprise was increasingly overloading, disrupting and depleting many of Earth's great biophysical systems. Here was a new, potentially serious dimension of risk to human well-being and health.

From this narrative we see that there are probable risks to population health whenever we exceed the capacity of the natural environment to stabilise, absorb, replenish or recycle. Intensifying the production of British beef by feeding cows recycled scraps of other cows, and thus violating nature's food chains, opened up a niche for an infectious agent. If global climate change intensifies the El Niño system, then droughts, tropical hurricanes and floods will increase in many regions. We can gain some perspective on likely future problems by considering some of the large-scale ecological experiences of past civilisations.

A polar bear for a bishop: carrying capacity and survival

The tragic story of Easter Island, one of the world's most remote specks of land in the south-east Pacific, encapsulates the dire consequences for humans of exceeding the natural environmental carrying capacity of a closed system.[5] Having settled the island in about 900 AD, the once thriving Polynesian population, the Rapanui, eventually denuded the island of forest. The trees were needed as rollers for transporting massive stone statues, the poker-faced *moai*, to their ocean lookout posts. Massive soil erosion ensued. Hence wooden canoes for fishing could no longer be built. From an estimated peak population of around 7,000 in the fifteenth century, numbers dwindled, conditions deteriorated, and warfare and cannibalism broke out. When Dutch explorers landed in 1722, there were fewer than 2,000 inhabitants – plus several hundred *moai*. By the nineteenth century, the survivors had dwindled to several hundreds.

A similar but less well known story comes from the other side of the world. The mysterious demise of the West Viking settlement in Greenland in the fourteenth century attests to the vulnerability of human societies to small shifts in environmental conditions if they are already living on the margins of viability. Which of the Four Horsemen of the Apocalypse bore down upon that remote settlement at the limits of European colonialism? Regional climate change, leading to malnutrition and culminating in acute famine, is the most likely.

Global temperatures began rising in the ninth century AD as the Medieval Warm period arrived. The Norse began to expand their settlements around the North Atlantic: from northern Scotland, to the Faroe, Shetland and Orkney Islands, to Iceland and, a hundred years later, to Greenland. The Norse colonisation of Greenland, established around 985 AD and eventually totalling about 4,000 persons, lasted for five centuries. The eastern settlement was initiated by the renegade viking Erik the Red.[6] With a real estate developer's flair and considerable poetic licence, Erik called the great ice-bound continent 'Greenland', to entice further settlers. There were indeed several grassy but treeless fjord-like havens around the south-western coastline. The eastern settlement was towards the southern tip of Greenland, four days sailing westwards from Iceland. The western settlement was 500 kilometres further up the west coast of Greenland, at Godthabsfjord. Each location had sufficient pasture for grazing and for the production of fodder for winter. It was difficult to grow cereals: the climate was cold and the soil was thin. The settlers got by with cows and sheep, along with some goats and pigs. The diet was supplemented with caribou, fish, seal, snow hare and some seasonal berries. Walrus ivory and polar bear skins were exported. Timber, iron nails and corn were imported.

Contemptuous of the primitive Inuit 'skraelings', whom they considered akin to trolls, the colonists learnt little about the wider possibilities for acquiring local foods. Had they, for example, adopted the Inuits' toggling harpoons, they could have hunted harp and ring seals all year round rather than just the harp seals during the warmer months. Indeed, compared to other contemporary Norse settlements in varied environments around Europe, the Greenland settlers displayed an unusual rigidity. They struggled to recreate a little Norseland with unchanged styles of clothing, housing and diet. Later, both the east and west settlements became more fervent in their religious practices. Christianity had only recently arrived in the Scandinavian region, after struggling northwards in Europe during the Dark Ages. The settlements paid their tithes to the Church in walrus tusks. The eastern settlement then petitioned the Norse king to send them a bishop in return for a live polar bear. Since bishops had become plentiful around the royal court in twelfth-century Norway, and since polar bears were a prestigious novelty, the deal was readily concluded. A stone cathedral with stained-glass windows was duly built. Its ruins remain there today. The bishop acceded to high office in the eastern settlement and assumed a large prime farming site for himself. Meanwhile, one presumes, the polar bear dined well in Norway.

In both Iceland and Greenland the settlers changed the landscape. Archaeologists have revealed that a loss of plant cover and extensive soil erosion occurred within several centuries, increasing the sensitivity of the area's pastures and cropland to climate variability. Computer simulations indicate that the western settlement was more vulnerable to the effects of temperature declines than the eastern settlement. Regional temperatures began falling during the fourteenth century and the climate deteriorated, as Europe's Little Ice Age emerged. Records from Iceland indicate an increase in sea-ice during the first half of the fourteenth century. The Inuit were moving south from above the Arctic Circle. The Greenland settlers were increasingly isolated, as sailing became more dangerous. A letter sent by the Pope took five years to be delivered. The western settlement perished mysteriously around 1350, and the larger eastern settlement vanished during the later 1400s.

The final collapse of the western settlement seems to have occurred abruptly. The zoo-archaeological analyses of the remains of animals and insects in association with human habitation are intriguing. In one of several well-preserved houseblocks there is chronologically layered evidence of inhabitants resorting to eating snow-hare and ptarmigan, of slaughtering lambs and young calves, and finally of eating the family dog. Meticulous study of the layers of preserved insects indicates that warm-loving faeces-feeding insects, long present in the inhabited houses, were abruptly succeeded by cold-dwelling carrion-feeding insects.[7] No human remains have been discovered. The fact that the front doors of the houses were left in place provides a clue since, in Norse culture, a family that was deliberately relocating would have at least taken the symbolically carved, spiritually significant, wooden doors with them. All the evidence thus suggests a rapid abandonment as food ran out, in late winter or early spring. Did they desperately board the boats and perish at sea?

Historians have not yet settled the matter. Did the climatic deterioration become irresistible by around 1350? Were there conflicts with the Inuit? Or was there a crippling decline in overseas trade as European consumers switched to high-quality ivory from African elephants in preference to walrus ivory? Recent analyses of Greenland ice-cores show that the extreme of cold in fourteenth-century Greenland occurred in 1349–56.[8] Although these were exactly the years when the Black Death reached Scotland and Scandinavia, there is no evidence of the bubonic plague having reached either Iceland or Greenland. On the other hand, the marked declines in harp seal and cod populations that occurred more recently in the region during the slight northern hemisphere cooling of 1950–75 indicate just how vulnerable the marine food yield would have been to the fourteenth century cooling. With the climate closing in on them, with their limited pastoral land degraded and with a limited repertoire of food sources, it seems likely that the balance of health, nutrition and survival was finally tipped against the West Vikings.

THE STORY of the West Vikings, like that of the Easter Islanders, may seem a rather extreme example. However, there are many other examples where human societies have pushed at the margins of environmental 'carrying capacity', leaving no buffering against the ever-present possibility of climatic-environmental reversals. An early example is the decimation of settlements along the River Nile 12,000 years ago as post-ice-age climatic fluctuations disrupted river flooding and vegetation patterns, causing violent inter-settlement conflict that is evident in fractured and shattered skeletal remains. Eight thousand years later a similar disaster occurred, when a prolonged drought brought the Old Kingdom of Egypt to its knees. The Pharaohs of the regrouped Middle Kingdom learnt a lesson, and took greater pains to defend agricultural Egypt against the vicissitudes of the Nile and its annual silt-bearing floods.[9]

After a thousand years of agricultural innovation and urban florescence the Mayan civilisation imploded early in the tenth century AD as a combination of global and regional climate cycles brought severe droughts to Central America. Several centuries later the pueblo-building Anasazi at the eastern fringe of the Colorado Plateau (Northwest New Mexico) disappeared as their tenuous water sources dried up.[9] For many centuries following the warmer and less populous Middle Ages, Europe suffered repeated acute famines during the Little Ice Age (approximately 1450–1850). The last great famines in Europe occurred in the nineteenth century.

These examples underscore the profound dependence of human wellbeing, health and survival upon environmental conditions and natural resources. Serious environmental disruption usually results in deprivation, disease or death typically mediated by pestilence, famine or conflict. Modern urban societies, both distant from and buffered from immediate exposures to most environmental changes, easily forget that a population's health depends crucially upon food supplies, fresh-water availability, local microbial ecology, reliable climatic patterns and shelter. Yet, as we shall see in later chapters, as urban populations expand and as the size of their 'ecological footprint' increases, so the risk increases of seriously exceeding Earth's aggregate carrying capacity.

The long story of human biological evolution, geographic dispersal and social development, and the associated patterns of health and disease, is a story of pushing back environmental limits. Non-human species must cope with local environmental vicissitudes by relying on their evolutionary endowment. Humans, however, have pushed back many environmental limits via spectacular cultural advances: tool-making, language, agriculture, animal husbandry, the harnessing of elemental energy, urban settlement, industrialisation, infection control, molecular biology and telecommunications. To support our growing numbers we have occupied more land and extracted more food and materials. Humankind now accounts for more than one-third of Earth's total photosynthetic product, either by direct and indirect consumption or by alienation of land.[10] Cultural evolution has thus hugely extended our control over diverse environments.

Within the past 80,000 years the anatomically modern species *Homo sapiens* has colonised non-polar habitats all around the world. This ability to migrate into new environments, buffered by cultural adaptation, has exposed human biology to various unfamiliar living conditions. This in turn has caused various genetic adaptations in body shape, skin colour and various metabolic capacities. Not suprisingly, some of these biological adaptations have had health consequences in recent times in populations that have, again, changed their place and style of living. Examples include fair-skinned Celts developing skin cancers in sun-drenched northern Australia, darker skinned South Asians developing vitamin D deficiency in less sunny northern Europe, and lactose-intolerant Asians discomforted by Western-style dairy foods.[11]

Over time, changes in human culture, social arrangements and, more generally, in human ecology have been the dominant influence on population disease profiles and survival. The drive to increase food supplies has frequently resulted in unintended changes in local ecosystems – changes that have usually then rebounded against human wellbeing. For example, when irrigated croplands turn salty, as happened in Mesopotamia 4,000 years ago, or when natural food supplies are over-harvested, then malnutrition and starvation occurs and civilisations may collapse. Inter-community warfare broke out among the Maori in New Zealand several centuries ago over the food pressures caused by wiping out the bonanza of large, flightless, edible moas within half a millennium after settlement.

These experiences tend to be the rule, not the exception. It is a characteristic of humans to seek to control and change the environment. We are what the ecologist Bill Rees calls 'patch disturbers'.[12] Our natural style as hunter-gatherers has been to exploit and deplete local patches, then move on to another. The size of the disrupted patch has increased over time. The early Australian Aborigines, from around 50,000 years ago, gradually transformed the landscape with 'firestick farming' and tropical forest burning which resulted in pine forests and rain-forest being replaced with eucalyptus trees and mallee scrub. Agriculture and forest manipulation by the North American native population extended over one-third of the continent by the fifteenth century. Today, however, the rate of human impact on the environment has increased dramatically and the biosphere is showing the strain.[13] Some types of environmental strain, such as stratospheric ozone depletion, human-induced climate change and accelerating widespread biodiversity losses, we have not previously encountered. We have, too, been careless with food-producing ecosystems on land and at sea, and their future capacity to feed several extra billion people is now in question. If the bruising environmental impact of 6-plus billion humans upon the biosphere persists, we can expect to encounter some larger-scale health setbacks in coming decades.

The ways in which these large-scale changes to our biophysical and social environments can affect patterns of health can best be understood within an ecological framework. First, though, we should try to define 'health'.

What is 'health'?

Defining 'health' is not much easier than defining 'time'. Health, in the non-human natural world, is no more than a means to an end; good biological functioning is a prerequisite to reproductive success. The level of biological functioning is a product of genes, life history and current environment. The genetically based component of reproductive performance is often referred to as Darwinian 'fitness': that is, the individual's innate capacity to contribute his/her particular genes to the population's next generation. In the human species, to complicate matters, reproductive capacity is modulated by cultural and socioeconomic influences. Reproductive 'fitness' is not necessarily the same thing as 'health'. The parental animal that instinctively sacrifices itself to defend its offspring, the bearers of its genes, suffers poor health (serious injury or death) but has high Darwinian fitness.[14] Conversely, a woman who avoids pregnancy may increase her personal health by avoiding the hazards of reproduction, but she reduces her Darwinian fitness. Nevertheless, throughout nature healthier individuals generally have better reproductive potential.[15]

Health can also be addressed as a collective property of a population. Indeed, this book is primarily about the determinants of patterns of health and disease in populations. Since healthy populations tend to out-perform, to out-compete, less healthy populations, let us also look briefly at the extent to which genetically based variation in Darwinian fitness can also be a property of groups. Within 'social' species such as bees, within-group cooperation can increase the average probability of survival and reproduction of individual members. As we shall see later, one particular selection pressure that probably favoured the evolution of the large human brain during the early Pleistocene was the need for greater cooperation in seeking food supplies, including the hunting of animals. A strain of early humans in which the 'cooperation' gene had become prevalent would function better as a group, and they would tend to out-reproduce other less cooperative strains. Nevertheless, much of the selection pressure in relation to that gene would have acted at the individual level: those individuals less able to participate in group activity would have been marginalised in the survival stakes. True group selection is unusual in nature: inter-individual variation yields much quicker changes in gene frequency than does inter-group variation.[16]

The notion of collective health can also be applied to whole ecosystems. Over the past decade the concept of 'ecosystem health' has been paid increasing attention by ecologists.[17] The attributes of ecosystems such as diversity, vigour, internal organisation and resilience are the criteria of healthy systems. Conversely, indices of 'ecological distress' or of reduced 'biological integrity' can help us identify ecosystems that are prone to decline or collapse.

Now, in humans, what is the relationship between good biological function and health? Nature, with its Darwinian agenda, may not be interested in how we feel or look – but we, via consciousness and culture, certainly are. We imbue 'health' with personal and social meaning. We aspire to health, wealth and wisdom, not just as functional means but as desirable ends. Nevertheless, in culturally diverse human societies the preferred form of health as an 'asset' may differ. René Dubos has pointed out that the state of human biological 'adaptedness' to the circumstances of an ancient agrarian society differed from that required by the nineteenth-century industrial revolution, and differs from that required in today's automated age.[18] When hunter-gatherers turned to agriculture, over the course of several thousand difficult years, the fossil record suggests that their health initially deteriorated. They experienced more food shortages and more nutritional deficiencies, their growth was stunted, dental decay and arthritic disease increased, and life expectancy declined a little. Yet, as we shall see in chapter 7, this agrarian transformation of human ecology allowed shorter birth spacing and hence an increase in fertility. Their reproductive 'fitness' thus increased, even as their health apparently decreased. Molecular genetic analyses of European populations show that Middle Eastern farming populations gradually expanded through Europe, overwhelming and replacing the slower-breeding hunter-gatherers.

The interplay between nature and culture, in humans, is well illustrated by the relationship between maternal health and reproductive success. In large-brained humans, the demands of fetal brain development draw upon the pregnant woman's nutritional reserves. Further, in order to enable passage of the large fetal brain, birth in humans occurs at a markedly 'premature' stage relative to non-human primates. Therefore, the adult woman in traditional society must continue to care for and breast-feed the helpless new-born baby for several years. Human reproduction and extended breast-feeding thus takes an unusually great toll on the woman's biological reserves. Traditional cultures have long understood that births need to be sufficiently spaced for a woman's 'vitality' to be preserved and replenished. Hence the wonderfully varied social taboos and within-marriage relations that different cultures use to modulate human conception. In some developing country settings, contraception is used much less to reduce the number of births than to space them. These practices affirm that the woman's health and vitality is both a means and an end – a biological means to successful reproduction and, therefore, a culturally reinforced end that is achieved by deliberate birth spacing.

There are, of course, no guarantees of good health in the natural world. The ceaseless interplay between competing species, groups and individuals; the ubiquity of infection; the vagaries of climate, environment and food supplies; and the presence of physical hazards – these all contribute to the relentless toll of disease, dysfunction and death throughout the plant and animal kingdoms. Nevertheless, within enlightened human society, we aspire to shared good health as an important social goal. Yet, there are inevitable differences in health status between individuals because of genetic susceptibilities and the occurrence of random events. Indeed, as René Dubos reminds us: 'The concept of perfect and positive health is a utopian creation of the human mind. It cannot become reality because man will never be so perfectly adapted to his environment that his life will not involve struggles, failures, and sufferings.'[19] While this utopian idea has inspirational value, he says, it can become a dangerous mirage if its unattainability is forgotten.

Birth, health, disease and death are part of the landscape of life. There are good times and bad times in the ongoing life of all populations as physical circumstances change, as disasters occur, and as natural environmental stocks increase and decline. The interplay between these stocks of resources and the flows of births and deaths determines the population's prospects. To survive, a population must be able to maintain its numbers across generations. To thrive and extend its range, it must be able to increase its numbers and expand into new territory. Expansion can be achieved either by occupying new terrain that meets that species' environmental requirements (of temperature, types of food, etc.) or by adapting to the new environment. Humans, with their omnivorous eating habits and brain-powered cultural ingenuity, are supremely adaptable. The ensuing chapters explore this story of *Homo sapiens* over many millennia as new frontiers have been encountered. But first we should clarify the notion of 'ecology' and its relevance to human health and disease.

Seeking an 'ecological' perspective

The word 'ecology' (from the Greek *oikos*, meaning household) was coined by the German biologist Ernest Haeckel in 1866. Ecology refers to the interconnected relationships between populations of plants and animals and between them and their natural environment. There is an emphasis on integration, interdependency, and feedback processes, all within a systems context. Ecological systems can be studied at different levels of organisation: individual organisms, populations, biotic communities, ecosystems, biomes, the biosphere and the ecosphere. The *biosphere* is that part of our planet where living organisms exist. At its limits it extends 10 kilometres above sea level and 10 kilometres below sea level. It is a thin and discontinuous film over Earth's surface, with a maximum thickness equivalent to no more than two-thousandths of the planet's diameter. The *ecosphere* consists of the biosphere and all of the inanimate systems and processes with which living things interact, such as the climate system, fresh water and oceans.

Ecology is the broadest and most inclusive of the natural sciences. The human dimension of ecology, says the *Oxford Dictionary*, encompasses 'humans' habits, modes of life, and relationships to their surroundings'. To understand the foundations of human ecology requires knowing something of the biological evolution of hominids, that branch of the primate family leading to the *Homo* genus. We must explore how hunter-gatherer social behaviour developed to maximise group wellbeing and survival, perhaps guided by natural selective forces that favoured cooperation and altruism. This perspective highlights the dependence of human groups and societies on the natural world, as the source of food, raw materials and of the many cleansing, recycling and stabilising 'services' of nature.[20] We can also understand from our ancestral past something of the foundations of childhood emotional and cognitive development, including children's fascination with domestic and caged animals, with tree-climbing, and the bedroom fear of nocturnal predators.

Part of the downside of Western science and culture has been the lost sense of human participation in and dependence upon nature. Ideas in Western culture, reaching back to Plato, have posited Man as the pinnacle of creation, the culmination of the Great Chain of Being, the centre of the universe. Ptolemaic astronomy maintained Earth's central position in a cosmos of theologically ordained perfect spheres, circles and epicircles. The corresponding centrality of humankind was essential to the Church's teaching and political power. The flowering of Late Renaissance science proclaimed the power of systematic observation, of reducing a complex real-world whole to researchable parts, of understanding the clockwork-like mechanisms of the world. The seventeenth-century views of Francis Bacon and René Descartes prevailed: empiricism, reductionism and material determinism would yield new understanding and control over nature. Here, at last, was the modern means of realising the Old Testament's exhortation: 'and God said unto them [Adam and Eve]: Be fruitful, and multiply, and replenish the earth, and subdue it; and have dominion over the fish of the sea, and over the fowl of the air, and over every living thing that moveth upon the earth.'[21]

In the realm of astronomy there were some particularly unsettling stirrings in the sixteenth and seventeenth centuries. Copernicus, Galileo and Kepler eroded the ecclesiastically endorsed view of the cosmos. They adduced evidence that the Earth circled the sun; the moon, viewed by telescope, was pockmarked; Jupiter had its own four moons; and planetary orbits were eliptical, not circular. Further crippling challenges to the dogma of a human-centred cosmos followed. Two centuries later, Darwin argued that we and other living creatures were not custom-built by a creator, but were the changeable products of an amoral and dispassionate process of natural selection. The human species was part of this continuing process of biological evolution, with no biblically certifiable birth-date and no guaranteed permanence. Then, early in the twentieth century, Freud (resurrecting a debate from classical Greek philosophy) queried the supremacy of individual free will and rationality.[22] The self-defining and executive decision-taking role of our 'ego', he said, is liable both to subversion by darker ancestral drives from the recesses of the midbrain, the id, and to being overruled by the socially conditioned, higher-minded, superego.

We have therefore passed through the twentieth century knowing that our planet is but a peripheral speck in a vast and violent universe, that there is a certain serendipidity about the origins of the human species and an uncertain future for it, and that human rationality is beset by inner fears, urges, prejudices, inhibitions and the echoes of childhood. We have also learned of the unpredictable and complex nature of the world around us. Newtonian physics suffices to plan moon-shots and to help pedestrians avoid being hit by a bus, but Einstein, Bohr and Heisenberg have shown us the surprising relativities, non-linearities and uncertainties of the cosmic and atomic worlds. Today, we are gaining insights into the phenomena of chaos ('ordered disorder'), complexity, and the self-organising properties of the systems and assemblages of the natural world.[23] We are thus complementing the 'selfish gene' perspective with a clearer understanding that cooperative activity, at various scales and via the realisation of emergent properties, can confer survival advantage.

We are duly acquiring an ecological perspective on humankind within the world at large, as scientists engage increasingly in integrative types of thinking. Yet there is a novel tension in the contemporary situation. At the other extreme of scale, we are unlocking the secrets of life itself. For half a century we have understood the basic genetic code – the four-letter molecular alphabet that comprises four nucleotide bases (designated as A, T, G and C). These, in runs of several thousands, are arrayed on chromosomes as 'genes' – with each triplet of nucleotides coding for a specific amino acid. Each gene thus specifies the assembly of a particular protein (made up of amino acids), and those proteins then do the cell's metabolic work or act as messengers or hormones to influence other cells. We now have the laboratory tools to catalogue the entire genome of an organism. We have begun with yeasts, worms and fruit-flies. Humans, with around 35,000 genes, have approximately two orders of magnitude more genetic material than do protozoan yeast cells and invertebrate organisms. We have now catalogued the full genetic sequence of a 'standard human'. We may next learn to repair genes by correcting molecular 'spelling errors'. We can already transfer whole genes between totally dissimilar species – such as taking the anti-freeze gene from cold-water flounder fish and inserting it into the genome of strawberries to make them frost resistant. Expectantly but nervously, we stand on the brink of a 'post-genome' society in which we face the possibilities of therapeutic cloning, of as-yet-unimagined transgenic organisms, of purpose-built DNA vaccines, of genetic therapy, and of personalised genetic bar-coding that may facilitate a risk-minimising individual lifestyle.

These technological triumphs aside, we are still struggling to come to terms with humankind's place within the biosphere. The idea of 'ecology' remains a relatively novel perspective. Western culture has fostered the illusion of humans as being apart from nature, rather than being a part of nature. Darwin's more egalitarian and ecological view of the human species was readily applied by others to a frankly competitive view of human society. In the ruthless struggle for existence, they said, only the fittest individuals survive to breed. It was Herbert Spencer, not Darwin, who coined the phrase 'survival of the fittest': if nature is red in tooth and claw then 'fitness' in humans must entail conquest, dominance and hierarchical relations. Here were the origins of social Darwinism and of the eugenics movement. The concomitant values of these early twentieth-century ideas were elitist, not egalitarian; they were controlling, not participatory. It has taken us another hundred years to become serious about trying to understand human biology, culture, social relations, health and disease within an ecological framework.

ECOLOGY IS a way of observing and thinking about the complex natural world; it is integrative, not disaggregative. Three decades ago, Paul Shepard, the first academic to be appointed a professor of human ecology, wrote:

> Truly ecological thinking [has] an element of humility which is foreign to our thought, which moves us to silent wonder and glad affirmation. But it offers an essential factor, like a necessary vitamin, to all our engineering and social planning, to our poetry and understanding. There is only one ecology; not a human ecology on one hand and another for the subhuman . . . For us it means seeing the world mosaic from the human vantage without being man-fanatic. We must use it to confront the great philosophical problems of man – transience, meaning, and limitation – without fear.

Shepard's proposition is that the ecological perspective highlights our dependence upon the natural world. It helps us see the limits to human intervention in nature, and the likely consequences of such interventions. In that final sentence he indicates that the human brain and consciousness are the product of biological evolution – and that they mediate a programmed connectedness of the human organism to the natural world.[24] We can thus understand, says Shepard, the inner human needs for contact with wilderness, with animal species and with symbolic place. To depart from the conditions, the rhythms, and the interdependencies of the natural world is both to stunt our own human essence and to risk damaging the environment's life-supporting systems.

For many decades ecology remained a fringe discipline in the life sciences. About 30 years ago, I bought a book entitled *The Subversive Science: Essays Toward an Ecology of Man*.[25] The central message of this mysteriously titled book was that we needed to rethink our ideas about humankind's role within the world at large, in order to regain an ecological perspective on the nature and needs of human biology and society. The subtext was a critique of the consumption-driven, high-throughput, environmentally damaging economy of the industrialised world. In the early 1970s ecology was 'subversive' in its challenge to the scientific-industrial complex and to the economic development orthodoxies of the day. After all, the 1950s and 1960s had been a time of optimistic anticipation of continuing economic growth. Indeed, US President Harry Truman had proclaimed in 1949 that this was to be the 'age of development' – for both 'developed' and 'undeveloped' nations. To assert that humans, too, were subject to ecological interdependence and that there were limits to the ecosphere's capacity to supply, replenish and absorb, particularly under the expanding weight of human numbers and economic activity, was to confront those assumptions.[26] The ecological perspective challenged techno-industrial enthusiasm for such things as controlling nuisance species with pesticides. It challenged the appropriation of vast tracts of space and surface for military and technological ends during the intensive mid-life of the Cold War.

Ecological thinking was also 'subversive' in transcending single scientific disciplines. Ecology is a synthesising science. It embraces the complex interplay between animate and inanimate components; it studies dynamic, non-equilibrial and non-linear natural processes. Ecological ideas necessarily lack the crispness of definition, simplicity of process and precision of measurement that characterise much of the physical and chemical sciences. To an ecologist, the world is neither deterministic nor randomly unpredictable; rather, it is a world of contingent probabilities within mutually adapted, self-ordering systems. Ecologists say to monodisciplinary scientists: give me your parts and we will assemble a greater whole. To many scientists, with their finely honed reductionist skills, these ideas are unfamiliar, unsettling and threatening (as, indeed, they are to most research-funding agencies).

As the twenty-first century dawns, we can hope to become more aware of the need to reconfigure our social and economic values and practices. It is evident that we cannot continue taking gross liberties with the natural world if we wish to sustain its life-supporting capacities for future generations – nor, indeed, if we are serious about seeking a decent life for all members of current generations. With today's technologies it is not even remotely possible that the impending 7, 8, or 10 billion humans could live at the level of consumption and waste creation that exists today in rich countries. Earth is too small. If we do not respond constructively to the ideas of ecology, then we can hardly avoid living in a world of declining natural capital, of persistent poverty for many people, of increasing political tensions, and of increased risks to our health and survival.

Population-level influences on human health

Thinking ecologically about health and disease requires us to consider the circumstances, experiences and dynamics of groups and populations. We know that personal health is influenced by day-to-day circumstances such as exposure to influenza viruses, food-purchasing choices, physical activity, alcohol consumption, sexual indiscretions, and urban air quality. Meanwhile, the health profile of the population at large reflects influences within a larger frame. As the British epidemiologist Geoffrey Rose pointed out in the 1980s, the question 'Why did this particular individual develop disease X?' is fundamentally different from the question 'Why does the population have an unusually high (or low) rate of disease X?'[27] That is, it is one thing to explain the occurrence of individual cases of some particular disease within a population; it is another thing to explain the distinctive *rate* of that disease within the population.

To address that second type of question requires an ecological perspective, an understanding of what has happened to the population at large. Such a perspective illuminates how the experiences of the population, how its changing relationship to its own social history or to the ecosystems upon which it depends, affect the pattern of disease. Examples abound. Breast cancer inci-

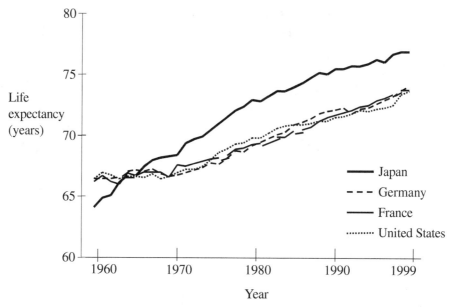

Figure 1.3 Increases in life expectancy in men in Japan and three other developed countries, 1960–99. Note the crossover by Japan in the mid-1960s, with further gains until around 1980, after which the survival advantage of approximately 3 years has persisted.

dence has risen in developed societies as the age of childbearing has been deferred, prolonging the exposure of 'immature' breast tissue to cyclical stimulation by female sex hormones. In mid-twentieth century, the incidence of polio in developed countries rose sharply and in subsequent decades rates of childhood asthma rose. Both rises apparently occurred in response to social modernisation which, via greater domestic hygiene and reduced family size, diminished the normal immune-stimulating exposure to infectious diseases in early childhood. Between 1960 and 1999 life expectancy in Japan increased markedly, starting clearly below European countries and ending above them (see Figure 1.3). Why? The rise occurred despite the fact that smoking rates were increasing rapidly and the traditionally healthy Japanese diet was Westernising. Maybe the adverse health consequences have not yet been fully realised? Meanwhile, Japan's gains in providing health-care were no greater than elsewhere. Was there a generalised beneficial effect of increasing prosperity? Did the egalitarian distribution of personal incomes in Japan foster social cohesion, access to resources and reduced life stress?

These examples suggest that some important health-determining factors operate essentially at the population level. This notion warrants additional exploration at this stage. Whereas the breast cancer, polio and asthma examples can be understood in terms of the impact of the particular shift in human ecology upon individual biology, the Japan example may operate via a more population-based process. Can we elucidate this latter type of factor further?

An interesting example is 'herd immunity'. If, within a population, the proportion of individuals immune to a particular infection is sufficiently large then the infection cannot sustain itself. Herd immunity for measles, for example, occurs when 95% of individuals are immune – in which case the other 5% are spared exposure to the virus. Herd immunity is a type of 'emergent' property of the population; it arises and acts at the group level. You, the individual, cannot have herd immunity. Similarly, among high-income countries with little difference in average personal income, the average life expectancy within each country differs according to how steep the income gradient is within that population.[28] The steeper the gradient the lower the average life expectancy. Of course, the greater the number of poor persons, the more their individual deficits in health status will lower the population's average. But this only explains part of the population's lowered life expectancy. Via some other collective processes at the population level, the income gradient affects material conditions and various psychosocial experiences that influence the population's health profile.

Another example is that of the extra toll of deaths caused by heatwaves in urban populations. At the population level, it is the design of the city – the amount of green space, the orientation to prevailing winds, the size and closeness of buildings, and aspects of building design (such as presence of air conditioning) – that determines how many excess deaths occur during a heatwave. Large cities, as aggregations of concrete, masonry and steel, display a 'heat island effect'. The heat they absorb during the day is released locally at night, thereby depriving inner-city residents of the nocturnal cooling that occurs in leafy suburbs and the countryside. Meanwhile, at the individual level, it is the elderly, the very young, the sick, the frail, and the housebound poor that are the most likely to die during a heatwave. Note, then, that we can ask two quite distinct, complementary, questions: (i) What are the characteristics of the individuals most likely to die during a heatwave? and (ii) What are the characteristics of the urban habitat that affect the death rate during a heatwave? As we shall see in more detail in chapter 9, in the extreme heatwaves of 1976 and 1995 in Britain the excess mortality rate in London was 50% greater than in the country at large, after adjusting for slight urban–rural differences in age composition. Recognition that London is a more hazardous habitat during a heatwave, or that different types of people live in London compared to those living elsewhere, is part of an ecological approach to understanding these variations in the magnitude of the heatwave impact.

None of these examples gainsay the basic fact that, for each affected person within the population, there are specific factors that determine that individual's risk of illness. Rather, the point is that there is another, larger-scale, level of influence on the overall profile of disease within the population. Those macroscopic influences include geographic and environmental influences on human biology and health. The rates of some diseases vary by latitude, for example. Rates of ulcerative colitis, rheumatoid arthritis, multiple sclerosis and some types of congenital anomalies (such as spina bifida) tend to increase with distance from the equator. In contrast, skin cancer rates in fair-skinned populations in Australia and the United States are markedly higher at low latitudes in those countries. Seasonal affective disorder (a recurrent winter depression) occurs most often in colder and less sunlit climes: in Europe, rates are relatively high in Finns and Scandinavians. In the United States, heatwaves cause death rates to rise more in northern urban populations, who are less used to dealing with heat, than in southern populations.

Some such geographic gradients may be explained by differences in cultural behaviours. Coronary heart disease death rates, for example, are generally much lower in the south of Europe than in the north. This may reflect the 'Mediterranean advantage' – the types of food and wine consumed in southern Europe, especially (although this is not certain) the unsaturated vegetable oils and the various antioxidant compounds – in fresh vegetables and red wine. The geographic gradients in many other diseases, however, reflect the influence of external physical environment. The latitude gradient in prostate cancer – one of the most common cancers in men, and increasingly frequent as populations survive to older age – may reflect the geographic gradient in ultraviolet radiation exposure. Sunlight greatly influences production of vitamin D within the skin, and this vitamin appears to stabilise cells in the prostate gland against cancer-prone behaviour.[29]

Within this ecological frame we can also consider the larger-scale environmental disturbances such as the potential impacts of global climate change upon patterns of mosquito-transmitted malaria, or upon local crop yields and hence human nutrition. The relationship between environmental geochemistry and health also fits within this same frame. For example, iodine deficiency in local soils and foods is a widespread and serious health problem around the world.[30] The fact that 1 billion of today's 6 billion people live in iodine-deficient

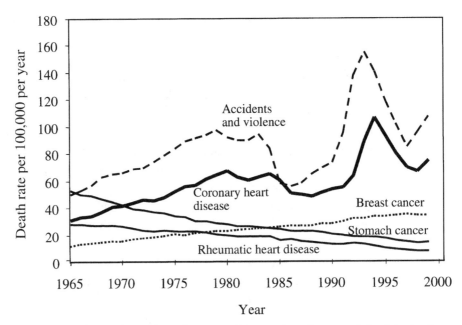

Figure 1.4 Trends in death rates (age-adjusted over time) from selected causes of death in Russian women aged 30–59, 1965–99. Note the decline in deaths from accidents, violence and coronary heart disease following the Gorbachev anti-alcohol campaign – and the surge in those causes of death following the collapse of communism.

local environments, often in mountainous or semi-arid regions of poor countries, reflects again how human populations have pressed against various natural environmental limits. As is discussed further in chapter 5, those populations are at risk of endemic goitre, reproductive failure and cretinism in their children.

On another plane, many influences on patterns of population health arise from the political and economic realms. The collapse of communism in Russia and its Central and Eastern European satellite countries in the late 1980s precipitated a wave of social and economic upheavals and, in some countries, a marked decline in life expectancy. In Poland and the Czech Republic life expectancy increased in the early 1990s, while in Hungary and Bulgaria it did not. Russia experienced something akin to the statistics of civil war – a loss of seven years in male life expectancy between 1989 and 1995.[31,32] Subsequently, Russian life expectancy has recovered some of that lost ground.

The Russian experience is captured in more detail in Figure 1.4, showing death rates in women aged 30–64 between 1970–98. Most remarkable are the very labile graphs for deaths from coronary heart disease, accidents and vio-lence. These show a decline in the late 1980s that apparently reflects the success of Mikhael Gorbachev's anti-alcohol policies, followed by a dramatic rise in the early 1990s as post-revolution economic disorder and loss of social cohe-sion ensued. (Heavy consumption of alcohol has various adverse effects on blood pressure, heart muscle function and blood clotting tendency, which would increase the likelihood of fatal heart attack.[32]) In the meantime, there has been a steady rise in breast cancer (probably reflecting the impact of the progressive deferral of fertility in earlier decades) and a steady decline in both stomach cancer and rheumatic heart disease mortality. Those two declines most probably reflect the lessening of early-life exposure to particular infec-tious bacterial agents (*Helicobacter pylori* and *Streptoccus pneumoniae*, respec-tively) within the Russian population beginning in the second quarter of the twentieth century. The insensitivity of these latter three causes of death to social and economic turmoil is a clear indication that their causation may largely reside in experiences earlier in life.

More fundamentally, poverty is an indisputable root cause of illness and disease. Indeed, in an increasingly unequal world (where the several hundred richest individuals today have a combined income equal to the world's poorest 3 billion people) one must conclude that the global economy is, in some ways, acting to the detriment of the health of large parts of the human population. In later chapters we will look at how patterns of health have been affected by the external imposition of 'structural adjustment' upon developing country economies. There are important, related questions about how the World Trade Organization's promotion of globally deregulated trade and capital investment is affecting gains and losses in the realms of social wellbeing and population health.

Overall, then, human culture, ecological relations, geography, environ-ment and politics all affect the profile of human population health and disease. So, also, do certain variations in genetic predisposition between populations. However, there is relatively little genetic diversity between regional populations or major racial groups.[33] This presumably reflects the fact that ours is a young species with a capacity for cultural adaptation that has greatly buffered the selection pressures of local environments. *Homo sapiens*, with a versatility conferred by its large and complex human brain, is clearly not a niche species. As we shall see in chapter 3, the sheer diversity of environments colonised by humans has resulted in various innate popula-tion differences in morphology, physiology and biochemistry. Some of these, interacting with environmental factors, contribute to the pattern of diseases in today's world.

Conclusion

In closing this chapter we should recognise a seeming contradiction. Life expectancies have been increasing for at least several decades in most countries, rich and poor. Yet simultaneously the ecosphere has come under unprecedented pressures and the stocks of many natural resources have declined. Have humans, extraordinarily, broken free of the constraints of nature and found how to sustain gains in life expectancy even as they disrupt the natural world?

From the nineteenth century, beginning in Western industrialising countries, gains in food sufficiency, sanitation, vaccination, education, the strengthening of civil institutions and democratic processes, and, later, the advent of antibiotics all contributed to lower death rates. These gains arose out of social modernisation, technological advance and wealth accumulation which, in turn, required vast inputs of materials and energy. Forests were cut down, coal was burnt, and arable land was overworked. Material expectations began to rise, mass production led to mass consumption, media advertising converted wants into needs, and eventually leisure became widespread. During this modernising process life expectancy approximately doubled.

In today's rich Western countries, the average personal use of energy is about one hundred times greater than in the world's poorer populations. Further, large amounts of material are consumed and wastes are generated. In the compelling metaphor proposed by Bill Rees, the 'ecological footprint' of industrialised societies is huge.[34] The Netherlands depends on an area of Earth's surface 15 times greater than its own national area to support its way-of-life. This, for the moment, is a subsidy that the world's rich can both afford and obtain. Thus, the populations of rich countries have, in part, attained their historically unprecedented life expectancies by creating wealth from the environmental resources of other less powerful populations or by 'borrowing' against the environmental capital of future generations. Populations in developing countries are, to varying extents, now also doing likewise.

An ecologically literate banker would disapprove of this long-term deficit budgeting. Any business whose 'profitability' depended primarily on borrowings and on the exhaustion of capital would face eventual bankruptcy.

However, with the convenience of orthodox economics, we have blindly 'externalised' most of the actual environmental and social costs of our high-consumption modern lifestyle. We continue to emit vast quantities of greenhouse gases, to commandeer much of the world's cereal crop for meat production, to over-fish the oceans, and to deplete biological diversity. Further, today's mighty surge in population within the Third World will translate, to some extent, into tomorrow's surge in materials and energy consumption.

The technological optimists and cornucopians may claim that we have finally thrown off nature's constraints. There is, they say, nothing misleading in the combination of gains in life expectancy and the accumulation of material wealth. Indeed, this merely continues a recognised historical relationship. The more sobering interpretation, however, is that unless we achieve a transformation of technology and a circular conserver economy, future gains in health and wealth can only be achieved by further consumption and degradation of Earth's natural ecological and physical resources. This is a high-risk strategy in a world that is, in most respects, a closed system.

To understand the forces shaping that future, we can learn much from human history and prehistory. There has been a shifting pattern of human disease and survival over time. Our extant genes, from the survivors of ancient, testing journeys, are the genetic variants that have not been washed from the sands of time by the relentless tides of natural selection. During those ancient journeys and the subsequent evolution and spread of culture we, the dominant species on Earth, have extinguished species, altered landscapes, disseminated infectious agents and other 'pest' species, transplanted crop and livestock species, and, now, begun to change the composition of the world's atmosphere. These genes, journeys and environmental impacts have shaped much of the course of human biology, health and disease.

The following chapters explore the origins and recent patterns of human biology and health. They discuss how human population health and survival depend upon stable and productive ecosystems and cohesive societies. Later chapters explore how our expanding footprints are now leading us into an uncertain future, as we put increasing pressures on our habitat and assume greater control over genetic processes. With an appreciation of the evolutionary basis of human biology and of the dependence of human wellbeing and health on an intact ecosphere, we will be better placed to achieve a sustainable way of living.

2

Human biology: the Pleistocene inheritance

Homo sapiens is the sole survivor in the branching succession of several dozen hominid species. That lineage split off from the ancestral chimpanzee line around 5 million years ago. By 2 million years ago there appear to have been about half a dozen hominid species in Africa. Some were vegetarian australopithecines; others were meat-eating hominines (the early *Homo* genus). Over most of the ensuing period there were always several *Homo* species in existence at any time. Until around 30,000 years ago *Homo sapiens* shared much of Eurasia with its Neanderthal relatives, a separate species. Today, however, all other hominids are extinct. We are the first of the hominid species to exist in isolation. This is a rare situation; natural selection normally fosters within-genus diversity. Our demise would, in a single stroke, eliminate the hominid line from the evolutionary repertoire – along with the hard-won, unique, attributes of complex cerebral consciousness and cumulative culture.

The hominids emerged in response to the profound changes in the cooling, drying climate and environment of eastern and southern Africa as Earth entered the Pliocene epoch, from around 5 million years ago. There were new opportunities for an upright-walking vegetarian primate that could forage in the spreading woodland and savannah, while retreating to the trees in times of danger. Enter the hominids: first the ardipithecines and then, from around 4 million years ago, the australopithecines. Subsequently, some time around 2.3 million years ago as further global cooling occurred, the *Homo* genus appeared. These early humans had distinctive biological and social attributes and a capacity to survive without recourse to the forest. Relative to the australopithecines they had longer legs, smaller jaws and larger brains.

As the local environment and vegetation continued to change there must have been a continuing struggle to find edible and nutritious plant foods, and to avoid their toxins. This search for food in a labile environment may well have contributed to the selection pressures favouring an enlarged hominid brain, along with free and dexterous upper limbs. Other selection pressures would also have acted on the hominids. Life in lightly wooded terrain would have entailed more exposure to the sun; and this would have caused more dehydration, to which heavily-sweating primates are prone. There were the physical perils of bipedalism, as evidenced by the numerous healed long-bone fractures in (more recent) hunter-gatherer skeletons.[1] There was increased on-ground exposure to feline predators. These selection pressures on hominid biology and survival yielded several branches of speciation, featuring different specialisations.

We are not sure of the structure of the hominid family tree. Palaeo-anthropologists repeatedly redraw it as, slowly, more fossils come to light.[2] A handful of fossils exist, stretching over about 2 million years from 4.5 to 2.5 million years ago. Lucy, found in northern Ethiopia, is the most complete, and the most famous, of the few discovered *Australopithecus afarensis* fossil skeletons. She dates from 3.2 million years ago. Fragments of several predecessor hominid species have recently been found in north-east Africa. We know rather more about the *Homo ergaster* and *erectus* species, dating from around 1.7 million years ago, soon after the beginning of the Pleistocene (Figure 2.1). Those two hominid species followed the transitional *Homo habilis*, a primitive stone tool maker, and were the first great out-of-Africa dispersers. They occupied much of Eurasia from about 1.2 million years ago, and the erectines reached Java and northern China around 900,000 years ago.[2] The *Homo* genus was beginning to succeed as a radical new evolutionary experiment.

WE KNOW VIRTUALLY nothing about the health experiences and life expectancy of the early hominids. *Homo erectus* fossils from sites in Africa and Asia indicate an average age of adult death of around 25 years. However, such averages can mislead – the distribution of ages-at-death is strongly skewed towards younger ages. Studies of skeletal remains in more recent hunter-gatherer populations of North and South America indicate that at least half the fully grown individuals died before age 20 years. Extrapolating this to the erectines, in order to maintain numbers quite a few adult females must have survived into their fourth decade and completed a reproductive lifespan in which they bore five to six children.

With their relatively short life expectancy, hunter-gatherers would have had little chance to experience the chronic noncommunicable diseases that dominate our modern lives – heart disease, diabetes, cancer and dementia. Besides, many of those diseases are an expression of a mismatch between human biological inheritance and current way of life. Studies of today's few remaining traditional hunter-gatherer communities reveal a virtual absence of raised

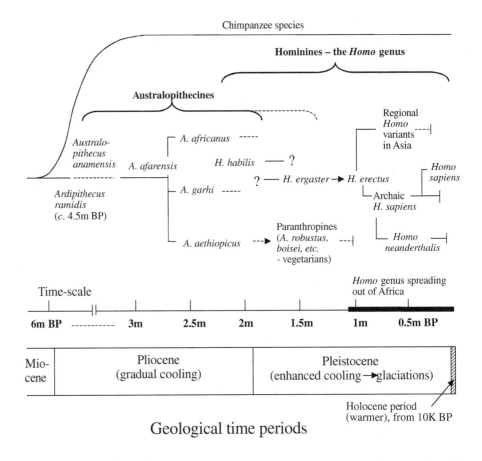

Geological time periods

Figure 2.1 The hominid family tree. This is subject to continuing revision as new finds are made and as fossil features are reexamined. The main storyline, connecting the australopithecines with the hominines, has been elaborated and consolidated over the past three decades. Unusually for a genus, the *Homo* genus today has only one surviving member species: *Homo sapiens*.

Debate persists over the extent to which the evolution of later *Homo* species, especially our own species, occurred in Africa. An enduring minority view asserts that earlier species radiating out of Africa, particularly *Homo erectus*, then evolved in 'multiregional' fashion to yield similar strains of modern humans. On that view, gene flow between regional populations across the Eurasian super-continent ensured continuing genetic overlap. Nevertheless, reply the critics, such convergent biological evolution is implausible – and not evident elsewhere in nature.

Today there is a rapid decline in other species of apes – the chimpanzees, gorillas and orangutans. The human species, by its own actions as deforesters and hunters, may yet end up as the only survivor of the great ape family.

blood pressure, obesity, heart disease and diabetes in middle and late adulthood. This mismatch between our Pleistocene-attuned biology and our current way of life has been amplified over the past century as urban sedentariness, dietary excesses and various socialised addictive behaviours (alcohol consumption and tobacco smoking) have become prominent features of modern human ecology.

Contemporary humans are the inheritors, from the past 2 million years of biological evolution, of what Paul Shepard called humankind's 'wild Pleistocene genome'.[3] *Homo sapiens* and its several predecessor *Homo* species evolved in, and for, their own particular environments. The parsimonious process of natural selection does not provide a species with biological capacity surplus to current circumstances. Its logic is that of adaptive response, not anticipation. We should therefore enquire, for example, how a human biology attuned by the Pleistocene diet to an intake of moderate amounts of plant oils and animal fats, predominantly unsaturated, will cope with an increased and more saturated dietary fat intake.

That issue will be explored in later chapters. The challenge here, while acknowledging the paucity of direct evidence, is to explore how those intensive several million years of hominid evolution left imprints on human biology that affect the probabilities of health and disease today. Now this is not to say that the biological legacy of the Pleistocene is the only source of modern genotype-environment mismatch, and consequent disease, in humans. Bipedalism, for example, dates back over 4 million years, well into the Pliocene. Some resultant features of the human skeleton remain poorly adapted for upright walking. First, the awkwardly curved lower back and the hip and knee joints must now support, on two legs, a body weight originally borne on four legs in combination with a straight, horizontal, backbone. Lower back pain is one of the most prominent causes of disability and lost working days. Vertebral osteoarthritis is evident in prehistoric hunter-gatherers.[4] The frequent damage to footballers' knee-joint ligaments and cartilages reflects a joint that is poorly adapted to the sudden twisting movements of a freed-up upper body. Human biology, from hips to haemoglobin molecules, has an evolutionary lineage that extends back well beyond the Pleistocene.

Before examining the human evolutionary story in more detail it is appropriate to review the natural selection process. That process and its product, biological evolution, underlie all of nature's ecological systems and relationships, upon which we humans depend.

Natural selection

Our planet formed from cosmic debris around 4.5 billion years ago as one of four smaller, solid, inner planets of the solar system. Sometime during the ensuing billion years, self-replicating assemblages of molecules arose. Here were the first stirrings of 'life'. We can never actually be certain how earthly life began. Living forms may even have reached this planet from elsewhere in the cosmos, arriving perhaps as molecular templates or single-cell stowaways embedded deep within impacting asteroids. However, although life on Earth was once thought to have been a freak, perhaps unique, occurrence, the more recent view is that, given a propitious physical and chemical environment, life *will* emerge via the self-organising properties of matter, assemblages and systems.[5]

Over long time, life becomes more complex and more diverse. Charles Darwin's profound insight was that species have evolved principally via natural selection. There is no metaphysical purpose, no implied improvement, in this process of natural selection. The process is the logically inevitable consequence of natural genetic variation within a population when limited environmental resources necessitate competition. The three essential elements of natural selection are variation, competition and differential reproductive success. Those individual organisms with above-average success in survival and reproduction contribute more genes to the population's evolving gene pool than do less successful individuals. Thus do necks become longer, tail-feathers brighter, flowers more colourful, seeds more drought-resistant, bacteria more antibiotic-resistant and early dairy-herders more lactose tolerant. Darwin's Galapagos finches had diverged and then speciated via their adaptation to the varied microenvironments of the individual islands. Occasionally a quantum leap occurs as a genetically distinct sub-set detaches itself from the parent stock, occupies a new niche, and launches a new species. In this way, quite recently, the simian immunodeficiency virus became the human-infecting virus, HIV.

Within any population of plants or animals, individuals vary in their biological functioning and this may affect their reproductive capacity. This biological variation arises from both genetic and environmental causes. In sexually reproducing organisms, genetic variation arises via random mutations to genes in the parental diploid germ-line cells that produce, by meiosis, the haploid sperm and egg cells.[6] Mutated genes that are compatible with survival and reproduction may persist within the population; they are called 'alleles'. The alleles comprise the menu from which natural selection makes its pragmatic choices. The genetically variant individuals that are marginally better attuned to the prevailing environment will reproduce more plentifully.

In nature both sexual and asexual reproduction occur. Bacteria reproduce mostly by asexual reproduction, transmitting entire intact genomes between generations. They must therefore rely on the occurrence of fortuitous gene mutations and on the random acquisition of genes from passing plasmids and other microbes, as the means to achieve biological (phenotypic) variation. Sexual reproduction yields greater phenotypic diversity in offspring because of the random shuffling of parental genes (alleles) that occurs during meiosis, yielding the haploid gametes. The wonder of sexual reproduction is that this mixing of parental genes (strictly, alleles[7]) maximises the diversity of offspring while maintaining stable gene frequencies within the population and allowing every gene an equal opportunity of phenotypic expression. Meiosis thus confers genetic stability and fairness within the population, while producing rich phenotypic diversity upon which natural selection can then act. This, notwithstanding other popular enthusiasms, is the *real* triumph of sex.

This brief description of natural selection implies that, in the natural world, the individual organism is the main locus of reproductive competition and, therefore, of biological evolution. This is discomforting to some people. Talk of 'selfish genes' and of the genetically self-serving basis of 'altruistic' and 'virtuous' behaviour in humans and other animals challenges cherished notions of social obligation and higher moral imperatives.[8] However, there are tantalising new ideas from the realm of 'complexity theory' about the self-organising properties of collectivities. Complexity theory proponents claim that Darwin only told part of the story of biological evolution. They argue that a fundamental property of all assemblages, whether of molecules, genes, cells, organisms or social groups, is to self-organise, to achieve more complex states of order.[5] Collectivities thus have emergent properties that cannot be foreseen from knowledge of the basic unit. Simple examples of emergent properties include mass hysteria and the rippled surface of a wind-swept sandy beach. More grandly, this view leads us to James Lovelock's notion of Earth as a superorganism, Gaia, with self-stabilising properties that arise from the feedback-rich interplay between populations of organisms and their biological and physical environments.[9]

These ideas of self-organising complexity, of emergent properties, are receiving more attention in the realm of ecology. A basic emergent property of complex living assemblages is their capacity to maintain themselves in a non-equilibrial state. That is, living organisms resist the tendency to degrade, to undergo an increase in entropy. These ideas are also beginning to extend the framework of our understanding of life, health and disease. Nevertheless, since they currently depend more on mathematics and computer modelling than on empirical evidence, we will here give greater weight to orthodox Darwinian evolution.

IN ANOTHER SENSE, however, natural selection *is* only part of the story. Over time, other cross-currents can significantly affect population gene frequencies. Most new genetic mutations, even if they affect some anatomical or metabolic characteristic, are actually 'selection neutral' – that is, they confer no advantage and therefore do not affect reproductive success. A process of random genetic drift, however, ensures that some neutral mutations persist and increase within the population while others disappear. Further, there are 'bottlenecking' and 'founder' effects. When groups split off from a large population and initiate a small and physically isolated population (as occurs, for example, when islands are colonised), the sub-set of genes may, by chance, be unrepresentative of the parent population gene pool. These random processes of genetic drift and genetic bottlenecks thus supplement the decidedly non-random process of natural selection.

Genetic bottlenecking is well illustrated by the surprisingly small number of human lineages (as assessed by mitochondrial DNA analyses) that originally radiated out of Africa from around 80,000 years ago, or that colonised Australia around 50,000 years ago and the Americas 30,000–15,000 years ago. Linguistic and molecular genetic analyses indicate, for example, that just three or four extended family groups originally settled arctic North America, drifting across the temporary and chilly land-bridge of Beringia, with at least one of them subsequently radiating further south.

Other genetic bottlenecks occur when population size declines catastrophically. For example, many centuries ago the Ashkenazi Jewish population living in the Baltic region was subjected to murderous persecution. The few hundred survivors, the progenitors of today's Ashkenazi Jews, apparently contained several persons with a rare genetic mutation: the BRCA1. Today the frequency of the BRCA1 cancer gene is about eight times more common in the descendants of that Jewish population than in the general European population, and may account for around one-third of their breast cancers. A similar genetic bottlenecking must have occurred when Iceland was settled, in the ninth century AD, resulting in a greatly elevated frequency of the other major breast cancer gene (BRCA2) in that population. The Finns, descended from a breakaway group of the original Eurasian settlers on the Hungarian plains, have several dozen other minor genetic disorders not found in other populations, and are free of the cystic fibrosis gene.

THE SPEED of biological evolutionary change depends on the generation time of that particular species and on the intensity of the selection pressure. Perceptible genetic change in human populations can occasionally occur over hundreds of years, but it usually takes very much longer. At the other extreme, populations of bacteria, with a generation time measured in hours, can develop antibiotic resistance in a matter of months or years. Staphylococci, streptococci and pneumococci have developed resistance to most of the antibiotics directed at them over the past several decades. The genetically labile HIV virus, dodging attack by immune cells and anti-viral drugs, produces thousands of new genetic variants within an infected person every day. The virus may thus achieve drug resistance within days to weeks.

We may think that the heavy overlay of culture in human societies, conferring protection against early death in some while imposing social inequalities in health on many others, would have slowed and muddied the waters of natural selection. But for most of the approximately 150,000 years existence of *Homo sapiens* only a minority of each generation reached adulthood and managed to transmit their genes to the next generation. Infection, starvation and physical hazard culled the majority, often soon after birth. Wherever infant and childhood mortality rates are that high, then natural selection can operate very strongly. Today's infant mortality rates in wealthy countries, of less than 10 deaths per 1,000 live births, are very recent and unusual.

If there had been much biological evolution since humans dispersed out of Africa, it would be evident mainly as variation between regional populations, reflecting the divergent selection pressures they had encountered. However, only about 10–12% of all human genetic variation is due to differences in gene frequencies *between* regional populations and their major subgroups, whereas almost 90% of the variation is between individuals *within* populations. Relative to many other dispersed species, there is rather little inter-population genetic variation within the human species. During the long ancestral period of *Homo sapiens* in Africa many neutral or biologically unimportant genetic variations (such as ABO blood group) arose. Nevertheless, there is about ten times as much genetic variation in our closest surviving primate relatives, the two species of chimpanzees, as there is in *Homo sapiens.* This is further testimony to the shortness of our existence as the modern human species: a mere 8,000 generations.

Climate, environment and hominid evolution

Prehistory is not merely something that human beings passed through a long time ago: it is something which, properly apprehended, allows us to view our contemporary situation in a perspective more valid than that encouraged by the study of our own parochial histories. (JGD Clark, 1961)[10]

The modern human species, *Homo sapiens*, has spread worldwide, beginning from approximately 80,000 years ago. We are nearly certain that our species originated in Africa, not just because of the accumulated palaeontological evidence but from the increasing weight of molecular genetic evidence.[11] From modest origins in eastern Africa, when the estimated total population of *Homo sapiens* at any one time may have numbered around 50,000, our species has subsequently multiplied 100,000-fold to 6 billion. This huge increase is a remarkable achievement for a single species. With a unique capacity to share, discuss and evaluate experience and to accumulate knowledge, our species has substantially supplemented basic human biology with culture and technology. Hence, humans can survive in a very wide range of environments. In contrast, other species are much more constrained by their biology. For them, nature sets the bounds: they live or die in response to fluctuations in their local environment.

Can we explain the origins of this distinctive capacity, achieved via cognition and cumulative culture, to modify or sidestep many of nature's constraints? Palaeoanthropologists, fortified with new knowledge about ancient trends in world climate, terrain, and tectonic drift, suspect that hominids evolved in response to unusual environmental selection pressures.[2] In particular, the complex human brain may be a product of climate change over the past several million years. Appreciation of this story requires an excursion, first into the long climatic-environmental backdrop to hominid evolution, and then into the emergence of the *Homo* genus.

EARTH IS NOW colder than it has been for several hundred million years. The last great cooling occurred around 250 million years ago, at the end of the Permian era, when the continents coalesced into Pangaea, drifting over the southern polar region. The resulting change in global climatic dynamics caused a great refrigeration that extinguished nine-tenths of life forms. That great natural extinction, the third of five that have occurred since the advent of vertebrate life a half-billion years ago, created vast new openings for the emerging reptile and dinosaur families in the much warmer Triassic and

Jurassic periods. Then just 45 million years later, the fourth great extinction episode occurred. Located in time between the Triassic and Jurassic, it was probably caused by several million years of global heating as tectonic rifting broke up the great single land-mass Pangaea, and the resultant massive vulcanism released vast amounts of carbon dioxide into the atmosphere. Palaeobotanical research indicates that the concentration of carbon dioxide may have soared four-fold to over 2,000 ppm (compared with the recent pre-industrial concentration of 280 ppm). This probably raised global temperatures by around 4 °C.[12] Approximately 95% of plant species are estimated to have died out, along with many of the animal species that depend on them.

Following the fifth great extinction which despatched the dinosaurs 65 million years ago, in a catastrophe that was probably caused by an asteroid impact, Earth underwent a long period of cooling. Isotopic evidence from ancient sediments indicates that this cooling dates from around 40–50 million years ago. That was when the Indian and Asian tectonic plates collided, causing the mighty Himalayan mountain range to begin forming. This, in turn, caused a great increase in regional rainfall from the moisture-laden monsoonal air swirling in from the equatorial Pacific. It is thought that this rain would have washed out much of the atmosphere's main heat-trapping greenhouse gas, carbon dioxide. Meanwhile, the concurrent rise of the North Atlantic ridge in the ocean floor reduced the flow of warm ('Gulf Stream') Atlantic water into the Arctic ocean, thus causing northern polar cooling. Palaeoclimatologists think that both these massive regional processes contributed to a prolonged era of global cooling. By 20 million years ago Antarctica and South America had separated. Around 12 million years ago the great East Antarctic ice sheet began to form, followed 6 million years ago by the West Antarctic ice sheet. (It is that latter ice sheet that is at some risk of breaking up and sliding into the ocean should global warming continue for several centuries. That would raise the sea level by around 6 metres.)

The dessication of equatorial regions associated with cooling and polar ice formation caused the eastern African terrain to change. Open woodland and savannah began to replace forest, and around 6 million years ago an ecological niche opened up for an ape able to survive mostly out of the forest. But life on the open ground, and with a somewhat unfamiliar plant food supply in a climatically varying world, was probably precarious for the early ape-like hominids.

In 1871 Darwin made the famously controversial proposition, in *The Descent of Man*, that humans were descended from apes. One Victorian lady is reputed to have confided to a friend: 'My dear, I pray that it is not true, but if it is true, I pray it will not become widely known.' Many eminent biologists of the day took comfort from the assumption that the initial divergence must have occurred tens of millions of years ago, in the early Miocene. This allowed a pleasing interval to separate the God-fearing human species from the grunting ape. However, in the 1960s, the power of 'molecular phylogeny' radically changed these older ideas.[13] Comparison of the molecular structure of the DNA of chimps and humans indicates that the two genuses diverged just 5–6 million years ago. The gorilla line appears to have split off several million years earlier. In terms of genetic proximity, Jared Diamond argues that humans are the 'third chimpanzee', alongside the common chimpanzee and the pygmy (bonobo) chimp.[14] Indeed, early on, there was nothing remarkable about the upright-walking australopithecine foragers. Their numbers were small; their lives were risky. They were *not* 'pre-humans'. They were well adapted, by evolution, to the environmental circumstances of the time.

Meanwhile, Earth continued to cool. This cooling trend steepened from around 2.5 million years ago. It is from this time that the fossil record indicates the emergence of the *Homo* genus from the australopithecine line. Then, around 1 million years ago the world attained a critical threshold temperature. This triggered a succession of glaciations of 50,000 to 100,000 years duration, interspersed with brief interglacial warm periods, over much of Eurasia and North America. Repeatedly, ice-sheets several kilometres thick have blanketed Scandinavia, Britain, northern Europe and Canada, with tundras extending much further south. Indeed, since the most recent of these glaciations began receding from around 15,000 years ago, northern Finland has risen by almost a kilometre, after having been pressed deep into Earth's mantle by a massive ice-sheet during the preceding tens of thousands of years.

During the eight major glaciations of the past million years, *Homo erectus* was beginning to spread throughout Eurasia (see Figure 2.1). The enlarging human brain and its byproduct, primitive culture and stone-tool and firestick technology, were gradually opening new doors to the future. Within the past half million years or so the early (archaic) form of *Homo sapiens* appeared in Africa. Meanwhile the Neanderthals were becoming established as the dominant hominid species in Europe and adjoining West-Central Asia. Then, from around 150,000 years ago the African fossil record indicates the emergence of the modern species of *Homo sapiens*. Subsequently, following the last interglacial period, some of those direct ancestors of ours began to disperse out of northeast Africa and radiate around the world.[2,15]

Much more recently, the rapid post-glaciation temperature rise of around 5 °C between 15,000 and 10,000 years ago caused great environmental change and the loss of many edible species. This environmental upheaval presumably contributed to the need for rudimentary agriculture in the Middle East and elsewhere. That radical shift in human ecology, via settled living, property and commerce, set in train the sequence of urbanisation, industrialisation and social modernisation that has brought us to today's condition.

Those later stages of the story are the subject of the following chapters. The rest of this chapter looks in more detail at the three main periods of hominid evolution, with particular emphasis on changes in diet. Those three periods are:

- The era of australopithecines during the Pliocene, 4–2.5 million years ago.
- From 2.5 million to 150,000 years ago: the early *Homo* species (hominines) in the Pleistocene, through to the emergence of the modern human species, *Homo sapiens*.
- From 80,000 to 10,000 years ago: the modern human species during its dispersal out of Africa and before the advent of agriculture.

The australopithecines

As the eastern African forest fragmented and savannah and woodland spread, 5 million years ago, new selection pressures favoured walking upright, supplementing fruits and berries with seeds and tubers, and maintaining on-ground security via group cohesion and primitive communication. Accordingly, the hominids underwent a rapid speciation – through the heavy jawed, low-browed, ardipithecines (over 4 million years ago) and australopithecines (approximately 4–2.5 million years ago) to the *Homo* genus. Survival must have been precarious. Life on the ground entailed new hazards to health. Being eaten by large-fanged predator cats was the most obvious. The paired holes in fossil skulls of hominids that exactly match the size and spacing of the canines of sabre-tooth tigers leave little doubt about the existence of this hazard.[16] Once out of the trees, these early hominids would also have encountered various new infectious agents, including ground-dwelling parasites such as hookworms.

In 1994, a promising candidate for a very early hominid was reported from Afar in northern Ethiopia. Teeth and bone fragments of seventeen individuals of a newly identified species *Ardipithecus ramidis* were found in fossilised volcanic ash dating from 4.4 million years. Pleasingly to palaeontologists, this species had various transitional features between ancestral chimps and the celebrated 'Lucy', *Australopithecus afarensis*. Lucy had been previously discovered in the Afar region also, in the 1970s, and has been dated to around 3.2 million years ago. The teeth of *Ardipithecus ramidis* have enamel of intermediate thickness; the base of the skull has an architecture consistent with upright walking. An extra lumbar vertebra appears to have been acquired (five, versus the three or four in apes), imparting added flexibility and uprightness. The hominid lumbar vertebrae have a large (horizontal) surface area, appropriate to bearing loads. However, we have no direct knowledge of the evolution of soft tissues, of metabolic pathways, or of patterns of thought and cognition.

Lucy type fossils have now been widely found in Ethiopia, Kenya and Tanzania, occupying a period from around 4 million to 2.5 million years ago. These bones indicate that here was an australopithecine of around 1.2 metres in height, about two-thirds the height of modern humans. The brain volume was around 450 cc, about one-third that of modern humans. Lucy's lower face protrudes less than an ape's and the canine teeth are less prominent. The arms are proportionately longer than a human's, but shorter than a chimp's. The thumbs are smaller and were, presumably, less versatile than the distinctively opposable human thumb. Analyses of foot bones suggest that these creatures were well advanced on the path from prehensile feet, with semi-independent movement of the slightly curved large toe, to upright-walking feet.

In 1974, Mary Leakey made one of palaeontology's most marvellous finds, in Laetoli, Tanzania. She uncovered a solid-cast impression of the footprints of a small band of three Lucy-australopithecines, made 3.7 million years ago in volcanic sludge. An evocative life-size copy of the cast is on view in the Kenya National Museum in Nairobi. There appear to be two sets of adult footprints and a child's footprints. Perhaps the little australopithecine band and the owners of the other criss-crossing footprints – the three-toed hipparion (a small horse-like creature, now extinct) and the hare – were all fleeing from the same volcanic rumbling, 3.7 million years ago. If so, then the littlest australopithecine, apparently stepping playfully in its parent's footsteps, was quite oblivious of danger. Such proto-human behaviour anticipates the familiar parent-and-child footstep-following games played on sandy beaches by modern humans.

From these australopithecine fossils it is clear that hominids became bipedal upright-walkers and chewers of coarse vegetation long before they became big-brained. Contrary to the assumption that sustained Britain's infamous Piltdown hoax in the first half of the twentieth century, hominid evolution was not brain-led. The evolutionary challenge that occurred in eastern Africa was for an ape descendant that could make a living in the open terrain of savannah and woodland, with occasional recourse to the trees for security. This presumably put an early premium on certain physical attributes: mobility, the capacity to see above the grass and shrubs, liberated forelimbs able to carry food back to the safety of the forest edge, and large wide molars suited to grinding grass-seeds and tubers that had not been part of traditional ape cuisine.

Changes in the australopithecine diet

As the climate continued to cool, it may have become more difficult to find a high quality diet in the increasingly sparse conditions. This environmental pressure on the australopithecines would have favoured a more complex brain. Finding below-ground tuberous vegetables, edible seeds and occasional animal foods is more difficult than being an arboreal forest-dweller picking fruit, berries and leafy tips off trees. These hominids therefore needed to learn where to look and dig for plant foods. They needed to be able to scavenge for meat without falling prey to carnivores. They needed to remember, to plan and to share foods from diverse sources. In the absence of abundant food, and lacking fangs, claws or speed, a quicker-witted brain with extra memory was a survival asset.

This question of the australopithecine diet is relevant to many of the contemporary considerations of human health and disease. Yet the evidence remains contentious. Since those early hominids were versatile eaters, there are few clues from their basic dental or mandibular anatomy. Patterns of wear and abrasion on teeth attest to the dominance of coarse plant foods – while obscuring any more subtle evidence of eating soft plant foods and meat. Fossilised gastrointestinal tracts, of course, do not exist.

As the tropical vegetation thinned and the African landscape became more arid during the prolonged global cooling of the Pliocene, the survival benefit gained from supplementary high-quality meat protein would have increased. Here is where science and ideology can clash; modern vegetarians cherish the image of an ancient vegetarian ancestry. However, there is no doubt that apes occasionally eat meat. Jane Goodall's pioneering studies of chimpanzees in the 1970s included descriptions of their frenzied group hunting rituals, culminating in the capture, killing, dismembering and eating of hapless young capuchin monkeys. If chimps have always eaten some meat, then it is possible that the common ancestor that we humans share with chimps may have been an occasional meat-eater too. But meat is not easy to come by, and the early australopithecines probably derived no more than around one-tenth of their daily food energy from meat from small prey and other opportunistic sources. Since they lacked stone tools, wooden spears and well-coordinated language-assisted hunting skills, those early australopithecines would have found it difficult to scavenge much meat from other predators' left-overs.

The last reported hominid fossil find of the twentieth century, in northern Ethiopia in 1999, yielded *Australopithecus garhi*, dated to around 2.5 million years ago.[17] This species is believed to be descendant from the Lucy australopithecines *Australopithecus afarensis*. Contrary to prevailing beliefs about transitional protohuman species (hence the 'garhi', meaning 'surprise' in the local dialect) this species appears to have been at least an occasional meat-eater. The archaeological evidence comes from the stone choppers and antelope long bones at an immediately adjacent site, the latter bearing the distinctive cut-marks and hammer indentations characteristic of butchering and marrow extraction. From other fossil evidence it is known that a profusion of herbivore grazer species was evolving on the expanding savannah, as grasses replaced trees in a cooling environment. These ungulates were a timely dietary option for hominids, brandishing their crude stone choppers.[18] This would fit with archaeological evidence from the succeeding early *Homo* era indicating that much of the animal protein eaten by hominids necessitated cracking open long bones and skulls. Early humans could thus glean food that was inaccessible to non-hominid predators.

There was something quite unusual about the predatory capacities that were evolving in early humans. Their physical and mental attributes enabled a versatile and non-specialised predation. This meant that each species of prey was expendable: when one species was hunted to extinction attention was switched to the next. Humans thus became the great casual exterminators. Unconstrained by the penalty that applies to the specialised carnivore, dependent on just several particular prey species, hominids can kill to extinction. The archaeological evidence and the more recent historical record indicate that humans have done it often. (Today we are doing it most obviously to the oceans' fisheries.)

The fossil evidence tells us that the evolutionary path from australopithecine to hominine entailed brain enlargement and a retraction of the protruding face and muzzle. *Australopithecus garhi* had a brain one-third the size of a modern human's, a projecting muzzle, and an adult height of approximately

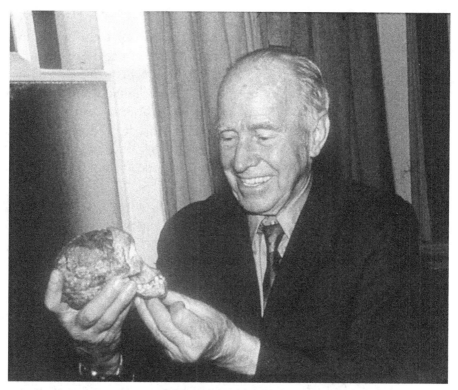

Figure 2.2 Raymond Dart, in later life, holding the skull of *Australopithecus africanus* which he discovered in South Africa in 1924. This predominantly vegetarian species is a strong contender as ancestor for the *Homo* genus. It dates from 2.5 million years ago. Recent evidence from Ethiopia suggests that some late australopithecines of that era were primitive tool users, scavenging meat from carcasses.

1.5 metres (male) and 1.2 metres (female). The evolutionary path also involved a full commitment to upright walking, with loss of the prehensile tree-climber's feet, a lengthening of the legs and a lessening in the forward tilting of the pelvis, and a shortening of the arms.

Another part of this palaeoanthropological story not only relates anatomical evolutionary responses to the great changes in climate and the hominid diet of 2–3 million years ago. It also illustrates the vicissitudes of scientific opinion and the pernicious effect of scientific fraud. In 1923 Raymond Dart, a young Australian, was appointed professor of anatomy at the University of Witwatersrand in Johannesburg. In 1925 he published a paper in the eminent scientific journal *Nature* in which he described the fossil skull of a young hominid from a limestone pit in South Africa.[19] The skull was dated at around 2.5–3.0 million years ago. Dart named this hominid species *Australopithecus africanus*, meaning 'southern ape' (see Figure 2.2). This, he proposed, was the long-sought missing link between apes and the *Homo* line. The skull, which he informally called the Taung Child, displays the typically apish low-brow cranium. It has a distinctively humanoid jaw, with smallish, flattened, grinding molars appropriate to a diet of tuberous vegetables, seeds and berries. The incisors are smaller than those of apes. Presumably they were not used primarily for tearing unpeeled fruit or raw meat; nor were they needed for aggressive display.

Dart's proposition was an affront to the prevailing assumption that the evolution of early humans was 'brain-led'. This cherished assumption had seemingly been confirmed by the discovery of Piltdown Man in 1912 in England. The fraudulent Piltdown skull combined a modern high-brow cranium with a modern ape jaw. Dart's conclusion that *Australopithecus africanus* was the ape-to-human connection was therefore rejected. Indeed, Dart's idea remained unaccepted for nearly thirty years, until the exposure of the Piltdown hoax in the 1950s, along with the important new fossil discoveries made by Louis and Mary Leakey in eastern Africa. Raymond Dart was at last vindicated.

By century's end it remained uncertain which of the australopithecines of around 2.5 million years ago were the progenitors of the *Homo* genus.[17] Was it the predominantly vegetarian *Australopithecus africanus* lineage of southern Africa, or the occasionally meat-garnering *Australopithecus garhi*, descended from the Lucy lineage of eastern Africa? Or was it some other environmentally challenged australopithecine lineage?

Hominine evolution in the Pleistocene

The hominines emerged as the cool Pliocene slid towards the even cooler Pleistocene epoch. As Earth continued to cool, the landscapes changed and traditional plant foods receded. One branch that evolved from the late australopithecine lineage, the paranthropines, remained vegetarian. Their biological energies were invested in large jaws, massive jaw muscles, and huge grinding molars. They relied particularly on tuberous vegetables. They survived for another million years until further climatic and dietary changes eventually rendered their attributes inadequate. The other branch, the hominines, took to meat-scavenging and hunting. They were the product of an evolutionary branch that invested in cognition rather than mastication: smaller jaws and shorter intestines, but larger brains. They are our ancestors.

The earliest representatives of the hominines yet identified are *Homo rudolfensis* and the better-known *Homo habilis*, the 'tool-maker'. Their position in the family tree remains uncertain. Once the Pleistocene had begun, 1.8 million years ago, and *Homo ergaster* and then *Homo erectus* appeared, our genus was firmly established. Brain size was increasing, legs were lengthening and stone tool-making was routine. The glass-encased near-complete skeleton of a young adolescent *Homo ergaster/erectus* male, the Turkana Boy from 1.6 million years ago, is on display in the Kenya National Museum.[20] Medical students would find his proportions similar to those on view in their anatomy museums.

In that cooler and drier Pleistocene world plant foods became more sparse.[21] Meanwhile, grazing animals on open grassy savannahs proliferated. Climate-induced changes and the associated fragmentation of habitats caused further speciation of large mammals, producing a much greater diversity than we contemporary urban zoo-visiting humans might imagine. The fossil record from eastern Africa shows a rapid increase in ungulate grazers, particularly gazelles from around 2 million years ago. Anthropologists think that early humans probably came to rely on meat for around one-quarter of their daily calories. Meat intake not only provided energy; it supplied the full range of amino acids (the building blocks of proteins) and some important micronutrients (such as trace elements and vitamin B12) that were deficient in a vegetarian diet. In those precarious dietary circumstances, a modest meat intake would have significantly aided survival. It would also have consolidated cooperative hunting and food sharing. Here, most probably, was strong positive feedback on the rapid evolution of the human brain.[22]

The evidence for this shift to carnivory is indirect. The fossil record from Pleistocene cave floors reveals animal long bones with systematic cut marks – recently supplemented by the above-mentioned evidence of earlier meat-eating by *Australopithecus garhi*. The isotopic content of fossil human bones indicates the consumption of grazing animals, as revealed by the distinctive ratios of carbon isotopes. Among the fossil record of the early Pleistocene, further circumstantial evidence comes from the bones of Hominid Number '1808' from Koobi Foora, in northern Kenya, also on display in the museum in Nairobi. This was an adult *Homo* female dated to 1.7 million years ago. The bones show multiple ossified blood clots where the fibrous outer lining pulled away from the underlying bone. This indicates that she probably suffered from the haemorrhagic consequences of hypervitaminosis A after eating vitamin A enriched liver.[23] (It also seems likely that she was cared for by others during her painful disability and subsequent recovery, during which the sites of bleeding formed into bony scar tissue.) From at least around 1.2 million years ago there is evidence from cave floors of the domestication of fire. The increasing use of stone tools and fire must have facilitated the trapping, killing and butchering of animals and the edibility of meat. Fire was also used to render various plant foods safe to eat by denaturing their toxic proteinaceous chemicals (their natural defence against animal predators).

As anthropologists collect more information about hunter-gatherer diets, and re-examine the reports of diverse studies from the nineteenth and twentieth centuries, it appears that animal foods typically account for over two-thirds of total caloric intake. Approximately half of that comes from muscle meat, and half from (mostly unsaturated) fat. The evidence, while still contentious,[24] points increasingly to a Pleistocene in which early humans became serious hunters and big meat-eaters. From late in the Pleistocene, the lifelike cave paintings of southern France and northern Spain dating from 20,000–40,000 years ago – when the last ice age was peaking and glaciation was creeping southwards in Europe – record explicitly the hunting of various large animal species. Perhaps the artists' motivation was to reflect, in celebratory but primitive technicolour, their dietary dependence on those animals.

The enlarging brain: thinking versus digesting

Getting, eating and digesting food and then efficiently metabolising the nutrients are crucial to survival. Much of human biology reflects the natural selection pressures of dietary modifications over 2 million years of climatic and environmental change. Simple examples include the lower jaw becoming lighter, as the emphasis moved from grinding and chewing towards cutting. This was further facilitated by the use of fire to soften plant foods and to cook meat. The incisor teeth were re-modelled, alongside the now smaller and flatter canines, to form a 'slicing' row. Two less simple examples, for which the evolutionary explanations are necessarily less certain, are those of the increasingly complex, enlarging, human brain and the modulated role of insulin in optimising the use of dietary glucose. Compared to other primates, modern humans clearly have a much larger brain and a markedly smaller colon (large bowel). Those two acquisitions may well reflect the shift from vegetarianism towards meat-eating. Indeed, as we shall see below, it is likely that the evolution of those two organs entailed a reciprocity, a trade-off.

The need to hunt animals for food was a new demand on humans. One novel way to compensate for the lack of claws, fangs and speed was to share knowledge, to plan, to cooperate strategically and to use recognisable call-signs. The habilines and the early erectines had, palaeo-anthropologists think, no open syntactical language. In the same way that our large-brained babies begin to say 'Dadda' and 'Mumma', without syntax, the erectines, pointing at a gazelle, must have learnt to say something like 'Gagga' to each other. We do not actually know when hominid 'language' began.[25] Those uncertainties aside, it is likely that cognitive skills and coded verbal communication became increasingly important around 2 million years ago as reliance on hunting for food increased. The enhanced social cohesion resulting from the use of fire for warmth, nocturnal security and prolonged group interaction may have further impelled the emergence of early language in the Pleistocene. Some corroboration for this view comes from evidence of an increasingly prominent indentation due to Broca's area, the brain's language centre, in erectine fossil skulls. The erectine who could imagine better the outcome of a particular hunting situation, who could string together three primitive words to convey the essence of the stalking strategy, and who could convey the emotion of cautious optimism to hunting partners would be more likely to bring back meat for the family. Selection pressure would thus have favoured more complex, hence larger, brains.

The extremely rapid evolution of the human brain, entailing a tripling from 450 cc to 1,450 cc in 2 million years, may have been further accelerated by the unusual climatic-environmental fluctuations of the Pleistocene and its resultant dietary insecurities.[26] Human cultural evolution has not just liberated human biology – it has helped to shape it. The early making and use of stone and wooden tools placed a heightened premium on fine and gross motor coordination, and hence the elaboration of the cerebral cortex. Likewise, the advent of early language as a means of enhancing social cohesion and of transmitting various categories of information must have greatly accelerated the later stages of evolution of the brain.

Brains, however, are metabolically expensive. The modern human brain accounts for only 3% of adult body weight but it requires about 20% of daily basal energy requirements. The erectine brain, approximately half the size of ours, would have used 10–15% of bodily energy. The australopithecine brain ran on even lower energy input. Marginal gains are the currency of natural selection: there is no selection pressure in favour of surplus, just-in-case, capacity. So, where could the extra energy for a larger brain be found? One solution would have been to make metabolic savings elsewhere. A shift from needing a large colon to digest and ferment voluminous starchy plant foods to eating meat, with simple efficient absorption of nutrients, allowed evolutionary contraction of the bowel.[27] Since the bowel, like the brain and liver, is a metabolically expensive organ, this contraction would have freed up energy for increased brain activity.

This gain in the relative size of the brain necessitated another difference between humans and other primates. To attain such a brain size without requiring a re-engineering of the human pelvis it was necessary to defer much of the brain growth and maturation until after birth. Hence the human neonate is essentially helpless for much of its first year of life. This contrasts with new-born monkeys and chimpanzees who are very soon able to clutch their tree-climbing mother's body. Once australopithecines had become committed ground-dwellers, this process of brain enlargement coupled with delayed maturation became an evolutionary option. Tree-climbing was out; the freed-up upper limits were available for carrying a baby. However, we can only guess when the process of immature birth actually began. It is fairly certain that it existed within the *Homo* line from early in the Pleistocene. Intriguingly, the fossil evidence suggests that the human brain underwent two particular surges in size, the first from around 1.8 million years ago and the other occurring several hundred thousand years ago. The stimuli for these surges, perhaps changes in the dietary environment, remain undetermined.

Handling metabolic energy: the insulin response

As the hominid diet changed, so the body's handling of the basic energy sources – glucose and fatty acids – evolved. Insulin, produced by the pancreas, modulates the storage and mobilisation of these simple metabolic fuels. Hence, insulin plays a crucial, central role in bodily metabolism. The australopithecines would have required sufficient insulin sensitivity to control the raised blood glucose levels resulting from their high consumption of carbohydrates. These were mostly complex carbohydrates from starchy root foods, along with some simpler sugars from wild fruits and berries. Under the influence of insulin, excess glucose would have been deposited as energy stores in muscle, fat and liver cells. Insulin would also have stimulated the australopithecine liver to synthesise fatty acids as an energy-storage currency for deposition in fat cells.

During the chilly and somewhat arid Pleistocene, as human survival became increasingly reliant on meat consumption, the intake of plant-food carbohydrate may have declined to around 100 grams per day (compared to a typical 300 grams in today's hunter-gatherers).[28] Given the crucial role of carbohydrate-derived glucose as a metabolic fuel, evolutionary pressures would presumably have acted to modify insulin action in order to maintain sufficient glucose in the blood. In particular, natural selection would have favoured those individual women best able to supply sufficient glucose to the glucose-dependent brain in the developing fetus and in the neonate during lactation.[29] Further, in the large-brained *Homo* genus, around 10% more total dietary energy would have been required per unit of maternal body weight during pregnancy and lactation relative to the requirement of the smaller-brained australopithecines. One evolutionary strategy to assist the mother to bear these energy costs of nourishing a large fetal and neonatal brain would have been to reduce insulin sensitivity – particularly since the brain is the one organ able to take up glucose without the assistance of insulin. Indeed, the evolution of a 'selective' insulin resistance (discussed below) would have ensured that more glucose was available to fetus and neonate, while also allowing the mobilisation of fats from energy storage tissues.

A further influence on insulin action may have resulted from the greater intake of n-3 ('omega 3') fatty acids from animal sources following the increase in meat intake. These particular polyunsaturated fats occur at high levels in meat from wild, grass-fed animals. Recent studies have shown that n-3 fatty acids enhance the diffusion and action of insulin.[30] To counter the resultant enhanced clearance of glucose from blood, natural selection may have imparted a further increment of insulin insensitivity. This selection pressure probably acted particularly on the proto-Amerindians migrating through northeast Siberia and across the (temporarily exposed) Beringian peninsula into Alaska, several tens of thousands of years ago.[31] Their diet as they traversed these chilly grasslands consisted mainly of land and marine mammals and fish, with sparse plant foods; their carbohydrate intake would therefore have been low and their n-3 fatty acid intake high.

These speculations, as plausible as they might be, cannot now be directly tested. Nevertheless, the accrual of knowledge and the advent of molecular genetic testing is beginning to fill in the picture, by corroboration if not by direct evidence. Formal interest in the biological evolution of insulin metabolism in hunter-gatherers dates from the influential idea of the 'thrifty gene'. In 1962, the population geneticist J.V. Neel proposed that the extremely high rates of diabetes in certain populations, when exposed to Western dietary abundance, was due to their having a 'thrifty genotype rendered detrimental by progress'.[32] Neel reasoned that various hunter-gatherer and small-island populations had, over thousands of years, experienced fluctuating feast-or-famine conditions. This setting would have favoured survival of the 'thrifty' individuals who had a 'quick insulin trigger' and were thus able to store energy efficiently. When, subsequently, the descendants of those populations found themselves in permanent 'feast' settings, as in today's Westernised dietary environments, the typically metabolically 'thrifty' individuals would continue to store energy and thus become obese. This process, Neel said, would exhaust the capacity of the pancreas to produce insulin, leading to insulin deficiency, excess glucose in the blood, and diabetes.

In the 1960s that was a reasonable argument. It accorded with reports of elevated rates of diabetes in several increasingly obese groups, such as the Pima Indians in Arizona, Nauruans and urban-fringe Australian Aborigines. However, there were three objections to Neel's thesis. First, anthropologists think it unlikely that hunter-gatherers experienced more famines than did subsistence agrarians. Second, relatedly, there was little evidence of differences between populations in their innate tendency to become obese. Third, the subsequent recognition that there were two main types of diabetes – IDDM (insulin-dependent diabetes mellitus) and NIDDM (non-insulin-dependent diabetes mellitus) – made it clear that NIDDM, the type at issue here, generally occurs too late in life to preempt reproduction. Hence, the lesser incidence of NIDDM in European populations could not have been contributed to by any reproductive detriment due to the rise in prevalence of obesity since mid-nineteenth century.

In 1982 Neel substantially modified his hypothesis, stating that the primary genetic defect in diabetes-prone populations was 'selective insulin resistance'.[33] This, he reasoned, had evolved in primitive hunter-gatherers to optimise the utilisation and storage of energy from meat-based diets. This selective decrease in insulin sensitivity affected carbohydrate but not fat metabolism. This would allow the sparse intake of glucose to remain in the blood as an immediate fuel, while allowing the liver to synthesise fatty acids from meat-protein for storage in adipose tissue. The latter step was necessary since muscle meat from wild animals contains very little fat. This 'selective insulin resistance' hypothesis is very plausible: such selectivity occurs in various diabetes-prone human groups and in individuals with impaired glucose tolerance or with frank diabetes. Further, the experimental lowering of carbohydrate intake induces selective insulin resistance in both humans and experimental animals[28] – a finding that may be relevant to the low-carbohydrate diet of Pleistocene hunter-gatherers.

In summary, then, meat-dependent hunter-gatherers may have reached the end of the Pleistocene, around 15,000 years ago, with a reduced insulin sensitivity by comparison with their australopithecine ancestors. That lessened insulin sensitivity may, as we shall see in the next chapter, be relevant to the ready occurrence of diabetes mellitus in many of today's regional populations.

Dispersal out of Africa

Ex Africa, semper aliquid novi. (Out of Africa there is always something new.)
(Pliny the Elder, *c.* AD 23–79)

From around 80,000 years ago, the modern human species, equipped with stone tools, spears, fire and basic language skills, began radiating out of northeast Africa into regions often less suited to the blueprint of human biology. Scientists continue to debate exactly when our ancestors first made their Out-of-Africa debut.[2] It occurred relatively early in the Wurm glaciation, which spanned from approximately 85,000 to 15,000 years ago. Environments and food supplies were changing under the cooler conditions. Humans had by then acquired an adequate technical, cerebral and communications survival kit to wander far. The aridity at low latitudes associated with the glaciation thinned the forests of West Asia, South Asia and Southeast Asia, and this probably facilitated the spread of human groups at the frontier.

The radiation out of Africa was not a mass phenomenon. The much lesser genetic heterozygosity in non-Africans relative to Africans has led population geneticists to estimate that as few as several hundred individuals may have initially drifted out of the northeast corner of Africa. This was the movement of a fringe group whose world ended somewhere near the visible horizon. They had no map, no destination. Like animal species everywhere, they were merely 'testing' the boundaries of their habitat. In the case of the human species, this experiment in habitat enlargement had spectacular results. Whereas *Homo erectus* had occupied much of Eurasia, *Homo sapiens* eventually occupied virtually the whole (non-polar) world.

Initially humans colonised the Arabian peninsula and eastern Mediterranean. In that latter region, as the climate fluctuated on a time-scale of centuries, they played a type of 'musical chairs' with outlying populations of cold-adapted Neanderthals whose heartland was in Europe, and whose branch of the human family had split from our lineage around a half-million years earlier. Dispersal continued throughout the prolonged Wurm glaciation. By

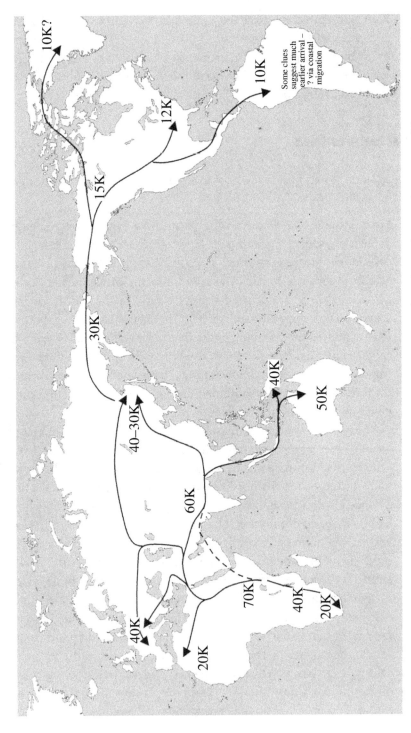

Figure 2.3 The major dispersal routes by the modern human species *Homo sapiens* during the past (approximately) 75,000 years. The sea level was 100–140 metres lower during the most recent (Wurm) glaciation, which extended from around 85,000 to 15,000 years ago. Dispersal dates are only approximate, and derive from studies of fossil humans and stone tools. The dates shown here are averaged from several sources.

around 50,000 years ago, modern humans had spread to Australia via the coasts, waterways and islands of Southeast Asia. They also spread to eastern Asia and to the steppes of Western and Central Asia. Meanwhile from around 45,000 years ago, *Homo sapiens* ventured westwards out of West Asia and the grassy Central Asian steppes and entered forested Europe.

Europe was already occupied by the Neanderthals.[34] Although popularly stigmatised as 'low-brow', they had a brain capacity as large as *Homo sapiens*. Where they fit in the family tree remains contentious. It seems likely that they originated from an offshoot of *Homo erectus*. They successfully occupied Europe and parts of Central Asia and the Middle East for several hundred thousand years. The Neanderthals were well equipped for living in predominantly glacial and frosty Europe, being stocky, large-boned, fire-using, cave-dwelling, meat-eating humans. The Neanderthals, however, were no match for the modern *Homo sapiens*. These presumably lighter-skinned modern humans had superior language skills, a more sophisticated cognition, a lighter build, and, perhaps, a quicker-footed mobility. They had a refined 'Levallois' stone technology, and made use of bone, ivory and wood. Like the Neanderthals they were serious carnivores. Out-competed, the Neanderthals died out around 30,000 years ago. They have left some tantalising clues. There are hints of rudimentary culture. They may have strewn the bodies of the dead with flowers before entombment under rocks. Healed long-bone fractures suggest social support for the disabled. Some later evidence of the decorative use of lightly carved teeth and ivory pieces suggests that they may have imitated the newly arrived moderns, or traded with them.

During the Wurm glaciation there were several particularly cold periods during which the heightened glaciation caused sea levels to drop to levels approximately 150 metres lower than today. Those may well have been the times when the ancestral Australian Aborigines island-hopped to the great south land and, later, when humans first drifted across the Beringian land-bridge to North America. By around 15,000 years ago the early Amerindians were drifting south through Canada between receding ice-sheets, heading towards the unexpected bonanza of the meat-laden temperate plains of North America. Throughout this dispersal, humans were eating plenty of animal foods. Depending on geographic location, they were also eating a variety of plant foods: tubers (especially yams), fruits, berries, some leafy vegetables, and occasional nuts and seeds. The prominence of animal foods, the diversity of plant foods and the range of their structural and nutritional composition, meant that the human diet was becoming rather different from the early *Homo* diet in eastern Africa.

As modern humans entered unfamiliar physical, dietary and microbiological environments around the world they underwent various biological and cultural adaptations. Eventually, responding to the climatic-environmental upheavals during the retreat of the last ice age from around 15,000 years ago and the extinction of various large animal species (partly natural, partly due to increasing human predation), along with the gradual build-up in human numbers, certain hunter-gatherer groups experimented with ways to increase food supplies via seed-grass cultivation and animal herding. Here, precariously, were the beginnings of a radical change in the human economy, in social relationships and in patterns of settlement. The consequences for human nutrition, infectious disease, warfare and conquest – the Four Horsemen of the Apocalypse – were enormous. The profile of human health and disease was about to be transformed. Increased food-yield per unit of land allowed population growth. Concepts of property emerged; food surpluses were tradeable; urban populations emerged, with ruling, priestly, warrior, trading and artisanal classes. Several millennia later, powerful city-states arose in several centres in Mesopotamia, the eastern Mediterranean, China, the Indus Valley and Mesoamerica. Much later, coastal and sea-faring migration from East Asia led to colonisation of the islands of the western Pacific and, later, Hawaii, Tahiti, Easter Island and New Zealand.

Over the course of 100 millennia, modern humans had thus either found, or had modified and then maintained, life-supporting ecosystems from equatorial forest to subpolar ice. Over many tens of thousands of years, the bony evidence indicates that the average life-span had changed little. Healthy individuals of all ages were at continuing risk of starvation, infection, and accidental or violent death. As in other animal species, our human ancestors usually died before middle adulthood.

Conclusion

Natural selection, ever blind to the future, and driven by the environmental challenges of the Pleistocene, gave a chance to a species of big-brained generalists with an unusual cleverness and versatility. This was a species able to survive in a great diversity of environments. The evolution of consciousness and language probably proceeded in parallel, as humans acquired social intelligence, then technical intelligence and natural history intelligence. What our forebears discovered they then discussed, thought about, and remembered.

Over the past 40,000 years or so, this new knowledge, these new ideas, were transmitted increasingly to succeeding generations via moral homily, legend or song. Here were the origins of 'culture'.

This grand, unplanned, experiment of nature could easily have failed at some time during those testing years. The *Homo* lineage could have become extinct. However, once the seemingly safer shores of the warmer Holocene were reached 10,000 years ago, and with diversified investments of humans now present in all continents, the outlook has never looked in doubt. The modern human species has not merely survived; it has, so far, succeeded spectacularly.

3

Adapting to diversity: climate, food and infection

It is approximately one hundred years since scientists first understood the basic currency of heredity: the discrete, non-divisible gene. In the 1860s Gregor Mendel discovered 'particulate' inheritance with his studies of garden peas in a monastery in Brno (in today's Czech Republic). However, his published findings were ignored by mainstream science for several decades.

Tantalisingly, Mendel's discovery was the crucial clue that eluded Charles Darwin, whose great work *The Origin of Species*, had been published in 1859. Darwin could only imagine, unsatisfactorily, that inherited characteristics were somehow transmitted by blood-borne 'gemules' that blended parental characteristics. But, over several generations, this blending would dilute the originally selected phenotypic character. Mendel's findings provided the answer. He crossed a wrinkled-pea plant with a smooth-pea plant and found that some offspring plants were wrinkled and some were smooth. There was no blending: each plant was either one thing or the other. Mendel inferred that each such character-specifying 'gene' comprised alternate all-or-nothing versions that were the irreducible units of inheritance. These alternate versions we recognise today as alleles.

We each carry a unique combination of genetic alleles and a few newly arising non-lethal mutations. Indeed, each of us is one of nature's little experiments, on stand-by for testing against the possibility of unexpected environmental change. Some genes influence susceptibility to particular disease processes. Susceptibility, however, is not predestination; the health outcome usually depends on interactions between genes and environment. There are some well-known major single-gene diseases with simple Mendelian inheritance, such as cystic fibrosis. Yet even those major genes are modulated by the action of other genes and environmental factors. Cystic fibrosis can thus affect individual children in very different ways. Much more common are complex disease-related traits that are influenced by many different genes. For example, at last count well over a dozen genes had been implicated in the 'causation' of obesity. The rapid advance of molecular genetic research is revealing complex polygenic influences on many diseases, ranging from Alzheimer's Disease and adult-onset diabetes to the various genes that affect the severity of infectious disease.

Those gene variants (alleles) that have come to predominate are likely to have conferred reproductive advantage in the past, even if no longer. This seems clear enough for genetically-influenced characteristics such as body shape and skin pigmentation, for which strong regional climatic selection pressures have apparently operated. However, as discussed in Chapter 2, population gene profiles differ because of several historical processes: (i) differential selection pressure; (ii) random genetic drift; and (iii) accidental 'founder effects' in small colonising groups – such as have imparted the high prevalence of retinitis pigmentosa (a form of visual impairment) to the inhabitants of the southern Atlantic island of Tristan de Cunha.

SOME OF HUMANKIND'S genetic variation has arisen over the 150,000 years of existence of *Homo sapiens* in response to ancestors colonising a very wide range of physical, dietary and microbiological environments. For example, we saw previously that humans may have inherited from their meat-eating Pleistocene predecessors a lower insulin sensitivity than had previously been needed for a mostly vegetarian diet – and less than would subsequently be needed for carbohydrate-based agrarian diets. Agrarianism, therefore, is likely to have further modulated the genetic basis of this metabolic characteristic. As discussed later in this chapter, the inter-population differences in insulin sensitivity affect the pattern of diabetes around the world, in conjunction with dietary changes and obesity levels. There are other genetic traits that vary between regional populations and which can also result in gene-environment *mismatches* if there has been a change in culture or environment. Two contemporary examples are:

- Vitamin D deficiency due to sunlight deficiencies in dark-skinned immigrant children living at high latitudes. This has been a well-documented problem in South Asian children living in the gloom of inner-urban northern Europe.
- Sickle-cell trait in African-Americans who are no longer exposed to malaria. This condition causes considerable suffering and some deaths in early life, despite no longer conferring a survival advantage, in the absence of malaria.

An important question arises here: Just how fast can genetic adaptation occur in humans? Of course, the greater the selection pressure, the more rapid the adaptation will tend to be. Much of the repertoire of genetic resistance to malaria, a potential child-killer, has apparently evolved within the past several thousand years since early farming communities were first exposed to locally circulating human-adapted malaria.[1] Some other genetic traits have evolved in response to dietary changes since the advent of agriculture and dairy herding. Two examples are the lifelong ability to absorb milk sugar ('lactose tolerance') and the tolerance of gluten protein in wheat cereal. (Absence of the latter causes coeliac disease, an inflammatory bowel disorder.) Nevertheless, human biology is the product of a long evolutionary process. Most of our genes predate agrarianism; indeed most are of far greater antiquity than the Pleistocene. The trail of human biological evolution stretches back into the mists of geological time.

The three great environmental agents of natural selection acting upon *Homo sapiens* populations have been climate, food availability and infectious disease. Although they are each considered separately in this chapter, it is important to note that they have often acted in concert in the shaping of human biological evolution. Indeed, many of the cell-surface proteins that influence susceptibility to infectious disease agents – for example, the entry of viruses or bacteria into cells – are activated by vitamin and other micronutrient molecules. There have been many other nutrition–infection interactions in human evolution. One of the evolved defences against malaria, for example, entails a reduced enzymatic capacity for metabolising glucose, thereby denying energy to the malarial parasite.

Overall, infectious diseases, as potential child-killers, have probably been a more important agent of natural selection in humans than have either climate or diet. Some specific genetic mutations confer protection against a particular infectious disease, as does sickle-cell trait against malaria. Fifty years ago, the polymath British biologist J.B.S. Haldane noted that 'the struggle against disease, and particularly infectious disease, has been a very important evolutionary agent, and some of its results have been rather unlike those of the struggle against natural forces, hunger, and predators, or with members of the same species'.[2] He observed insightfully that large predators are nearly always outnumbered by their quicker-breeding smaller prey, and they therefore do not present the same population-level threat as can a rapidly proliferating infectious agent. Not only is the pressure on the target species less from the macro-predators, but it is more difficult to evolve anatomical defences against the predator than to evolve an immunological or molecular defence against a microbe. In Haldane's words: 'it is much easier for a mouse to get a set of genes which enable it to resist *Bacillus typhimurium* [the typhoid bacterium] than a set which enables it to resist cats'.[2]

The rest of this chapter will consider these three main agents of natural selection: climate, diet and infectious disease, with particular reference to diabetes and malaria in relation to the latter two agents.

Climate: skin pigmentation and immune function

Changes in the world's climate over the past several million years have shaped much of hominid evolution. Changes in the landscape and, consequently, in food sources propelled the move to upright walking, the move towards an omnivorous diet and the enlargement of the brain. Later, as *Homo sapiens* began dispersing around the world, local climatic conditions, particularly temperature, humidity and solar ultraviolet radiation levels, exerted further selection pressures on body shape, skin colour, hair type and various metabolic characteristics.

Scientists have long speculated about the evolutionary reason for population differences in skin pigmentation. Pigment is made by special cells called melanocytes in the lower layer of the epidermis. Fair-skinned people appear to have a genetically determined abnormality in the melanocytes' receptors for the hormone that normally stimulates melanin production in response to ultraviolet radiation. Instead, they produce a reddish pigment called phaeomelanin. The pink cheeks of the English (which elicited the derisory term 'pommes' – or apples – from the French) are the product of a conserved melanocytic mutation. Skin pigmentation protects the skin against direct solar damage, both acute and chronic, and it also modulates the action of ultraviolet radiation on several blood-borne vitamins circulating in superficial blood vessels. Within each particular climatic-dietary environment, natural selection has achieved an improvised balance between several competing needs of human biology.

The ancestral African human skin was probably less darkly pigmented than in the majority of contemporary indigenous Africans. Indeed, the original skin colour probably resembled the milk-coffee-coloured skin of Africa's Khoi and San people today. Molecular genetic studies indicate that the dark-skinned Bantu population of Africa may have migrated back into Africa tens of thousands of years ago from the coastal regions of south-east Asia. This region had been a prominent migratory route eastwards for early humans, when forests were less dense and shorelines more habitable. Jonathan Kingdon reasons that the many millennia spent, between 60,000–40,000 years ago, gathering marine food in south-east Asian tidal flats at times dictated by tides, not by time of day, must have necessitated frequent exposure to the midday sun.[3] Dark protective skin would have been the genetically adaptive response. That same darker pigmentation occurs in other groups thought to have descended from those coastal-dwelling Asians: Dravidians in southern India, Melanesians in Papua New Guinea and Australian Aborigines. However, other scientists question the role of climate and sunlight in the genetic differentiation of skin pigmentation. Jared Diamond, noting the contention between eight diverse theories of skin pigmentation, argues that sexual selection pressure may also have been particularly important.[4]

Whatever their exact starting colour, it seems clear that early European populations acquired lighter-coloured skins than their ancestors. One likely explanation hinges on the role of vitamin D in ensuring calcium-enriched bone structure.[5] Ultraviolet radiation converts blood-borne 7-dehydrocholesterol, made by the liver, into vitamin D as it passes through the capillaries beneath the skin. Vitamin D enhances the absorption of calcium from the gut. Since calcium is essential to the growth and development of bones, vitamin D deficiency results in bone-deforming rickets. Hunter-gatherer *Homo sapiens*, coming from the Asian steppes, moved northwards through Europe into less sunlit climes from around 40,000 years ago. A fall in vitamin D levels due to lessened solar exposure would have resulted in weakened, calcium-deficient bones. This would explain the above-average prevalence of rickets observed in the prehistoric bones of Denmark and Norway.[6] Indeed, deformity of the weight-bearing, calcium-deficient pelvis could have directly impeded reproduction, and this would have exerted a strong selection pressure in favour of lighter skin colour that maintained blood calcium levels. As for most plausible evolutionary explanations, no direct evidence is available for this particular suggestion.

Such biological adaptations often entailed trade-offs. There is, for example, a need to protect blood-borne folic acid (vitamin B6) against the damaging effects of ultraviolet radiation. Indeed, since folic acid is crucial for fetal brain and spinal cord development, there may well have been a strong selection pressure favouring the retention of skin pigmentation. An increase in pigmentation would also have reduced the risk of skin cancer.[7] However, since skin cancer is normally a disease of later adulthood it is usually assumed not to generate natural selection pressure (although the most life-threatening of the skin cancers, malignant melanoma, quite often occurs in early adulthood).

In the modern world, with much longer life expectancies, the influence of skin pigmentation on risk of skin cancer has become a more prominent health problem. The migration of lighter-skinned people from European climes to sunnier lower-latitude locations such as Australia, New Zealand, South Africa and the southern United States over the past two centuries has resulted in those 'Caucasian' populations experiencing a substantially increased risk of skin cancer. Australia has the world's highest reported rates of skin cancer. Not suprisingly, the rates are much higher in fair-skinned (Celtic) migrants from Britain and Ireland than in olive-skinned migrants from Italy and Greece.

Solar ultraviolet radiation also suppresses some facets of the immune system. The reason for this somewhat surprising effect remains uncertain. Perhaps it arose in hominids as they became increasingly reliant on finding food in open sunlit terrain, and as body hair receded for other reasons. The resultant sun-damaged proteins in the skin may have provoked local 'self-destructive' immune attack by T-cells (white blood cells), causing skin damage. Natural selection would therefore have favoured an adaptive dampening of the immune system occurring in response to solar exposure. However, since the same phenomenon is demonstrable in laboratory studies of rodents, who lack that sun-exposed food-gathering history, there must also be a more basic explanation of this immunosuppressive effect in mammals.

Humans have dispersed from tropics to polar regions, and are thus exposed to a substantial geographic gradient in ultraviolet radiation levels. If ultraviolet radiation significantly suppresses aspects of the human immune system, then this geographic spread is likely to yield different rates of various immune-related disorders at high and low latitudes. This, indeed, appears to be so for multiple sclerosis, an autoimmune disease.[8] In both northern and southern hemispheres, the rates of multiple sclerosis generally increase with distance from the equator. In Australia, for example, the rates increase approximately five-fold between north and south of the country. Several other autoimmune diseases, including type 1 (child-onset) diabetes and rheumatoid arthritis, appear to show latitude gradients, with their rates increasing with distance from the equator. Scientists still have much to learn about this fascinating relationship – one that may become more relevant over the coming several decades at mid-to-high latitudes in the wake of stratospheric ozone depletion. Meanwhile, the relationship illustrates well how environment can modulate the expression of underlying human biology, thereby influencing the risk of disease occurrence.

Diet: beans and genes

Phenotypically, 'we are what we eat'. Genotypically, we are to some extent what our forebears used to eat. As the hominid diet has changed over the past 2 million years, so human biology – jaws, teeth, gut size, enzymatic repertoire and metabolic handling – has evolved. Regional differences in the foods encountered by dispersing human populations have contributed to human biological variation. Those dietary differences have included exposures to plant toxins, and the levels of consumption of meat, simple carbohydrates, dairy foods, wheat flour and alcohol.

The impact of diet upon the human genotype is well illustrated by the population genetics research done by Luigi Cavalli-Sforza and colleagues. Their research includes an analysis of the main genetic gradients that span contemporary European populations, using the documented geographic variations in approximately 100 nuclear genetic loci.[9] The strongest gradient runs from south-east to north-west (Figure 3.1). This is the so-called 'farmers' genes' gradient, and it explains approximately 28% of the genetic variation in Europe.[10] It shows the genetic footprints of the ancestral farming populations, as they radiated out from the eastern Mediterranean, and spread north-west across Europe at an average speed of about 1 km/year, reaching Brittany and England about 4,000 years ago and Ireland 1,000 years later. This scenario accords with the contemporary gradient across the European population in gluten (wheat protein) intolerance. Coeliac disease, due to gluten intolerance, is much more common in the north-west than in the south-east of Europe. As discussed later in this chapter, it may also help us understand why European populations in general have an above-average sensitivity to insulin.

There is some scientific disagreement on this matter. Evidence from mutations in mitochondrial DNA (which, unlike the nuclear chromosomal genes, are not subject to meiotic shuffling, and hence are less sensitive to selection pressures) suggests that modern human genes began to enter Europe rather earlier, from around 50,000 years ago, and with a less strong subsequent influence from in-migrating farmers.[11] However, genetic techniques aside, various other independent archaeological and linguistic evidence appears to accord with Cavalli-Sforza's thesis of a major infusion of 'farmers' genes'.

The juxtaposition of the words 'beans' and 'genes' in this section's subheading invites a brief digression about the death of the Greek philosopher-mathematician Pythagoras in the sixth century BC. Like many fellow citizens of Croton, Pythagoras had inherited a genetic defect in the G6PD (glucose 6-

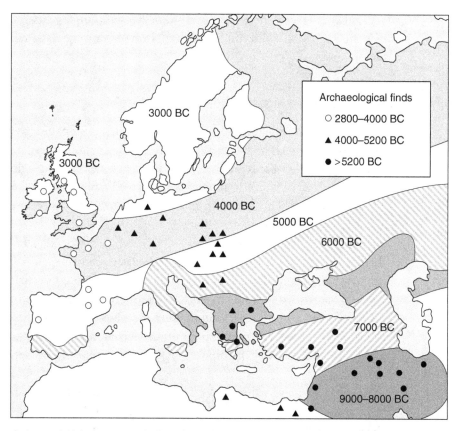

Figure 3.1 The spread of farming populations through Europe, from southeast to northwest, as revealed by genetic analyses and archaeological findings. The process occurred approximately over the period from 9,000 to 4,500 years ago. Genetic analyses indicate that this migration (represented by the successive shaded areas) was one of the strongest historical influences on the modern genetic gradients in Europe.

phosphate dehydrogenase) enzyme. This enzyme defect weakens the structure of the red blood cells, predisposing them to rupture, which can cause serious haemolytic anaemia. This genetic trait has persisted in Mediterranean populations because it gives some protection against falciparum malaria. In persons with this trait, eating the *Vicia faba* bean – or even inhaling its pollen – can cause a haemolytic crisis. It was fear of life-threatening contact with beans that reportedly led to Pythagoras' death. Having enraged the local populace (once again) with his outspoken political views, he then fled into the adjoining fields. However, he was confronted by a flowering bean-field that he was loathe to run across. His pursuers therefore caught and killed him. (Presumably Pythagoras realised that even if he had run around the right-angled boundaries of the field, his pursuers would still have caught him by running diagonally across the hypotenuse.)

Diabetes: the Pleistocene legacy?

Ancient medical texts refer to the sweet-tasting urine of patients with diabetes mellitus. The word 'mellitus' alludes to honey-like sweetness. Diabetes is a serious metabolic disease, characterised by excessive levels of glucose in the blood (hyperglycaemia). It seriously damages the blood vessels, kidneys and peripheral nerves. The two main forms of diabetes, mentioned in the previous chapter, are insulin-dependent diabetes mellitus (IDDM, or 'Type I') and non-insulin-dependent diabetes mellitus (NIDDM, or 'Type II'). In the former there is a lack of the hormone insulin; in the latter there is metabolic resistance (or insensitivity) to the action of insulin. IDDM tends to occur early in life, perhaps because of an unusual childhood viral infection of the pancreas that results in autoimmune attack on that organ, thereby impairing its production of insulin. NIDDM, the predominant type, occurs mostly in adults and entails a diminished sensitivity of adipose (fat) tissue, muscle and liver to the actions of insulin.

NIDDM (which I will refer to simply as 'diabetes') entails a range of metabolic and cardiovascular disorders, including hyperglycaemia (elevated blood sugar concentration), an abnormal profile of blood lipids, raised blood pressure and coronary heart disease. Diabetes occurs particularly in individuals who are overweight, especially those with 'abdominal' obesity.[12] Today, diabetes is markedly on the rise in urbanising Westernising populations everywhere, reflecting the general increase in the prevalence of obesity. This, in turn, is due to the combination of an increased consumption of energy-dense foods and a marked decline in physical activity. The World Health Organization estimates that, as populations age and as obesity becomes more prevalent, today's 140 million cases of Type II diabetes will become 300 million cases by the 2020s – that is, approximately 6% of the world's adults.

The central metabolic defect in diabetes is insufficiency of insulin – either its production or its action. This hormone, as we saw in chapter 2, orchestrates the metabolism of glucose and fatty acids, the body's main metabolic fuels and energy stores. Insulin is an ancient vertebrate hormone that has been conserved over several hundred million years of evolution. It has various functions. In addition to regulating the storage of glucose and fatty acids, insulin in humans also influences the renal excretion of sodium and nitrogen and the action of leptin, the satiety-inducing hormone secreted by fully stocked adipose tissue.

The prevalence of diabetes varies by more than ten-fold between major population groups. For example, rates are high in the Pima Indians of Arizona, Nauruans, Australian Aborigines and South Asian migrants in the United Kingdom. Rates are low in European populations and in many traditional rural populations. Some of this variation reflects differences in population levels of obesity. Some of it reflects genetically determined differences in susceptibility. For example, lean young male Australian Aborigines, living near-traditional lives, have a lower sensitivity to insulin than do young male European-Australians.[13] Similarly, the Pima Indians of the southwest United States are less insulin sensitive than is the general US population – and the trait tends to run in families.

Differentiating the effects of genes and 'environment' on diabetes is difficult. Studies in racially mixed persons, with parents or grandparents from populations at divergent risk of diabetes, demonstrate a clear genetic influence on the level of insulin sensitivity. On the other hand, the importance of environmental factors is evident from comparing genetically identical populations of Pima Indians that became separated geographically several centuries ago: the Arizona Pimas with their partly Westernised lifestyle have a very high rate of diabetes, whereas the Mexican Pimas, following a traditional agricultural life, have a low rate. The elevated rates of diabetes in urbanised Indian, Chinese and African migrants in Mauritius, relative to their populations of pre-migration origin, also attest to the importance of the social and dietary environment.[14]

It is not, however, a matter of genes *or* environment. The critical determinant of diabetes risk is the interaction between genetic predisposition and environmental trigger. Indeed, without the environmental stressor (or 'trigger') the genetic predisposition may be rather unimportant. Various studies in populations at innately high risk of diabetes – the Yanomami Indians of South America, several North American Amerindian groups and Australian Aborigines – show that in the absence of obesity the prevalence of glucose intolerance is very low, and clinical diabetes is non-existent. The conclusion from this is important. It is that, irrespective of their genotype, non-obese populations living in energy balance with their local dietary environment do not display significant metabolic abnormalities. In other words, the clinical disease, diabetes, is predominantly a manifestation of an imbalance in way of life.

This is not to exclude other contributory explanations to the modern pattern of diabetes in the world. Much recent research has shown that suboptimal development of the human fetus, due apparently to maternal undernutrition, leads to persistent adaptive metabolic adjustments. This metabolic reprogramming of the undernourished fetus can be regarded as an 'environmental' process, and has prompted David Barker and Nick Hales, in Britain, to call it the 'thrifty phenotype' phenomenon. The fetus, they argue, acquires greater insulin insensitivity in order to optimise immediate developmental outcomes, especially brain development, that require sufficient glucose in blood.[15] These low birthweight babies (especially if undernourished in the later stages of pregnancy) are at increased risk of diabetes in adult life, particularly if, in adulthood, the individual becomes overweight. This phenomenon could help explain the rapid escalation in diabetes rates in various traditional societies undergoing rapid Westernisation, such as Nauruans where more than half the adults over age 30 years have had diabetes in recent decades. (The fact that the Nauruan rate appears now to be declining could indicate that the problem is partly one of cultural transition, reflecting the decline in prevalence of low birthweight in later generations. Less probably, it could also reflect an actual differential reproductive success between those women with and without diabetes.) Even so, there is still debate about the extent to which there may be a shared genetic determination of both birthweight and particular metabolic characteristics such as insulin sensitivity.[16] Finally, it remains clear that, notwithstanding birthweight, the diet, physical activity and body-weight in adult life are potent determinants of an individual's risk of diabetes.

AS TODAY'S POPULATIONS urbanise, change lifestyles and migrate, variations in diabetes rates are becoming more apparent. There is an intriguing contrast between European populations in which only a minority of obese persons eventually develop diabetes, compared to over half the obese persons in various high-risk non-European populations.[17] That and other evidence indicates that European populations with their lower susceptibility to diabetes might be the metabolic exception, rather than the rule.[18] This inverts the various earlier constructions that were based upon J.V. Neel's influential 'thrifty gene' hypothesis from the 1960s (see chapter 2). It suggests that heightened insulin insensitivity may be the general human legacy of the Pleistocene era. Perhaps, then, non-European populations are the genotypically faithful standard-bearers from our Pleistocene ancestors' struggle to survive in the high-meat and low-carbohydrate dietary circumstances of a cooler world. In other words, heightened insulin insensitivity was the 'background' genotypic condition from which just a few neolithic populations, particularly the early farming proto-Europeans, later diverged.

For this to be plausible there must have been a selection pressure, specifically in early European agrarians, for relaxation of the Pleistocene insulin resistance. This could not have been a pressure to avoid obesity-associated life-shortening since Europe's rural masses and urban poor subsisted, with no prospect of obesity, until the twentieth century. If the genetic disposition to insulin insensitivity has been selectively lessened in European populations, then it must have been by some other route. We have no direct evidence on this matter. However, it is likely that the distinctive chronology of farming and dairy herding in the ancestral European populations played a central role. After the last glaciation ended, around 15,000 years ago, dietary environments began to change. Large mammals were either naturally migrating, dying out, or had become over-exploited by increasingly successful late stone-age hunters. In the middle-eastern region, as human numbers continued to increase, hunter-gatherers were forced to increase their consumption of wild grass seeds – the forerunners of barley, wheat and oats. As is discussed in much more detail in chapter 5, systematic harvesting and cultivation gradually emerged from around 10,000 years ago, first in the Middle Eastern 'Fertile Crescent' and later in various other population centres around the world.

Agriculture markedly changed the nutrient profile of the diet. The 'low glycaemic index' palaeolithic diet, inducing a slow and modest rise in blood glucose after feeding, was superseded by a more glycaemic neolithic diet. Animal foods and fibrous plant foods were substantially replaced by cultivated cereal grains, lentils and tuberous vegetables. This much greater reliance on starchy carbohydrate foods, especially mashed and ground cereal grains with their more rapidly absorbed sugars, would have required greater insulin sensitivity.[19] European populations, whose ancestors came from the world's oldest agrarian centre in the Middle East, have the world's longest history of farming. They also have lower rates of diabetes than all other major population groups. We can identify three such categories of non-European populations who are at apparently higher innate risk of diabetes:

(1) Many populations that have never farmed (e.g., various Amerindian groups, Eskimos and Australian Aborigines) are at particularly high risk of diabetes.

(2) Those who began farming either relatively recently or only partially (e.g., West Africans, Japanese and the Pacific's Polynesian and Micronesian

horticulturist populations who originated from East Asia around 2,000–3,000 years ago) also tend to have elevated rates. (In the United States, diabetes rates are much higher in African-American than in European-derived populations; rates are also high in African-Caribbean populations.)

(3) Although rates of diabetes remain generally low in China, the rates in overseas Chinese populations, with higher levels of obesity, are elevated.[14] The Chinese were also early agriculturists, but their agrarian diet differed from the European diet in at least one important respect. The same distinction may also apply to South Asians, among whom the diabetes rates are high in urbanised populations even though agriculture began quite early in both northern and southern India.

The provisional thesis that emerges is that the genetic adaptation of populations to diets of differing glycaemic load over the past 10,000 years has imbued them with different levels of insulin sensitivity. The least sensitive are Amerindians, Polynesians and Micronesians; the most sensitive are the Europeans; and in between are many other populations. The lack of standardised information about the prevalence of both diabetes and obesity in many populations impedes conclusive analysis. Nevertheless, Europeans appear to be distinctly more insulin sensitive than other populations. Yet the extra few thousand years of farming seems hardly sufficient to account for this disparity in insulin sensitivity. How else did Europeans differ? The next section suggests an answer.

The lactose tolerance factor

Middle Eastern farmers were the first to domesticate wild plants. They also made the radical breakthrough of herding and then domesticating goats, sheep and, later, cattle. From around 7,000–8,000 years ago these agrarian communities began consuming milk and milk products. The result, today, is that genetically based tolerance of lactose (milk sugar) is much more prevalent in European than in most non-European populations. In Scandinavia, for example, nearly all persons are lactose tolerant, whereas in East Asian populations nearly all are lactose intolerant.

Human infants can digest the lactose in breast-milk and thus absorb its component simple sugars, galactose and glucose. In nature, this intestinal enzymatic capacity becomes redundant after weaning and, in accordance with natural selection's principle of energy conservation, the activity of the lactase enzyme is greatly reduced after the age at which, prehistorically, children were normally weaned: four years. However, the introduction of dairy foods into the early Middle Eastern agrarian diet created a selection pressure that favoured retention of lactase, both to capture the energy available from lactose and, presumably, to avoid the aversion to nutrient-rich milk that would result from the uncomfortable bloating caused by lactose intolerance.[20] In situations of subsistence farming, such marginal gains in energy availability can be crucial to survival. The 'mutant' gene for lactase retention behaves as a simple dominant gene. Assuming that the gene conferred a 5% advantage in reproductive success (a high but plausible figure) population geneticists estimate that the lactose tolerance trait would have become predominant within about 7,000 years. During that time, approximately 350 generations, the gene frequency would have increased from a single new mutation to around 90% of the population.[21]

As farming populations spread north in Europe into less sunny climes, so the body's ultraviolet-powered production of vitamin D – and hence intestinal absorption of calcium – would have declined. However, lactose tolerance facilitates calcium absorption from dairy foods. Since calcium is essential for healthy bones, this additional selection pressure is likely to have favoured lactose tolerance. This may partly explain the lactose tolerance gradient in Europe today, which ranges from around 50% in Greece and Italy to around 97–99% in Denmark and Sweden.[20] Indeed, this selection pressure would have been amplified further in Scandinavian populations because of their unusual reliance on dairy foods in a colder climate where cereal production was often difficult.

Dairy foods are traditionally not consumed by East Asians, Pacific islanders, Australian Aborigines and Amerindians. In several African tribes (the Tussi, Fulani and Hima) lactose tolerance has been traced by molecular genetic analyses back to the ancestral Middle Eastern sources of those migrating tribal groups. When agrarian-herders radiated outwards from the Fertile Crescent thousands of years ago, some diffused south-west into the Nile Valley and on into sub-Saharan Africa. In some other cultures, such as India, Tibet and much of Africa, fermented (i.e., lactose-depleted) milk products such as yoghurt and buttermilk are consumed by the predominantly lactose-intolerant population.

The picture that thus emerges is that the proto-European farmers consumed a diet unprecedentedly high in simple sugars, from stone-ground cereals, other cultivated plants and whole milk. We can speculate that this unusually high glycaemic load would have intensified the selection pressure to remove excess glucose from the blood by relaxing the ancestral Pleistocene

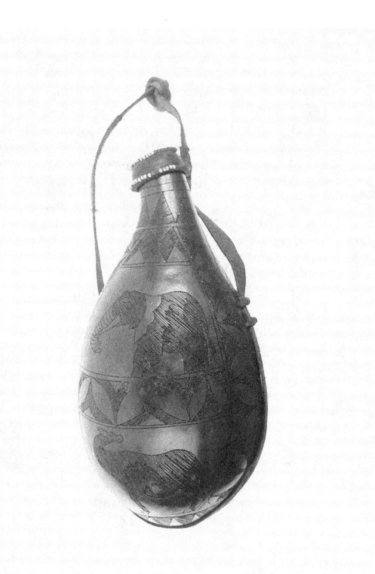

Figure 3.2 Decorated gourd milk container, from Kenya. The Masai are one of several tribal groups in Africa whose ancestors migrated into north-eastern Africa from the West Asian region, as cattle-herders and milk consumers. They, along with Europeans, are one of the few human populations with a high level of lactose tolerance – a capacity to absorb milk sugars.

insulin insensitivity. In accord with this idea, an inverse, crude correlation has been identified between the rates of lactose tolerance and diabetes in more than 40 different populations around the world.[22] Populations with little or no exposure to dairy foods (i.e., low lactose tolerance) tend to have high rates of diabetes (i.e., high insulin insensitivity). European populations lie at the other extreme of the scatter-plot of data, with high rates of lactose tolerance and low rates of diabetes.[23]

This thesis about the role of typical total glycaemic load does not preclude there having been other selection pressures on insulin sensitivity in hunter-gatherers and early farmers. Famines occurred severely in some regions, and food sources changed as new environments were entered. As mentioned in chapter 2, the diets eaten by the proto-Amerindians spreading across the temporarily exposed tundra of the Beringian land-bridge around 30,000–20,000 years ago must have been unusually high in meat and fat. The colonisers of the Pacific of several thousand years ago must have encountered food shortages and occasional famines, not just on their long ocean journeys but for several years after their arrival on islands with often limited agricultural potential.[24]

There is a final, important, point to emphasise again. Diabetic predispositions aside, non-obese populations living in energy balance with their local dietary environment do not display metabolic abnormalities. Such innate differences tend to be unimportant within the normal range of dietary intake with traditional patterns of physical activity. Any future increases in diabetes incidence in human populations around the world will be a signal that human ecology has deviated unduly from the conditions of healthy living.

Other selection pressures from novel foods

Plants, unlike animals, cannot retreat from predators. Hence they have evolved various deterrent, often toxic, chemicals. In their coevolutionary response, plant-eating species have acquired various detoxifying enzymes. Consequently, human populations around the world, with differing dietary histories, display innate variations in their enzyme profiles. Differences between major population groupings are particularly evident for the family of oxidative cytochrome P450 enzymes. These enzymes are active in liver cells, and four of the ten enzymes act primarily to detoxify ingested chemicals. As previously noted, however, this genetic variation in metabolic propensities between populations reflects a mix of active natural selection, genetic drift and some genetic bottle-necking in small founder groups. There is therefore an ever-present risk of over-interpreting the environmental 'causes' of interesting genetic variations between groups.

An important detoxification pathway is by acetylating the potential toxin. Humans segregate, genetically, into 'fast' and 'slow' acetylators. The former can drink coffee at 11 p.m. and be asleep by midnight; the latter (like me) are still awake at 3 a.m. The acetylation pathway metabolises various substrates, including caffeine, the anti-tuberculosis drug isoniazid and organic chemicals (arylamines) present in cigarette smoke and in cooked meat. However, we do not know what dietary substrate might have induced selection for the acetylator variants.

A person's acetylator phenotype is largely determined by the NAT2 (*N*-acetyltransferase) gene. The gene has, in effect, two alleles that confer fast or slow acetylation enzyme activity. There is considerable interregional variation in the frequencies of these two alleles. Since all the main single-nucleotide mutations of the NAT2 gene occur in all populations that have been studied, it appears that the mutations arose before humans dispersed out of Africa.[25] The tracking of several of the NAT2 single-nucleotide mutations follows the major routes of human migration. Fast acetylators are much more prevalent in eastern Asia (80–90%) than in Europe (30–45%), which, in turn, exceeds North African populations (15–20%). This broadly coherent gradient suggests that the ancient African 'slow' allele has subsequently been selected against in dispersing populations, perhaps in response to toxins in newly encountered plant foods that needed rapid detoxification.

Epidemiological studies in Western populations have consistently shown that slow acetylators are at increased risk of bladder cancer (because they deactivate certain chemical carcinogens too slowly to prevent their passage into the urine). Less consistently, it looks as if fast acetylators are at increased risk of cancer of the colon, especially if they frequently eat well-cooked meat (which contains chemical compounds produced at high heat that are precursor carcinogens).[26] There is occasional equity in genetic dispensations.

Infection

Infection, as we shall see in chapter 3, is one of nature's fundamental ways of life. All non-plant species live by expropriating, directly or indirectly, the products of plant photosynthesis. Plants are the 'producers'. There are basically five ways for a non-producer species to gain the energy and nutrients that it needs:

- Herbivores eat plants.
- Carnivores and omnivores (including humans) eat herbivores.
- Saprophytes, such as fungi, thrive on the decomposing bodies of the dead.
- Insect species feed on plants, blood, excreta, decaying matter and one another.
- Parasites – multicellular, unicellular and subcellular – extract their needs by infecting the living.

This interdependent recycling scheme comprises producers (plants), consumers, decomposers and – infecting each of these – parasites. When we talk about infectious disease we tend to lapse into military metaphors: we talk of infectious disease 'attack rates', of microbes and cancer cells as 'invaders', and of bodily 'defences'. Yet the point of a microorganism's struggle to survive is not to do harm to other organisms. The microorganism seeks merely to survive and replicate.

Human biological evolution, too, has pursued self-advantage. Defences against infection evolve in two ways. First, a human population, under constant pressure from an infective agent – especially those with a heavy fatal toll in childhood – tends to acquire a genetic resistance. In 1949 J.B.S. Haldane noted the overlap between maps of malaria and of sickle-cell anaemia in Africa, and deduced that the sickling trait must have evolved as a defence against malaria infection. He then proposed his more general thesis that natural selective pressures in childhood must have greatly influenced human biological evolution. Second, while the genetic 'mean' may thus change, continuing protection arises from the genetic variation between individuals in the protein 'marker' molecules on the surface of their cells. This human molecular diversity makes it difficult for an infectious agent to evolve a camouflage against immune detection by 'mimicking' the host's cell-surface proteins. Human antigenic diversity thereby confers a type of genetic 'herd immunity', a property of the population at large.

Malaria illustrates well the evolutionary and ecological dimensions to infectious disease, including the coevolutionary competition with one of its more recent host species, *Homo sapiens*.

Malaria: a redoubtable survivor

Malaria remains one of the world's great and dreadful diseases. It is currently endemic in over 100 countries, and two-fifths of the world population lives in malaria transmission zones. During the 1990s, the estimated annual number of cases rose from around 250 million to 400 million. The annual number of deaths attributed to malaria, occurring predominantly in children, is approximately 1 million. In the late 1990s the World Health Organization initiated a special 'Roll Back Malaria' programme, following the frustrations of the previous quarter-century during which eradication efforts failed widely. Resistance of the malaria parasite, the plasmodium, to anti-malaria drugs has increased widely in recent years, and the anopheline mosquito 'vector' that transmits the parasite has acquired increasing resistance to DDT and other insecticides.

There are two main species of the malaria parasite (plasmodium): *Plasmodium vivax* and *Plasmodium falciparum*. Although falciparum malaria requires warmer temperatures and therefore occurs less widely than vivax malaria, it is much more life-threatening. Its geographic range is also limited by its inability to 'hibernate' over winter in the human liver, as vivax can. The search for a vaccine and effective anti-malaria drugs has been repeatedly frustrated by the complexity of the parasite's life-cycle and by its great genetic flexibility.

Malaria is an ancient affliction of humankind. Coevolution has therefore brought about some mutual biological adaptation. Humans have acquired various genetic adaptations in haemoglobin structure and in the architecture and metabolism of red blood cells. These improvised evolutionary responses, based on the selective retention of randomly occurring molecular abnormalities, have thus far conferred more protection than have recent attempts to eliminate mosquito populations, to develop a vaccine, and to maintain successful prophylaxis with drugs. Over many centuries, human social adaptations to malaria have been hampered by ignorance about its nature. The mode of transmission, via mosquito, was only elucidated at the end of the nineteenth century. The long struggle with malaria is well illustrated by the experience of southern Italy.

Over 2,000 years ago, the colonies of Classical Greece in Sicily and southern peninsular Italy struggled against malaria. (The logo of my own institution, the London School of Hygiene and Tropical Medicine, is based on a Greek-Sicilian coin from that era commemorating the temporary retreat of malaria.) Subsequently, southern Italy was enfeebled by endemic malaria for many centuries. Historians describe the people south of Naples and on the islands of Sardinia and Sicily as chronically infected with malaria, and therefore malnourished, stunted and debilitated. Malaria sapped social initiative and economic energy; it distorted social relations by weakening the peasantry; it largely determined patterns of land ownership and daily farm-work patterns; and it eroded the vigour of community life. This ancient disease was thought of as King of the South.

Malaria ruled not just because of the warm temperatures; the landscape favoured the mosquito by its year-round provision of pools of surface water. The modest southern Apennine mountains have negligible snow cover and cannot sustain the summer flow of rivers. Instead, the seasonal rains cause river floods in winter and drying out in summer, both creating pools of standing water. This paradise for the anopheline mosquitoes was further enhanced by the accelerating deforestation of hillsides during the nineteenth century, with increased water run-off, as privatisation of land-ownership spread, as demand for fuel-wood and railway sleepers increased.

Until the early 1900s – soon after Britain's Ronald Ross and Italy's Battista Grassi had (competitively and separately) demonstrated that mosquitoes transmit malaria – it was widely believed that malaria was caused by telluric emanations from 'poisoned soil'. For example, turn-of-the-century records from British India show that the army medical corps exonerated the (immensely profitable) new irrigation schemes as a cause of increased malaria, attributing it instead to maladies of the soil. Similarly, Italian farm labourers of that time, living in villages on the non-malarious slopes, feared the nocturnal miasmatic malaria curse that lurked in the fields below.

Early attempts at eradication by land drainage and, after 1900, by mass medication with quinine were unsuccessful. Meanwhile, malaria provided a rallying point for political campaigning for land reform and the rise of unionism to protect the health of rural workers. In the 1930s, the fascist government sought to control malaria via better land management and intensive drainage to limit mosquito populations. These hardwon steps were soon nullified by the environmental mayhem of World War II. Livestock (the alternative source of blood for mosquitoes) were wiped out; adaptive social behaviours disintegrated; and the retreating German Army in 1944 flooded the fields. In Monte Cassino, south of Naples, the devastation resulted in a catastrophic outbreak of falciparum malaria. Infection rates of 100% occurred in many village populations among the rubble and watery debris. The resultant death rates depopulated parts of this brutally blighted countryside.

After the war came the widespread use of DDT. As elsewhere in Europe, DDT in combination with more vigilant environmental management and rapid treatment of malaria cases soon prevailed over the disease. Southern Italy thus became free of malaria within several decades.

Malaria: evolutionary origins

The evolution of malaria is a fascinating saga. Viewed from the present, we can see ready evidence of the evolutionary pursuit of self-interest: female mosquitoes obtain protein nutrients from the blood of humans and other vertebrates in order to reproduce; the malaria parasite has found intricate ways of accessing both human liver and blood cells and the mosquito gut to gain the nutrients it requires at each of its several life-stages; and all three species – humans, mosquitoes and parasites – have evolved intricate defences and subterfuges against one another.

The single-celled protozoan organism that causes malaria belongs to the ancient *Plasmodium* genus. That genus has done well in the post-dinosaur era. The plasmodium lineage that led to human malaria is thought to have infected ancestral primate species from around 50 million years ago. The close genetic relationship, today, of the malaria parasites in humans and African apes makes clear that human malaria is indeed an Old World disease in its origins. However, the wider profile of plasmodium-related parasites found today in invertebrates, reptiles, birds and mammals suggests the uncertain outlines of a much older story.[27]

How could this wonderfully fine-tuned and intricate two-host life-cycle of the malaria plasmodium have arisen via the evolutionary process? Well, as the neo-Darwinians keep reminding us, evolution does not work towards a 'goal'.[28] It proceeds opportunistically, and often gets by with improvisations. To be evolutionarily selected a biological variation does not have to work well; it simply has to work a bit better. For an emergent animal species that had to forage in daylight, an 'eye' with one-tenth the capacity of a modern mammalian eye to distinguish light and colour would have been better than having no eye. So, each biological species we see around us today is no more than the work-in-progress product of a sequence of sufficient responses to environmental pressures.

The malaria organism probably evolved from single-celled coccidia, several hundred million years ago.[27] The coccidia, originally free-living microbes, subsequently evolved a parasitic lifestyle inside the gut cells of ancient marine creatures. Here they fed and sexually reproduced, and their offspring were excreted to the watery outside world – where, with luck, another prospective host would ingest them. One branch of the coccidia, the Haemosporidia, evolved to spend part of their life-cycle in the host's blood stream. They diversified further into forms able to infect amphibians, reptiles and birds. Then a more novel step was taken: an evolutionary variant of the Haemosporidia took advantage of the transport opportunity provided by blood-feeding insects. When an insect fed on the blood of (say) a bird, the Haemosporidia in the ingested blood would reach a new host when the insect was eaten by another bird. Via this somewhat crude 'vector-borne' technique, the parasite achieved readier transmission between hosts. Later, the parasite achieved further gains in 'fitness' by deferring the sexual reproductive stage of its life-cycle until inside the blood-feeding insect. By thus using the insect's nutrients for its sexual reproductive stage the parasite multiplied its reproductive ability. The spore-like offspring would then congregate in the insect's mouth parts, and be injected in large numbers into the next potential host that the infected insect preyed upon.

The Haemosporidia then apparently differentiated into several 'families', including the Plasmodia. Although biologists debate the details, there is broad agreement that this type of parasite infected reptiles and birds during the dinosaur-dominated Mesozoic era. Malaria parasites are still common in reptiles and birds. In the post-dinosaur Cenozoic era they began to infect mammals including, before long, the ancestral primates. Mosquitoes may have become their preferred vector, from around 40–50 million years ago.[29]

The subsequent evolution of the malaria parasite in monkeys probably occurred mainly in tropical Africa and Southeast Asia, over tens of million of years. There are today many malaria species in monkeys. Three of the four species of plasmodium that infect humans came from simian origins 25–50 million years ago, according to molecular genetic studies. The origins of *Plasmodium falciparum* are less clear. Molecular genetic analyses indicate that humans acquired falciparum malaria directly from birds. This means that it is less well adapted to mammalian biology – which may account for its greater virulence in humans.[30] During the past 10 million years or so, various forms of malaria in Africa evolved within apes. Perhaps the early hominids, preceding the upright-walking australopithecines 4–5 million years ago, brought malaria with them from their arboreal existence. If so, malaria is one of humankind's 'heirloom infections' (see chapter 4). Or perhaps in those early foragers and later hunter-gatherers malaria began rather tentatively as a sporadic zoonotic (presumably ape-based) infection which became adapted to humans in Africa during the Pleistocene.[27,29]

Glaciation predominated during the Pleistocene, and had become more severe by the time *Homo erectus* first colonised Europe from around 1 million years ago. Malaria probably failed to establish a firm hold in that continent in prehistoric times. The more cold-tolerant *malariae* and *vivax* species may have survived around the Mediterranean coastline. The *vivax* species may then have evolved its distinctive capacity to lie dormant in the primate liver during the cold winter months, thereby gaining a competitive edge on other malaria species unable to survive year-round in cold climes. Over the past half-million years, Neanderthals and their predecessors may therefore have occasionally suffered the fevers, chills and sweating of malaria, during the brief interglacial respites when, for about 15,000 out of every 100,000 years, Europe's temperature increased by 5–10 °C. During those warmer times with their higher sea-levels, the formation of coastal and riverine marshes would have allowed anopheline mosquitoes to move into Europe.[31]

BEFORE THE CURRENT Holocene interglacial, from around 10,000 years ago, followed by the onset of farming and settled village life, malaria could not have become an endemic infection in humans. However, this began to change in western Africa as land clearance and early agriculture emerged around 4,000 years ago. Population geneticists think that vivax malaria must have entered African populations around that time since, among indigenous Africans, there is now near-universal genetically based resistance to this form of malaria.[32] Indeed, vivax malaria is now virtually absent from sub-Saharan Africa. Meanwhile, falciparum malaria became established in African populations. The spectrum of genetic defences against this potentially lethal form of malaria, which includes the well-known sickle-cell trait, is greater in African than in non-African populations.

Vivax malaria subsequently spread northwards, around the shores of the Mediterranean and into much of Asia, as larger, forest-clearing, farming populations emerged in southern China, West Africa, South Asia and Papua-New Guinea. The introduction of agriculture into Greece, from the Anatolian region around 7000 BC, may have enabled malaria to become established there. In subsequent millennia, it would presumably have accompanied the diffusion of farming populations across Europe. However, the earliest actual references to malaria come from Ancient Egypt. The Ebers papyrus from around 1500 BC mentions 'rigors', fever and enlargement of the spleen. Hieroglyphics on temple walls describe an intermittent fever following heavy flooding of the Nile. A thousand years later, Hippocrates, the Greek physician (who did a stint of training in Egypt) placed the documentation of malaria onto a firmer footing. He gave a clear clinical account of the disease and its environmental origins, especially the hazards of low-lying swamps and their effluvia and bad airs (hence, in later Renaissance Italy, the phrase 'mala-aria'). There was, of course, no formal notion of 'infection' in those days.

Over the ensuing 2,000 years malaria fluctuated in the European region. Falciparum malaria, which requires higher temperatures than vivax, probably did not penetrate far into Europe. Malaria appears not to have been much of a problem during the heyday of the Roman Empire – primarily because the dominant anopheline mosquito, *Anopheles atroparvus*, in Europe was an inefficient vector for human malaria (and, anyway, it preferred to feed on livestock). Later in classical times two new mosquito vectors became established in the Mediterranean region, one from North Africa and one from South Asia. Malaria thus became a serious problem during the decline of the Roman Empire. The subsequent history of malaria in Europe is obscure for many centuries. It may have contributed to the collapse of several of the Crusades in the Middle Ages. Because of the profusion of Olde Englishe names for variants of 'agues' and 'fevers', it is not clear when malaria became endemic in England, although it seems to have been endemic along the coasts and estuaries of south-east England in the fifteenth century.[33] The rapid growth in international sea trade in the sixteenth century facilitated the spread of the disease, and malaria re-emerged as a major problem in Europe in the seventeenth and eighteenth centuries. This, paradoxically, was a time of great cold (shown also in Figure 5.1).[34] Meanwhile, Europeans introduced vivax malaria into Latin America in the course of their conquests in the early sixteenth century. Receptive anopheline mosquitoes were naturally widespread in that continent. Subsequently, via the slave trade from West Africa, falciparum malaria was introduced to the Americas where it caused particular devastation in Brazil.

In the 1660s, the statistically minded London haberdasher, John Graunt, began to compile the Bills of Mortality, noting that the third most common cause of death was 'agues and fevers', and the eminent English physician Thomas Sydenham left precise descriptions which make clear that most such deaths were due to malaria. In the 1670s, King Charles II was an early recipient of an exotic treatment with an extract from the Peruvian cinchona tree, recently introduced to Europe by Spanish missionaries (and hence called 'Jesuits' powder'). This extract contained the alkaloid quinine, later to become the mainstay of malaria treatment. Meanwhile, various ingenious folk remedies for malaria emerged. Residents of the watery Fens district opted for opium from locally grown poppies and from opium-laced beer served in local hostelries.

During the nineteenth century, changes in farming methods and animal husbandry began to alter the ecology of malaria in northern Europe – where

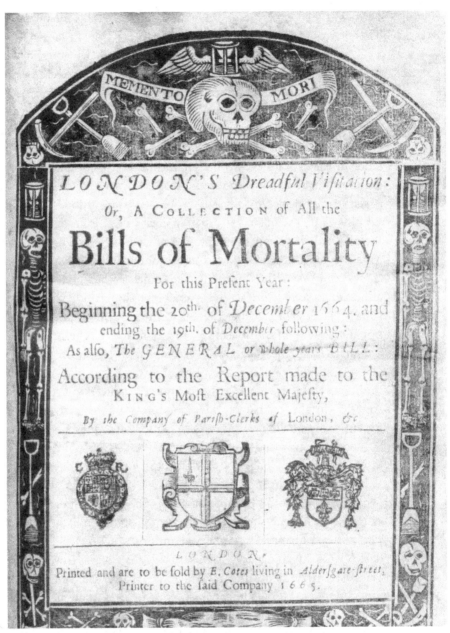

Figure 3.3 Frontispiece for the famous, pioneering, Bills of Mortality compiled by the statistically minded haberdasher John Graunt in London during the 1660s. This was a decade of resurgent bubonic plague, but malaria was also rife (it had killed Oliver Cromwell – who refused, on sectarian grounds, to take the one available remedy, the 'Jesuits' powder').

epidemic outbreaks were occurring as far north as Finland and northern Sweden. Forest clearance reduced mosquito habitat. The introduction of barns for cattle and sties for pigs led to a massive diversion of anopheline mosquitoes away from human targets. They relocated into the barns, and fed freely on unprotesting animals. Because the malaria parasite cannot survive in most farm animals, with their higher levels of sodium in blood, the cycle of infection and transmission was broken. The disease therefore receded.

In the tropical world, however, malaria remained a major killer. Following World War II, a massive effort was launched via the World Health Organization to eradicate malaria, using the new wonder-pesticide, DDT. The combination of spraying, surface water management, and rapid treatment of cases all contributed to the reduction of malaria in many countries and its elimination in some. By the 1960s Europe was essentially malaria-free. Likewise North America and Australia. But by the 1970s, the campaign had faltered. DDT-resistance was occurring in mosquitoes, the public was becoming somewhat reluctant to use DDT in view of its indiscriminate and persistent ecological impacts, and the malaria parasite was becoming resistant to drugs. Diverse strategies of vaccine development were tried, but without significant success. By the late 1990s the estimated annual number of malaria cases in the world was of the order of 400,000 per year.

Malaria is currently on the rise again. Increases in human numbers, mobility and peri-urban poverty, changes in patterns of land use, and the continued rise of drug and pesticide resistance are all contributing to this resurgence. The quarter-century of global warming since the mid-1970s may also have contributed, although, if so, this is not yet directly discernible. Overall, the ecological balance has, for the time being, tipped in favour of this ancient and versatile infectious disease.

Malaria: the struggle between parasite and host

The malaria parasite makes many different proteins over its several life-stages. Some of these antigenic proteins evoke a strong response from the host immune system in which white blood cells release cascades of both parasite-destroying chemokine molecules and antibody molecules. The balance between these two cascades determines how much collateral host-tissue damage occurs during the immune response. In previously infected persons, the inflammatory response is more muted and the risk to host tissues is less.

The hit-and-run acute infections, such as measles and chickenpox, have already passed to a new host by the time the body mounts an effective immune response. For many slower-acting infections, such as malaria and HIV, the key to the infectious agent's success lies in evading the immune system. Malaria illustrates well the extremes of immunogenetic camouflage, confusion and counter-measure that a parasite can achieve. For example, successive waves of malaria trophozoites, released by the liver, display differing surface antigens which confuse the host immune system.

The molecular arms-race between parasite and human host is further illustrated by the trophozoites' mode of entry into red blood cells, where they feed and multiply. On the parasite's surface there is a molecular protein protruberance, the tip of which the parasite must excise by enzymatic action before it can enter the blood cell. The human immune system produces an antibody, A, which by attaching to this protruberance prevents the enzymatic excision. However, another of the parasite's surface proteins stimulates the host immune system to produce a different antibody, B, which physically obstructs the binding of antibody A. The plasmodium thus subverts the host immune system to its own advantage. Having gained entry to the red blood cell, the parasitic plasmodium then takes action to maximise its chances of feeding on the amino acid constituents of the haemoglobin molecule. Infected blood cells are normally detected and destroyed by the host spleen. The plasmodium averts this fate by inducing the infected red blood cells to clump together as they pass through capillaries. These aggregated cells therefore lodge in backwaters of the vascular system, giving the plasmodium extra time to feed unmolested by the host's spleen. Falciparum malaria particularly induces these vascular blockages, resulting in life-threatening 'cerebral malaria'.

Malaria, as a potent child-killer, has evoked some very distinctive human genetic adaptations. The main genetic adaptations are thought to have arisen over the past 4–5 millennia, since farming populations in equatorial and northern Africa and in southern Europe attained sufficient size to sustain endemic circulation of the disease. However, there are uncertainties about this time depth; it could extend back much further.[35]

Africans are immune to vivax malaria because they have acquired the 'Duffy negative' mutation, which thwarts attempts by the vivax plasmodium to gain entry to the red blood cell.[36] Even more intense selection pressures have come from falciparum malaria. In Africa, the sickle-cell trait evolved; around the Mediterranean, Asia and Melanesia the several thalassaemia traits evolved; and in tropical and subtropical countries the red-blood-cell enzyme deficiency 'G6PD' evolved widely – and, as we saw earlier, affected Pythagoras.

In the well-known sickle-cell trait, the abnormal haemoglobin S distorts the red blood cell and hampers the parasite's attempts to feed and reproduce. Since SS homozygosity entails near-certain death in childhood, the SA heterozygous children must have a considerable malaria-surviving advantage over the 'normal' AA children for this abnormal S gene to be maintained. This trade-off between high-fatality (SS) and life-sparing (SA) genotypes is an example of a 'balanced polymorphism' – a biological cost-benefit equilibrium point. Simple calculation shows that in parts of Africa the mortality from falciparum malaria must have been as high as 25% in AA children. A similar mutation has arisen in Papua New Guinea, where falciparum malaria transmission is intense. This 'Melanesian ovalocytosis' also yields deformed red cells, partially resistant to invasion. Homozygosity is 100% lethal to the fetus, and yet the mutation persists in the population via a balanced polymorphism because of the benefit to the heterozygous individual. The dispassionate arithmetic of natural selection depends only on gene frequencies in populations: if more individuals gain than lose, then the relevant allele will prosper.

Human diversity: misplaced notions of 'race'

In discussing genetic variations between regions and populations, the fascinating but fraught concept of human racial differences arises. As is clear from this chapter, the human species has undergone many localised anatomical and metabolic adaptations to environmental pressures, and regional populations have also been subject to the vagaries of genetic drift and founder effects. However, modern molecular genetics has demonstrated that there are no clearcut 'racial' divisions; that humans everywhere exist on a genetic continuum. Nevertheless, the idea of 'race' is deeply embedded in the human psyche, and the horrors of ethnic cleansing persist in today's world.

These ideas have deep foundations in Europe and elsewhere. In the eighteenth century, Carolus Linnaeus (the founder of the modern taxonomy of plants and animals) gave formal expression to the popular notion of the Great Chain of Being. Later that century, the German naturalist Johann Blumenbach identified 'Caucasians', originating in Georgia, as the aesthetically ideal human type. He proposed four other races: Mongolian, Malay, Ethiopian and American. However, two related problems were evident in this hierarchical schema. First, the anatomical boundaries between races were manifestly blurred. Second, how might such blurring and variation arise in nature? After all, the Bible prescribed a creationist stasis.

In 1859, Darwin's theory of evolution offered a solution to this second problem: living forms evolved to improve their fit with the environment. Elitarians, including Darwin's cousin Francis Galton, seized upon and distorted the idea that certain classes of person within the population were naturally fitter.[37] Thus was eugenics born. It was soon reinforced by the new insight that Mendelian genes were discrete and unchangeable. This suggested that 'pure' human genes would breed true if admixture with other human genes were avoided. The eugenics movement flourished in the early twentieth century, seeking particularly to control the quality of breeding. A total of 25,000 Americans were sterilised to avert transmission of feeble-mindedness or criminality. The culmination of these ideas was racial genocide directed at preserving racial purity. The state, declared Hitler, had a duty to uphold nature's biological laws. The Aryan race must protect itself from erosion by inferior races. There was sympathy for this view well beyond German borders.

Since mid-twentieth century, the UN and other international bodies have sought to promote a sense of universality. Science, too, has changed its concepts and terminology: the human species is now recognised to be a network of interconnected breeding populations. But still there are darker shadows: the tribal massacres in Africa; the sporadic flickering of anti-Semitism in Europe and the United States; the continuing persecution of the Romani Gypsies (the Roma) in Europe;[38] recent essentially eugenic legislation in China and Singapore; and the recurrent controversy over 'race' and 'intelligence'.

This latter controversy has been most intense in the United States where hereditarian scientists substantially attribute black–white differences to genes, while environmentalists argue for the primacy of socioeconomic influences.[39] In fact, cognitive ability is as likely to be influenced by genes as are many other aspects of human biology. Indeed, *some* of the variation in intelligence between individuals *is* due to genetic factors, although recent twin studies suggest that well over half the variation is due to social-environmental influences. The flashpoint in the debate is the proposition that there are innate differences in average levels of intelligence between different *population groups*. However, the science on this topic is elusive. Just what is 'intelligence'? Are different dimensions of intelligence (linguistic, logical, visuospatial, etc.) suited to dealing with different environmental and social challenges? Anyway, can the measurement of 'intelligence' ever be standardised across diverse cultures? The hereditarian position is defective in several obvious respects: poor conceptualisation and measurement of 'intelligence', the selective use of evidence, and failure to allow for all-important social-environmental experiences.[39] The marked gains in average levels of IQ in successive generations of young Japanese after World War II have, most certainly, not been due to genetic change. Environment is paramount.

The idea of 'race' remains uncomfortably close to the surface of human affairs, and therefore of science. We need a new synthesis of biology and culture that both explains and celebrates human diversity, and which recognises diversity as an expression of the natural evolutionary essence of each and every species, including our own.

Conclusion

These opening three chapters have looked broadly at the evolutionary backdrop to human biology, and at the great diversity of environments and cultures within which humans have lived. In nature, health and survival play a central role in relation to reproductive fitness. Within human societies everywhere, patterns of health and disease are the product of antecedent biological evolution interacting with current social and physical-environmental conditions. That interaction is at the heart of 'human ecology', the dynamic process that describes and delimits the experiences of groups and populations.

Chapters 4–9 will explore how a succession of changes in human ecology have affected patterns of health and disease. Great changes have occurred in relationships between humans and microbes, in the production of food, in local environmental impacts (particularly industrialisation) and in longevity and fertility, followed more recently by the rise of modern mass consumption behaviours and by urbanisation and its social consequences. This is an ancient, and continuing narrative, chronicling the quest for survival, material advance and cultural evolution, and the attendant consequences for population health, in Earth's dominant species as it encounters and traverses new frontiers.

4

Infectious disease: humans and microbes coevolving

There will come yet other new and unusual ailments, as time brings them in its course . . . And this disease of which I speak, this syphilis too will pass away and die out, but later it will be born again and be seen again by our descendants – just as in bygone ages we must believe it was observed by our ancestors.

Girolamo Fracastoro *De Contagione*, 1546

This chapter brings us to the biblical Fourth Horseman, pestilence. Despite the rather naive optimism of Western science around 1970 – when the US Surgeon-General, for example, declared that it was time 'to close the book on infectious diseases' – this horseman continues to ride on.[1] Indeed, he has seemed to ride with new vigour over the past quarter-century.

During the 1990s there was much talk about the apparent 'resurgence and emergence' of infectious diseases. Americans were gripped by talk of 'coming plagues' and 'killer diseases'. There is a real basis for this concern, although not quite of the melodramatic kind suggested by these popular accounts. The main issue is not the emergence of exotic new infectious diseases such as Ebola virus disease – although the advent of HIV/AIDS reminds us of the ever-present possibility of new epidemic development. Currently, the greater problem is that various ancient infectious diseases such as tuberculosis, malaria and cholera are increasing again within the world at large, and others that may have been quietly circulating for some time (such as cryptosporidiosis, Lyme disease and hepatitis C) have only recently increased to the point of being noticed. A further increasingly serious problem is the rise of antibiotic-resistant infectious agents. These several developments reflect the endless coevolutionary interplay between microbes and their human hosts.

Indeed, the interplay may be more complex than that. Consider influenza: the avian influenza virus, present in several southeast Asian bird species, can infect pigs, ducks, horses and, eventually, humans. The recruitment of influenza viruses into the human circuit has been intensified over the centuries by the crowding together of pigs, poultry and humans. Today, in southern China, the intimate pig/duck farming culture creates a particularly efficient environment in which multiple strains of avian viruses infect pigs. The pigs act as 'mixing vessels', yielding new recombinant-DNA strains of virus which may then infect the pig-tending humans.[2] Every now and then, such a viral variant successfully enters the human population and is launched as a major new influenza pandemic. We had four such pandemics during the twentieth century, beginning with the catastrophic pandemic of 1918–19 when approximately 30 million people died.

The coevolution of humans and infectious agents has a long history. In human prehistory two profound transitions in this relationship occurred: the first when early humans became serious meat-eaters, thereby exposing themselves to various animal parasites, and the second when *Homo sapiens* spread out of Africa into new environments and climates where they encountered unfamiliar microbes. Since the advent of agriculture and animal husbandry, and the dawn of 'history' via written records, three other great transitions have occurred in the human–microbe relationship. First, the early civilisations of the Middle East, Egypt, South Asia, East Asia and Central and South America each acquired their own distinct repertoire of locally evolving 'crowd' infectious diseases. Second, later, over the course of a thousand years the ancient civilisations of greater Eurasia made contact, swapped microbes and painfully equilibrated. Third, from the fifteenth century onwards, Europe – now pre-eminent technologically and as a sea-faring power – inadvertently exported its lethal, empire-winning, germs to the Americas and later to the south Pacific, Australia and Africa.

Today, there appears to be an increased lability in the occurrence, spread and biological behaviour of infectious diseases. Is this history's Fourth Transition, as we globalise, urbanise, increase our mobility, and intensify our food production and our medical technological activities? Will a new equilibration arise as the post-genome era of molecular biotechnologies yields new ways to constrain the natural biological impulses of microbes?

Cholera and tuberculosis are two of humankind's oldest infectious disease scourges. Both have been increasing in recent decades – although we would not have predicted this a quarter-century ago. A brief account of these two diseases gives a foretaste of the larger story about the endless coevolutionary adaptations between humans and microbes.

Cholera

Every young epidemiologist learns that John Snow's inspired studies of cholera in mid-nineteenth-century London were major foundation stones of modern epidemiology. Those epidemiologists who visit London are drawn to Soho to look at, if not drink at, the John Snow Pub next to the site of the famous Broad Street pump – that epicentre of the 'Golden Square' cholera outbreak of summertime 1854. Students of epidemiology learn about the insightful comparisons of cholera death rates in sets of households that Snow made by capitalising on the intermixed neighbourhood supply of drinking water. In many streets, adjoining houses were supplied by two competing water companies, one drawing its Thames water from above the sewer outlets, the other from below. Combining his compelling demonstration of differences in cholera death rates between suburbs and between categories of households with astute biological reasoning, Snow inferred the presence of some specific infective particle in the sewage-contaminated drinking water. This was radical reasoning, three decades before the formulation of the germ theory. It challenged the prevailing theory that disease was caused by non-specific airborne miasmas.[3]

There is, however, much more that we can learn from the story of cholera. Its history has important evolutionary, social and ecological dimensions. Cholera is thought to be an ancient infectious disease. Severe outbreaks of cholera-like dehydrating diarrhoeal diseases are recorded in ancient Hindu, Chinese and Greek texts dating from 2,000 to 3,000 years ago.[4] Over the ensuing centuries it has flared up in South Asia, nurtured by large dense populations, poor sanitation, extensive surface water, warm temperatures and high humidity. Its ancestral homeland appears to have been in riverine and estuarine India, particularly in the great and populous river basins of the Ganges and Brahmaputra rivers. Indeed, a great many serotypes (genetic strains) of the *Vibrio cholerae* bacterium circulate today in those waters, but only one strain induces disease in humans. This it does by attaching to the inner epithelium of the gut, damaging the epithelial cells with its toxin, and thus inducing massive diarrhoea. The watery diarrhoea, of course, greatly boosts the vibrio's chances of transmission to another hapless human, even as it dehydrates its stricken host.

Like HIV and some other infections that initially circulated obscurely within a restricted area, cholera eventually shifted gears and assumed epidemic proportions when perturbed by intensified human activities. This occurred on a localised scale several times during the seventeenth century, and then more substantively in 1817, as British military and colonial activity in India increased. John Snow, writing in 1854, observed that cholera 'began to spread to an extent not before known; and, in the course of seven years, it reached, eastward, to

China and the Philippine Islands; southward, to Mauritius and Bourbon; and to the northwest, as far as Persia and Turkey. Its approach towards our own country, after it entered Europe, was watched with more intense anxiety than its progress in other directions.'[5]

Molecular genetic analyses indicate that, in the early 1800s, the cholera bacterium acquired a toxin-generating gene from a virus or plasmid. (The 'horizontal' transfer of genes occurs often between bacteria and the various self-replicating micro-packages of genetic material that pervade the microbial world.) The cholera bacterium thus became more virulent. The subsequent historical course of cholera has been dramatic. There have now been seven pandemics in each of which the disease spread through at least several regions and many countries. In the early 1830s cholera reached Russia, Western Europe and North America. In Russia the tsar had to quell an uprising by terrified peasants who suspected that the disease had been unleashed against them by the ruling classes to reduce their numbers.

The still-continuing seventh pandemic is the largest and longest ever. It began in 1961 and has engulfed Southeast Asia, the Middle East, Russia, Europe, much of Africa (where it has now become endemic for the first time), and the Americas. Its most recent major extension, in 1991, was into Latin America where it has subsequently caused over 1 million cases and around 12,000 deaths. We will consider, in chapter 11, why cholera has assumed such giant proportions in the late twentieth century. It illustrates well how the weighty processes of contemporary globalisation and the accompanying changes in human ecology can affect patterns of disease.

Tuberculosis

Tuberculosis is the stuff of tragedy and romance: Mimi's tiny frozen hand in Puccini's 'La Boheme'; the dying courtesan, Violetta, in 'La Traviata'; Frederic Chopin, hectic and emaciated, composing his final Mazurka; and the precocious, ill-fated Bronte sisters. *Mycobacterium tuberculosis* has been one of evolution's success stories. Around one-third of all humans alive today have been infected with the tuberculosis bacterium. Approximately 1 in 10 – or 200 million – of those have the active disease. At 2 million deaths every year, tuberculosis causes more deaths than any other single infectious agent except for HIV/AIDS. That, though, is not the main measure of the evolutionary success of *Mycobacterium tuberculosis*. Rather, the bacterium's success is in allowing the great majority of infected persons to survive for many years with active infectious disease, and thus infect others.

The tuberculosis bacterium acquired this facility over several thousand years of coevolution with humans. Because its transmission is via the relatively precarious airborne person-to-person route, the 'fitness' of the bacterium is increased by ensuring the long survival and mobility of infected persons. This differs from the 'fitness' needs of mosquito-transmitted diseases such as malaria, or water-borne diarrhoeal diseases such as cholera, where the immobilisation and serious illness of the infected person do not hinder transmission.[6]

Tuberculosis-like lesions have been identified in the lungs of ancient mummies from Egypt and Peru dating from several thousand years ago.[7] Indeed, lesions in skeletons from the Middle East indicate that tuberculosis may have afflicted humans from at least 6,000–7,000 years ago. *Mycobacterium tuberculosis* originates from an ancestral soil-dwelling bacterium which, genetic analyses suggest, must then have gained 'fitness' by evolving to infect various mammals and birds – and, much later, humans. *Mycobacterium tuberculosis*, from humans, and *Mycobacterium bovis*, from cattle, are genetically very closely related. The fact that *Mycobacterium bovis* has some capacity to cause human disease accords with the general thesis that the 'crowd' infectious diseases of humans arose by the acquisition of mutated infectious agents from cohabiting domesticated and pest animals. It looks as if the tuberculosis organism crossed the species divide, from domesticated cattle to humans, about 7,000 years ago. The passage of the bovine spongiform encephalopathy (mad cow disease) prion into humans sometime in the 1980s provides a novel modern reprise of this cattle-to-human microbial traffic.[8]

Gradual genetic adaptation to the human host has rendered the tuberculosis bacterium almost exclusively dependent on humans. Tuberculosis increased in frequency in Greco-Roman times. It subsequently began a long increase in Europe from the fourteenth century as its close relative leprosy, also caused by a mycobacterium, disappeared in that subcontinent. Recent studies in eastern Africa have shown that there is cross-reactivity in the human immune response to these two mycobacterial diseases, suggesting why a leprosy-ridden underclass in feudal Europe would have been somewhat resistant to tuberculosis. Subsequently, tuberculosis became endemic in Europe and then North America where, during the seventeenth and eighteenth centuries, the 'white plague' killed one in five adults. Indeed, the rise and decline of tuberculosis has occurred successively in regions of the world, peaking in England around 1780, in Western Europe around 1820, in Eastern Europe and Russia later that century, in the Americas early in the twentieth century, and it is still rising in Asia and Africa. The onset of epidemic HIV/AIDS within those latter regions has boosted tuberculosis further.

The tuberculosis bacterium continues to evolve, and has done so particularly in recent decades by adapting to antibiotics. Indeed, along with *Staphylococcus aureus* (which thrives in hospitals), tuberculosis has served notice on us that microbes can acquire simultaneous resistance to multiple drugs. Multiple-drug-resistant tuberculosis, which flared up in New York City in the early 1990s, has subsequently spread in Russia where the chaotic and crowded condition of prisons since the collapse of communism has provided an ideal incubation medium for tuberculosis. Meanwhile, human resistance to tuberculosis is no doubt continuing to evolve via genetic winnowing within susceptible human populations – such as Brazil's Yanomami Indians who first encountered European infections in the 1960s. Scientists think that Europeans carry several genetic legacies from their long struggle with tuberculosis.[9]

In a world where poverty persists on a wide front, in both poor and rich countries, tuberculosis will prosper. Paul Farmer has poignantly described the situation in Haiti, where the two infectious diseases that now kill the most people – tuberculosis and HIV/AIDS – are personified within that mystical culture as 'big and little sisters'.[10] These two diseases are today a major dual scourge of the world's poor.

Infection as a way of life

Throughout prehistory and history, humankind has encountered new and resurgent infectious diseases. We are surrounded and inhabited by microbes. Theirs is a world of fleetfooted genetic lability, of freely exchanged genetic material unrestrained by the formalities of sexual reproduction, and of agile ecological opportunism. These families of organisms have endured for aeons, during which they have honed their adaptive skills to deal with nature's antibiotics, nutrient shortages and hostile immune systems. We humans, evolutionarily, are newcomers. For the duration of their tenure on Earth humans will share the world with microbes.

Infection is a way of life for the potentially 'bad' microbes. As we saw in chapter 3, parasitic microorganisms derive energy or nutrients by colonising body spaces or the insides of body cells. But there is more than mere parasitism involved; often the relationship is of mutual 'symbiotic' benefit. Without nodules of nitrogen-fixing bacteria on their roots, legumes and certain other plants would not grow. Humans could not survive in an infection-free world; without infection the large bowel would cease to work. Indeed, during each human lifetime there is a succession of different bacteria in our bowels. Straight after birth we acquire a profusion of coliform bacteria (including the well-known *Escherichia coli*). After weaning, the bifidobacteria assume the ascendancy, outnumbering coliforms by about 100 to 1. We regard the bifidobacteria as 'good', because they ferment complex carbohydrates and contribute to the healthy function of the large bowel. Then, in later adulthood, the potentially 'bad' clostridial bacteria begin steadily to close the million-to-one gap that separated them from the bifidobacteria during most of adulthood. So, being infected is not the problem. Indeed, our bodies contain very many more bacterial cells (which are relatively small) than they do cells of their own.[11] No, the problem is infectious *disease* – that is, being adversely affected by an infecting agent.

If the microorganism is naturally virulent in humans (such as the cholera bacterium) or if the quiescent balance between host and microbe is disturbed, then a disease process ensues. This causes acute, chronic or perhaps fatal damage to host tissues. This 'disease' process, however, is not malicious. Rather, it is the product of the two conflicting 'fitness'-seeking agendas – agendas which, over time, may tend to converge via coevolution.[12] In part the disease reflects the biological response by the infected person, such as inflammation due to heightened blood flow and local tissue damage associated with the immune system's counterattack, or fever that seeks to over-heat and harm the infecting microbe. In part the disease is a manifestation of the process that the microorganism has evolved to ensure its own dissemination. Microbes, genetically programmed to enhance their own survival, therefore make us sneeze, get diarrhoea, scratch or develop open sores.

Nature's inventiveness in this regard seems limitless. Chickenpox, like other acute and highly contagious infections, can exhaust the local population's supply of non-immune individuals. This puts the virus at risk of dying out within that population. Therefore, in most infected individuals the virus surreptitiously takes cover within the nervous system, where it is beyond the routine surveillance of the immune system, and bides time for five to six decades. Then in some individuals in later adulthood it migrates along peripheral nerves to colonise the filamentous neural network that sensitises areas of skin. Inflamed blotches of skin called 'shingles' are the result. Scratching these itching lesions disseminates the virus into a population which, by this time, has been replenished with young susceptible persons. And so the cycle repeats. The rabies virus also exploits the immunological sanctuary that is afforded by the nervous system. It achieves its proliferative goal by migrating to the animal's brain, inducing deranged aggressive behaviour, and so achieving transmission to other canines – or, inadvertently, humans – via infected saliva from the bite of the rabid animal. Humans, of course, are a 'dead end' for the virus since they do not routinely bite one another.

The microbial world displays well the creative genius of nature, the improvised ingenuity of biological evolution. Anything goes – if it works.

FOR MUCH of the past century infectious diseases in human populations, particularly in wealthy countries, have been in retreat. We learnt to sanitise our cities, cleanse our water supplies, improve domestic hygiene, use antibiotics, control vector organisms and vaccinate. In the later twentieth century the developed world became rather complacent, naively welcoming the false dawn of a life mostly free of infectious disease. However, since the 1980s things have looked much less secure. Around 30 new and previously unrecognised infectious diseases have been identified since the mid-1970s, most spectacularly HIV/AIDS – but also including rotavirus, cryptosporidiosis, legionellosis, the Ebola virus, Lyme disease, hepatitis C, hantavirus pulmonary syndrome and *E. coli* 0157. Meanwhile, as already noted, others such as malaria, tuberculosis, cholera, bubonic plague, salmonellosis and diphtheria have rebounded widely.

Infectious diseases remain the world's leading killer, accounting for one in three of all deaths. Each year 17 million people, mostly young children, die from infectious diseases. Acute respiratory infections kill almost 4 million people; diarrhoeal diseases kill 3 million; HIV/AIDS kills 2.5 million, tuberculosis kills 2 million, and malaria kills 1.5 million. The discrepancy between rich and very poor countries is huge: infections cause 1–2% of all deaths in the former, yet over 50% in the latter. Indeed, among the world's poorest sub-populations infectious disease causes almost two-thirds of deaths. Diseases such as tuberculosis, leprosy, cholera, typhoid and diphtheria are pre-eminently diseases of poverty. As happened historically with tuberculosis, HIV infection seems now to be entrenching itself among the world's poor and disempowered, especially in sub-Saharan Africa and South Asia. Much of the spread of HIV has been along international 'fault lines', tracking the inequality and vulnerability which accompany migrant labour, educational deprivation and sexual commerce.[10] The ramifications of economic disadvantage have been further highlighted by some recent consequences of free trade agreements. For example, in the 1990s there were several outbreaks of hepatitis A and cyclosporiasis (a recently identified protozoal infection) in the United States caused by faecally contaminated strawberries and raspberries imported from Central America. The North American Free Trade Agreement had subordinated environmental and labour standards (such as providing toilet facilities for workers) to the demands of open competition and profitability. This, plus modern rapid air-transport, meant that within two days of the berries being picked, upmarket diners in New York acquired the same faecally transmitted infections as the dispossessed farm workers in Guatemala.

There has also been some good news. The smallpox virus, having neither a non-human host nor a vector organism in which to hide, was eradicated in the late 1970s. Polio, measles, guinea-worm and perhaps leprosy may soon each go the same way. Several new vaccines (for hepatitis A and B, for example) have been developed – and there is the promise of DNA vaccines which enable body cells in the vaccinated person to manufacture the DNA-specified antigen that induces immunity. Meanwhile, the gradual increase in the provision of safe drinking water is lowering risks of infectious diseases in many low-income and slum-dwelling populations. However, the good news will be limited unless there is widespread investment and refurbishing of public health systems around the world. Those systems, for various economic and political reasons, were widely under-funded, neglected or damaged during the later years of the twentieth century.

This continuing interplay between human culture and the microbial world is an ancient narrative. Today the plot is thickening. Antibiotic over-use, increased human mobility, long-distance trade, intensification of livestock production, large dam and irrigation projects, urbanisation, extended sexual contact networks, expanding numbers of refugees, and the exacerbation of poverty in inner-urban ghettos, shanty towns and in poor undernourished populations everywhere – all these trends have great consequences for infectious diseases. The clearance and fragmentation of forest have increased the exposure of Third World rural populations to various infectious diseases, such as the several newly encountered arenaviruses that cause haemorrhagic fevers in South American rural populations. On an even larger scale, as will be discussed in chapter 10, climate change and other global environmental changes will have further impacts on patterns of infectious diseases.

The narrative has not been confined to infectious disease in humans. In the 1890s, cattle infected with a morbillivirus were imported by Italian colonialists into Ethiopia. This initiated the twentieth century's devastating epidemics of rinderpest in domesticated cattle and wild herbivores in eastern and southern

Africa. Similarly, the export of cattle from West Africa by French colonists in the eighteenth and nineteenth centuries introduced tick-borne cattle infections to the Caribbean, where the infection has spread through the island chain and is now threatening mainland South America. In the 1990s, intensively raised pigs in Germany, Taiwan and Malaysia succumbed to mass viral infections. Malaysia's Nipah virus outbreak of 1998, apparently originating in infected bats, caused the deaths of thousands of pigs and hundreds of pig-handling humans. Algal blooms and other human-induced disturbances of coastal ecosystems have caused unusual infections in various sea-mammals, such as the manatees of the Florida coast.

Running through this story of the interplay between human ecology and the microbial world is a common and important theme. That theme is the fundamental role of cultural, social, economic and political conditions in modulating the ecological opportunities for infectious diseases. The Fourth Horseman has long followed in the footprints left by humans as they entered new terrain, disturbed the natural environment, altered their patterns of settlement, and changed their patterns of contact with one another.

FOR AN INFECTING MICROBE, the ideal is to achieve successful reproduction without having to expend extra energy on a host–parasite struggle. But since hosts are usually not that accommodating, compromises must be made and energy must be expended. We may not usually see it their way, but it's not easy to become a successful infectious disease agent. There are millions of microbial species out there able to take a chance on colonising a new host species. The process entails no intent; new infections arise by chance encounter – and mostly we are unaware of it.

Most of the microbes that try out potential new hosts fail. Success, too, may be short lived. The mysterious 'English Sweats' which ravaged the English population several times during the first half of the sixteenth century then seemingly simply disappeared. The new variant Creutzfeld-Jakob disease (CJD), a fatal neurological disorder apparently caused by the transmission of prions from 'infected' British beef, will in time probably disappear also, since there is no apparent possibility of person-to-person spread. However, a few human infectious diseases succeed in the long term. With this seemingly secure tenure they have become our textbook infections: measles, chickenpox, tuberculosis, typhoid, cholera, syphilis and so on. In nature, though, there is no permanent success. All species are at high probability of becoming extinct, either by termination or by replacement through speciation. The English Sweats disappeared. Smallpox, after several thousand years as a major infectious disease in humans has now been eliminated. Pinta, yaws, non-venereal syphilis, and, later, venereal syphilis display an intriguing evolutionary trail, in which each of the earlier forms has apparently evolved to the next.

Once colonisation of a new host species has been achieved, the infectivity and virulence of the infectious agent evolves in favour of genotypic variants better able to achieve sustained transmission. These genetic adaptations are of various kinds. For example, the outer antigenic surface of the infecting species evolves as immune surveillance by the infected host culls the detectable strains of invaders. Likewise, metabolic changes evolve in micro-organisms under the intense pressure of antibiotic use. As we have seen in the evolution of ancestral malaria (chapter 3), infectious agents also find new and improved ways of passage between individual hosts.

Along with the clear failures and successes in this evolutionary procession there are many microbial *arrivistes*, yet to establish their long-term credentials. The human immunodeficiency virus (HIV) has now circulated in human populations for several decades. It has, for the time being, become a success story. Time alone will confirm the durability of this viral infection.

Evolutionary origins of human infectious diseases

The historian William McNeill has described how human cultural evolution has repeatedly disturbed the biological equilibrium between man and microbe – and how in the fullness of time natural forces reestablish a new equilibrium.[13] The initial change in eastern African hominids from tree dwelling to ground dwelling brought a radical change in the microbial parasitic environment for the newly upright-walking australopithecines. Soil-dwelling hookworms and the tetanus bacterium would have been encountered, along with an unfamiliar constellation of low-flying mosquitoes. As the australopithecines were superseded by the bigger-brained *Homo* genus, the use of animal skins for rudimentary clothing and shelter, and a heightened reliance on eating meat, must have brought further contact with food-borne helminths (the various worms) and bacteria. More recently, our cousin species, the Neanderthals, occupied Europe and western Asia for much of the last quarter-million years. The few available palaeoanthropological clues indicate that they were familiar with dental caries and infective arthritis.

Humans have both 'heirloom' and 'acquired' infections.[14] The heirloom infections were handed on from primate ancestors when the early hominid line diverged. The simplest category would have been the lumpenproletariat of the bacterial world – the staphylocooci, streptococci and coliform bacteria that cause routine wound infections, throat infections and diarrhoeal diseases. Those infections may have been more lethal in the debilitating conditions of malnutrition and, in *Homo erectus* and in our Neanderthal relatives, the intense ice-age cold of northern climates. Our heirloom infections also include the non-pathogenic commensal bacteria that flourish in our mouths, stomachs and intestines. However, hominid foragers and, later, human hunter-gatherers, living in small, isolated and mobile groups, could not sustain endemic circulation of acute infectious diseases such as measles and influenza. Indeed, such diseases did not exist in humans until they evolved in response to the radical new opportunities afforded by neolithic settled agrarian populations.

Probably three other categories of infections affected these foragers and hunter-gatherers. First, certain viruses were able to persist or even lie dormant for decades, including the ubiquitous Epstein-Barr virus and various herpes and hepatitis viruses. Those viruses achieved unhurried transmission, sometimes by a process of reactivation after several dormant decades. Second, there would have been various chronic parasitic infections by protozoa and helminths (including tapeworms and pinworms). Through hard-won evolutionary toil, these persistent, mildly debilitating, infectious agents had learnt to damp down the human host's immunological response. Since they had time to achieve unhurried transmission across generations, from parent to child, they did not require large host populations. Third, zoonotic infectious agents would have been acquired incidentally from locally circulating endemic infections in wild animals. Some, such as simian malaria in monkeys and trypanosomiasis in antelope and buffaloes, require an insect vector for transfer from animal to human; others are acquired by direct contact. This category may have posed only a sporadic problem to hunter-gatherers, living in species-rich ecosystems, since these zoonotic microorganisms were not adapted to human biology. Scares in recent years over the Ebola virus and the Marburg virus, both acquired from animal sources, have reminded us of the occasional virulence of such agents when they transfer to humans.

Subsequently the tempo of change in the microbiological environment accelerated. Around 85,000 years ago the warmer interglacial interlude began to recede, and a cooler aridity returned to equatorial regions. Early modern humans began to drift from the deteriorating dietary environment of northeastern Africa into the lands of west Asia and beyond. As we saw in previous chapters, those ancestral moderns radiated east, north and then west, entering all continents except Antarctica. They would have encountered various new 'emergent' infectious diseases as they spread into these unfamiliar, though parasitically less dense, environments.

Early food-foraging groups remained small, comprising aggregations of no more than several hundred (during good seasons) at most. This meant that acute infections, sporadically encountered, could not be sustained as endemic infections. Among acute infections, only exceptional parasites able to withstand the dryness and temperature extremes outside the human body could survive long enough in the environment to infect itinerant hunter-gatherers. Recent research on the bacteria that cause infections of ears, noses and throats in Australian Aborigines indicates that those strains that reside longer in their human hosts (before being evicted by rival strains or by immune attack) can sustain endemic circulation in smaller groups of humans than can more ephemeral bacterial strains.[15] Measles, which remains transmissible for just several days, requires a local population of around half a million to have a sufficient supply of previously uninfected young people to enable the disease to become endemic. Acute contagious diseases of that kind were not compatible with small foraging bands of early hunter-gatherers.

From around 15,000 years ago a momentous change occurred. The long glaciation began to recede and Earth entered a prolonged, but erratic, warming phase. The fossil and pollen records show that this resulted in climatic stresses upon many species of edible animals and wild plant foods. In low to middle latitudes, humans responded by learning to grow plants and herd animals. Slowly the food yields increased. Conforming to a general law of nature, human population size expanded to the extent that available food supplies allowed.

The first historical transition: agrarian ecology

In various locations around the world, human life gradually became more settled and less nomadic. Villages, towns, and, later, cities appeared. These human settlements offered a major new ecological niche for infectious agents. For a start, humans made more frequent contact with one another, vector organisms such as mosquitoes were often abundant around such settlements, and the greatly enlarged human numbers afforded the security of continuous (endemic) transmission. This radical transition in human ecology greatly changed the pattern of human disease. This is evident from most of the palae-opathological studies comparing pre-agrarian and post-agrarian skeletal remains.[16] The early farmers were shorter, and shorter-lived, than their imme-diate hunter-gatherer forebears; they were generally less well fed and more exposed to infectious diseases.

While hunter-gatherers had been exposed to a limited spectrum of infec-tious and parasitic agents, in settled agrarian communities this spectrum was greatly widened by two main factors. First, human settlements were pervaded by their own accumulated waste and excreta, and this enabled the recycling of infectious agents, assisted by proliferating rodents and insects. Second, many new infectious agents were acquired from closely encountered animal popula-tions. The new opportunity afforded by large numbers of humans cohabiting with domesticated and pest animals multiplied the likelihood of occurrence of mutant strains of microbe, some of which successfully crossed the species divide.[17] This was the main source of today's familiar 'crowd' infectious dis-eases, acute viral diseases like measles, mumps, chickenpox, and influenza and bacterial diseases such as tuberculosis that we modern urban dwellers think of as part of the natural landscape. Smallpox arose via a mutant pox virus from cattle. Measles is thought to have come from the virus that causes distemper in dogs, leprosy from water buffalo, the common cold from horses, and so on. The list is very long, and the story continues today as we acquire from animal sources such infections as HIV and the Nipah virus. Historians consider that Asia, with early large agrarian populations, was the likely cradle of many of the infectious diseases that entered human populations from domesticated and pest animal species – whereas Africa was the cradle of vector-borne infectious diseases from wild animal sources, including malaria, dengue and African try-panosomiasis (sleeping sickness).

A few infective agents must have entered early settled populations more simply. For example, mosquito-borne yellow fever circulates naturally high in the forest canopy as a long-established infection of monkeys. As early agricul-turalists cleared the forests, so they would have brought the infected mosqui-toes down to ground level where they readily fed upon, and infected, this larger hairless primate. More generally, the clearing of land for agriculture has repeatedly put humans into closer contact with disturbed ecosystems, from which they have encountered many new mosquito-borne, tick-borne and rodent-borne infectious agents. Malaria most probably gained its foothold as a human infection from early forest-clearing and farming in western Africa.

When, later, irrigated agriculture evolved, so opportunities increased for water-breeding mosquitoes, for the water snails that spread schistosomiasis, and for the guinea worm.

Serendipity in cultural practice sometimes played a protective role. For example, in ancient Nubia, on the upper Nile, the method of storing grain appears to have provided villagers with natural antibiotic protection. Nubian fossil bones show little evidence of infectious diseases. Instead, under fluorescent examination they show an unusual content of tetracycline. Archaeologists think that the micro-environment within the Nubians' mud-walled grain storage silos promoted the growth of a tetracycline-producing mould, and that this conferred protection against many bacterial infections.

The same animal-to-human evolution of infectious disease occurred in other far-flung centres of agriculture and urbanisation. Chagas disease entered human populations several thousand years ago via the domestication of guinea-pigs by Amerindians, probably in Brazil. Along with the llama family and canines, the guinea-pig is the only other indigenous mammal that was available for domestication by Amerindians. Chagas disease is caused by a protozoan cousin of the trypanosome which, via infected tsetse flies, causes African sleeping sickness. It is transmitted via the triatomine bug, and infects a massive 15–20% of the population in the 'southern cone' countries of South America. It is an essentially untreatable infection that causes thinning and, often, rupture of the walls of the heart, colon and oesophagus. This may have been Charles Darwin's mysterious chronic disease: he recorded being bitten by a triatomine bug while in South America. Mummies from northern Chile, dating from more than 2,000 years ago, show incriminating evidence of organ damage and the presence of the triatomine bug itself. This blood-feeding bug lives naturally in the earthen walls of guinea-pig burrows and transmits the infection between guinea-pigs. It adapts readily to the earthen walls, thatching and floor mats of housing in poor rural areas, where it now also transmits the trypanosome between humans.[18]

This great shift in human infectious disease profile thus has its earliest origins in Mesopotamia from around 6,000–7,000 years ago, at the dawn of history. Before long, there were sufficiently large and dense human populations for the sustained endemic circulation of infectious agents and for recurrent epidemic outbreaks of those diseases able to take temporary refuge elsewhere. Their crops and herds, which were both increasingly dense populations, were also at risk of invasion by pathogens and pests. The historian Alfred Crosby remarks that farmers and herdsmen could drive away wolves and pull up weeds, but there was little they could do to stop infections raging through their densely packed fields, flocks and cities.[19]

We should note that the various mutant microbes that we acquired from animal sources have very much longer ancestries than this 'First Transition' story might imply. The mammals and birds from whom we have recently acquired so many of our infectious diseases are themselves late-stage hosts in these long-running narratives. Indeed, bacteria and viruses predate the evolution of multicellular life by a billion years or so, and must have spent aeons learning to infect one another, and acquiring an evolutionary facility to adapt to hostile biochemical warfare (i.e., nature's antibiotics). Their rapid generation time, immunogenetic lability and capacity to develop resistance give them a survival facility that we have only recently begun to fully recognise.

Towns and city-states: extending the first transition

Great civilisations began to appear in western Asia from around 5,000 years ago, during the warmer 'Holocene Optimum' period. They arose first in Mesopotamia, then in Egypt and, a little further east, in the Indus Valley. Large civilisations in eastern Asia, dominated by northern China, and in south Asia and Mesoamerica followed. Many of these great civilisations had signature epidemics which, for thousands of years, remained regionally confined.[13]

Such populations would, at last, have become large enough to sustain acute contagious diseases, such as measles. These were diseases that left their survivors with lasting immunity and, for their own survival, required a continuous supply of previously uninfected persons. Even so, the historical record is sparse. The best, indirect, evidence from Sumeria is a stone inscription describing epidemics and invoking the Goddess of Epidemics. Skeletal remains from the eastern Mediterranean region suggest an increase in infectious diseases in agrarian-based populations from around 4,000 years ago. However, assessment from bones alone is difficult since most infections leave no skeletal evidence. Ancient South Asia may well have been the cradle of many acute viral infections, such as smallpox. The large early civilisations of India that arose following the Aryan invasions from the northwest from around 4,000 years ago, and their later Asian regional contacts via Buddhist missionaries and extended political-cultural dominion, would have assisted the early urban circulation and dissemination of such diseases.

Egypt provides a near-unique source of ancient historical material because of the combination of dessicating aridity and the practice of mummification of the dead. Religious beliefs required the preservation of a recognisable body, to which the individual's spirit could readily return. Hence, from around 3000 BC, mummies were produced.[20] Parasitic infections are frequently found in mummies: hydatid cysts, flukes, roundworms and tapeworms.[21] Schistosomiasis, which infects an estimated one-fifth of Egyptians today, is evident in many mummies, often in calcified lesions in the urinary bladder. Immune-based tests reveal the presence of malarial antigens from *Plasmodium falciparum*. The evidence for tuberculosis and smallpox in early mummies remains equivocal. However, lesions in preserved bones from predynastic Egypt and from Middle Eastern sources suggest that tuberculosis was present from earlier millennia. Figure 4.1 shows the apparent marks of smallpox vesicles on the face (angle of jaw) of Pharoah Rameses V who died in 1157 BC. Microscopic examination of fragments of scabs and antibody tests have been suggestive but not conclusive.[21]

FROM AROUND 3,500 years ago there are clear references to epidemic diseases in the Bible. There were the plagues of Egypt during Israel's bondage, late in the pharaonic Middle Kingdom. One plague entailed 'sores that break into pustules on man and beast'. Another, more famous, killed the first-born Egyptian children on the night of the original Jewish Passover: 'and there was a great cry in Egypt; for there was not a house where there was not one dead'. After the exodus from Egypt, the Book of Deuteronomy records the subsequent divine injunction to Moses on Mount Sinai to exact a ransom to God from each of the newly liberated Israelites in order 'to avert plague'.

During these times, as city-states and civilisations came increasingly into commercial and military contact, so infectious agents were exchanged. The initial contact would often have caused violent epidemics. For example, in Deuteronomy it is recorded that the Hittites suffered in great anguish from the twenty years of pestilence that followed their importation and enslavement of Egyptian prisoners-of-war. The enslaved Egyptians would have carried with them an array of their more ancient civilisation's semi-socialised microbes. But among the less cosmopolitan, immunologically defenceless Hittites these alien microbes wreaked havoc, despite the anguished prostrations of the Hittite priests.

The first Book of Samuel tells of the conflicts, occurring in the seventh century BC, in which the Lord smote the neighbouring Philistines for their seizure of the Israelites' Ark: 'after they had carried it about, the hand of the Lord was against the city with a very great destruction. And He smote the men

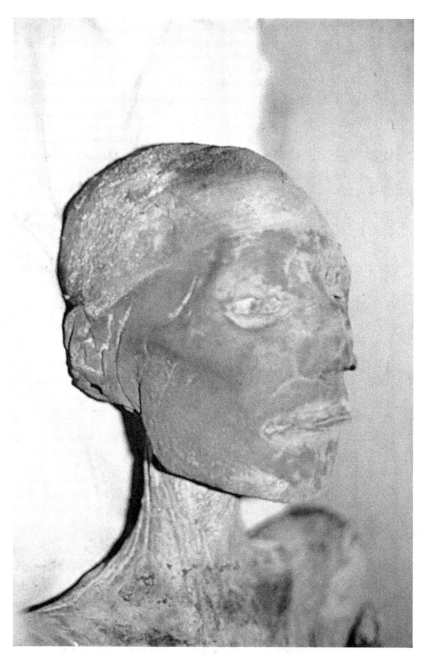

Figure 4.1 Head of Pharaoh Rameses V, from twelfth century BC, showing apparent smallpox vesicles on face (around jaw line). Immunological and electronic microscopic analyses of fragments of scabs have provided strong, but inconclusive, evidence of smallpox. (Reproduced with kind permission of J.E. Harris.)

of the city, both small and great, and they had emerods in their secret parts.'[22] This implausibly precise account records that 5,070 men were smitten 'with a great slaughter'. The embarrassingly located 'emerods', or tumours, have long tantalised historians. They could have been swollen lymph nodes in the groin, the telltale swellings of the bubonic plague. In penitence, the Philistines offered up 'golden mice'. Some historians have seen this as an allusion to the rodents whose infected fleas spread bubonic plague – although that would impute to the Philistines a knowledge of disease transmission several thousand years ahead of its time.

THIS, THEN, IS THE STORY up to around 2,500 years ago. Agrarian civilisations had by then begun to form in regions around the world. A spectrum of new infectious diseases was acquired in each region, and local exchanges between populations began. Initially, the impact of each of these new infectious diseases was probably devastating because of the immunological naivety of the human populations. Subsequently, both human host and infectious agent coevolved. Usually (but not always) the pathogen became less virulent; meanwhile, via the deadly but dispassionate process of natural selection, the intensely selected human population acquired some genetic resistance to the disease. These coevolutionary processes resulted in many of the erstwhile serious epidemic infections becoming the routine endemic infections that persist in the population and typically infect young persons: measles, smallpox, chickenpox, mumps, whooping cough and others.

The process did not occur evenly around the world. Various ancient texts, including the Sumerian *Epic of Gilgamesh* from 4,000 years ago, ancient court texts from Egypt and China, and the Old Testament, indicate that by the second millennium BC epidemic diseases were no longer dire enough to enfeeble the civilised societies in the Middle East and constrain their imperial ambitions. The diseases were evidently evolving towards an accommodation with their human hosts.[13] This, however, was not so in the peripheral, less consolidated, civilisations of the Yellow River and the Ganges Valley, nor in the Aegean-Mediterranean coastal region where, by around 500 BC, the ecological balance of infectious diseases remained less settled.

History's next two great infectious disease transitions occurred as large branches of the human family came into contact again, after tens of thousands of years of separation following the ancient hunter-gatherer dispersals. Each transition established a new infectious disease equilibrium between the interacting populations.

The second transition: contacts between civilisations

From around 2,500 years ago, trade, travel and regional warfare increased between the contiguous civilisations of Eurasia. Consequently, between south-east Europe, West Asia, northern Africa, South Asia and East Asia, ancient boundaries were breached and the pools of infection began to intermix. Historians think that many of the eruptive viral diseases (smallpox, measles, chickenpox, rubella and others) had their origins in the populous settings of South Asia. Early exchanges of infectious disease occurred between Egypt, the Middle East and Mediterranean Europe. Thucydides postulated that the mysterious and deadly Plague of Athens in 430 BC, which permanently weakened that city-state's civic prowess and military power after its glorious century, originated in Ethiopia. Some historians think that the bubonic plague, with its probable origins in the Himalayan foothills as an enzootic infection of wild rodents, may have reached Egypt from India via infected black rats in coastal shipping quite early. This makes it a possible candidate for the Plague of Athens. However, it is also possible that this event was the European debut of smallpox, measles or some other novel infection.

Two thousand years ago, the Roman Empire and China's Imperial Han Dynasty, at opposite east-west poles of Eurasia, began to make contact, via overland trade through Central Asia. Subsequently, epidemic convulsions began to occur as virulent, newly exchanged epidemics ravaged both populations. Most of the Middle East and India, however, with a longer history of regional trade and germ-swapping, apparently experienced few such serious epidemics. In the second century AD, the records indicate that both Rome and China were overwhelmed, and probably politically enfeebled, by pestilence. Smallpox entered the Roman Empire via troops returning from quelling unrest in Syria in the second century AD. The Antonine plague of Rome in 165 AD was the initial dramatic result, after which smallpox spread widely in the western empire, depopulating many areas. The Antonine plagues brought the hey-day of the empire, overseen by Emperors Trajan, Hadrian and Antoninus, to a close. The Roman imperial system never recovered from the combined impact of epidemics and the incursions of Germanic tribes. Meanwhile, the east–west trade linking Rome with China via the Silk Road periodically introduced smallpox and measles to China. This appears to have caused a catastrophic halving of the northern Chinese population during the third and fourth centuries AD.

The great Eurasian pooling process thus climaxed with several devastating exchanges of infectious disease between the great empires of Rome and the

Chinese Han Dynasty. The most spectacular example was the arrival of bubonic plague in the Roman Empire and its subsequent regional and transcontinental spread. Bubonic plague, caused by the bacterium *Yersinia pestis*, seems to have made its debut on the fringe of Europe as the frightful Justinian Plague of 542 AD in Constantinople, by then the capital of the Roman Empire. There is tantalising palaeoclimatic evidence that temperatures fell dramatically during the years 535–542 AD, in association with a massive volcanic eruption from the Krakatoa (Indonesian) region that shrouded the skies of Turkey, the Middle East, China, Japan and Korea for several years. Other studies have shown a relationship between climatic fluctuations, rodent behaviour and bubonic plague occurrence.[23]

The bubonic plague raged for several centuries throughout the declining Roman Empire. During the seventh century, plague ravaged the Arab world (just as newly proclaimed Islam was gaining momentum) and, via land routes or coastal shipping, reached China.[24] At about that time Buddhist missionaries from the Asian mainland introduced smallpox, plague, mumps and measles into Japan. Within India, the ancient epidemiological standoff between the Indus Valley civilisation of semi-arid northwest India with its Old World epidemics and the forest tribes of central-southern India with their retaliatory tropical repertoire of malaria, dengue (presumed) and cholera was breached. Early in the second millennium, further violent equilibrations occurred between Europe and the Middle East via the grand folly of the Crusades. Repeatedly the vast hordes of crusaders and their horses were culled disastrously by typhus, bubonic plague and other pestilences, all capped off by scurvy and starvation. In several crusades less than one-tenth of the original contingent reached their destination.

After many turbulent centuries, this transcontinental pooling resulted in an uneasy Eurasian equilibration of at least some of the major infectious diseases.[13] Meanwhile, in both Asia and the West, tuberculosis was on the increase, in response to the crowding and privations of urban life. As we shall see below, during the later Middle Ages in Europe many of the epidemic diseases evolved towards endemic, often less virulent, conditions. On the horizon, nevertheless, was a pestilential disaster.

The Black Death

The Black Death, in mid-fourteenth century, seems to have occurred because of an ill-starred conjunction of ecological and political circumstances. Historians continue to debate the reasons for the precipitate arrival of bubonic plague in

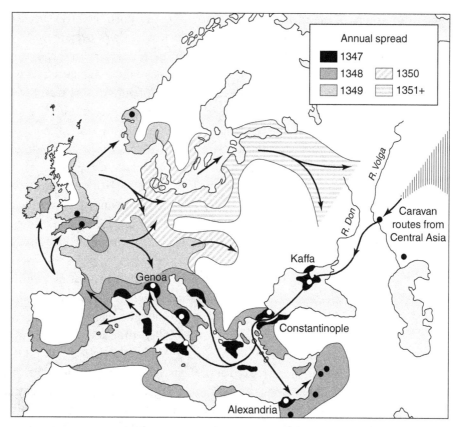

Figure 4.2 The approximate sequence of spread of bubonic plague (the Black Death) in Europe, between its entry from Asia in 1346 and its eventual spread, via the Baltic region, into Russia in 1352. Around one-third of the European population perished.

Europe and its rapid and deadly spread. The following seem likely parts of the story. A deteriorating, cooling, climate at the end of the 'Mediaeval Warm', associated with severe famines during the second decade of the fourteenth century and some continuing downturn in crop yields in Europe, had left a legacy of pockets of underfed and weakened segments of European populations. The combination of an epidemic of bubonic plague in China during the 1330s (perhaps associated with climatic disturbances of the wild rodent reservoir of plague infection in Central Asia), an increase in the caravan trade (with infected stowaway black rats) across the Asian steppes, and an attack by the Mongolian army on the Black Sea ports appears to have brought plague-infested rats to the eastern fringes of Europe in 1346. Indeed, biological warfare may have had its origins in the ensuing siege of the trading seaport of Kaffa. The Tartars reportedly catapulted their dead plague-stricken soldiers over the city walls. When plague broke out in Kaffa, the panic-stricken European merchants took to their boats and fled to Genoa, where the rats, fleas and plague bacteria went ashore.

From the central Mediterranean, the bubonic plague travelled northwards overland, and westwards around the shipping ports and up the Atlantic coast. Two years later it entered Britain; four years later it arrived in Scandinavia and then Russia. As the Black Death swept through Europe during 1347–50, it killed an estimated one-third of the population.[25] France was particularly badly affected, losing almost 40% of the population, whereas Scotland lost around 20%. Social, political and religious reactions to the plague were diverse and often bizarre. The cause of the dreadful disease was unknown. Blame was directed variously at noxious miasmas, emanations from rats, the wrath of God, astrological malalignment, or deliberately poisoned well-water (for which Jews were blamed and widely subjected to vicious pogroms, causing many to flee eastwards to Poland where King Casimir – perhaps influenced by his Jewish mistress – headed a more tolerant regime). Preventive measures were idiosyncratic: in Florence, they killed the cats and dogs; in Milan they locked the diseased in their houses; in Venice they closed the gates of the city. In Avignon, the pope retired apprehensively for several months into an isolated palatial chamber where a disease-purging fire burnt night and day. Meanwhile, self-appointed bands of flagellants paraded around the towns, whipping themselves in bloodied and penitent frenzy. This they did initially with the blessing of the Church. Later, however they were villified by Church authorities who had become fearful of their growing popularity.

The plague became a widely destructive Eurasian pandemic. Outbreaks occurred in Europe every decade or so throughout the next century. In China it contributed mightily to the estimated halving of the population during the fourteenth century, along with the destructive civil war against their Mongolian overlords. It probably helped to depopulate the vast fertile Eurasian grassland steppes and the fertile steppes of eastern Europe (the Ukrainian region). In Europe, the Black Death eroded both the orthodoxy and the authority of the established Christian Church, and the compensatory rise of secular city-state authority helped launch the ideology and energy of the Renaissance.

The bubonic plague smouldered on for the next five centuries in Europe, with particularly serious outbreaks in the seventeenth and eighteenth centuries. During the 1650s and 1660s plague outbreaks in Naples, Amsterdam and London killed an estimated 300,000, 50,000 and 70,000 people respectively.

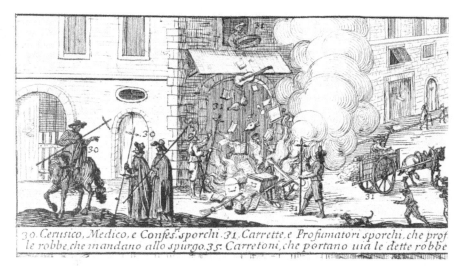

30. *Cerusico, Medico, e Confes. sporchi. 31. Carrette, e Profumatori sporchi, che prof
le robbe, che mandano allo spurgo. 35. Carretoni, che portano uia le dette robbe*

Figure 4.3 Disinfecting a house in Rome during the outbreak of bubonic plague in 1656. The belongings of the stricken family are being jettisoned and burnt. In the left foreground (item 30) are a surgeon, physician and priest.

Meanwhile, from the late Middle Ages, many of the other once-epidemic infectious diseases in Europe had become somewhat domesticated. This occurred via parasite–host coevolution (which included the selective survival of resistant strains of humans[26]) and via the acquisition of widespread adult immunity. Indeed, the 'urbanisation' of these diseases had led to their becoming predominantly endemic infections of childhood. The surviving adult European populations had thus acquired a huge constitutional biological advantage – one that would inadvertently but fortuitously facilitate their colonising ambitions. The coincidental introduction of Old World diseases to distant populations would lead to dramatic indigenous depopulation, cultural and socioeconomic disintegration, and the founding of great European empires.[27]

The third transition: trans-oceanic decimations

Christopher Columbus reached the Americas in 1492. Shortly after, the next great confluence of infectious disease pools began, as Eurasian and non-Eurasian civilisations made trans-oceanic contact. As biological warfare the catapulted corpses of Kaffa in 1346 might be apocryphal. But there is no doubting the potency of microbiological weaponry, albeit unplanned, in the

Spanish conquests of Central and South America early in the sixteenth century.[28] The surprisingly rapid victories over the powerful Aztec and Inca civilisations by tiny and tawdry bands of Spanish conquistadors were largely due to the germs they carried. The Amerindian populations' total lack of experience with these diseases and the absence of appropriate social and health-care infrastructure heightened their vulnerability to these 'virgin population' epidemics. Smallpox, measles and influenza cut great and instant swathes through hapless, immunologically naïve, Amerindian armies and townspeople. Smallpox was the great exterminator, except in Brazil where, a century later, malaria did most of the depopulating. During the remainder of that century these acute infectious diseases killed around 90% of the native populations – and presumably demoralised the remainder, who saw only the wrathful hand of divine retribution being directed against them.

This third transition was thus predominantly a dissemination rather than an exchange. There appear to have been few serious infectious diseases in the pre-Columbian New World.[29] Evidence of infection (with the possible exception of syphilis and tuberculosis) is unusually rare in pre-Columbian skeletal remains, although other evidence from burial sites indicates the presence of intestinal worms and protozoa. The extensive Amerindian populations were the descendants of populations from the Siberian region that had migrated through the frozen environment of Beringia 20,000 years earlier. As mentioned earlier in the chapter, the ensuing central and southern American civilisations had no large dense herds of wild animals to domesticate (in contrast to Europe and Africa), and therefore no ready herd-infection sources of potential human pathogens.[27] Thus, despite the massive size and density of the Aztec and Inca civilisations, fed on the abundant yields of their maize and potato agriculture and each totalling an estimated 25–30 million, these populations had remained relatively free of 'crowd' infectious diseases.

Syphilis, caused by the spiral-shaped *Treponema pallidum* bacterium, was seemingly Europe's main disease legacy of the 'Columbian exchange'.[29] However, debate continues as to the possible alternative origins of syphilis. Was it, for example, a home-grown newly evolved venereal variant of a spirochaetal skin infection, of the kind familiar to the physicians of mediaeval Europe? Majority opinion among palaeopathologists is now that the skeletal treponemal lesions of pre-Columbian Amerindians are probably not due to syphilis.

Subsequently, other European settlements in California, Louisiana and Canada acted as seeding points for Old World infections that spread destructively into North American Indian populations. For example, a great pestilence of some kind spread from the French settlement of Nova Scotia into the New England region – conveniently, just three years before the Plymouth Pilgrims arrived in Massachusetts Bay.[13] On 22 May, the first governor of the Massachusetts Bay Colony, John Winthrop, declared: 'For the natives they are neare all dead of the small Poxe, so as the Lord hathe cleared our title to what we possess.'

Meanwhile, back in Europe, the period from 1490 to 1648 (the year of the Treaty of Westphalia) was scarred by warfare, religious schisms and fast-moving epidemics. These included typhus (introduced from the Middle East), the mysterious English sweats, influenza and syphilis. In the sixteenth century, syphilis – the subject of the quotation at the opening of this chapter – was a severe, deforming and disabling disease; its virulence declined in later centuries. Subsequently, as the Little Ice Age approached its nadir and Europe became increasingly war-torn and epidemic-ridden, the social turbulence and strife of the early 1600s laid the foundations for a miserable century. A district physician of Regensburg wrote in 1602:

There was a severe winter, a cold April, a hailstorm in the summer. The wine was scarce and of poor quality. In this year, there was plague in the Palatine, through Saxony and Prussia. In Danzig 12,000 people died in one week. There was a smallpox epidemic in Bohemia; another in Silesia. In southern Germany there raged the terrible *Bauch kranheit* [probably an enteric infection]. There was a famine in Russia accompanied by pestilences of plague and typhus, and in Moscow alone 127,000 people are said to have died of pestilence.[30]

In the most benighted regions of Europe, almost two-thirds of the population died. During the Thirty Years War, from 1618 to 1648, the population in the warring region declined from around 16 million to 6 million. Most deaths were from infectious diseases and starvation. Emigration occurred on a grand scale. These terrible years evoked widespread premonitions of Judgement Day. The loss of faith in establishment Christianity, along with the rise of entrepreneurial mercantilism and its challenge to traditional authority, hastened the Reformation during the later sixteenth and early seventeenth centuries. The next great outbreak of the bubonic plague occurred in the 1660s in a demoralised Europe struggling to cope with cold temperatures and sporadic famines. Warfare disseminated typhus throughout Europe, establishing it as an endemic infection in eastern Europe. One hundred and fifty years later, typhus helped to devastate the remnants of Napoleon's ill-starred Grande Armée as it limped back from Russia.[31]

Trans-Atlantic slavery and South Seas explorations

In the seventeenth century the trans-Atlantic slave trade introduced the deadly falciparum malaria and yellow fever to the Americas.[32] Those diseases, as we saw in chapter 3, further ravaged Amerindian populations, as well as European settlers, in the tropical lowlands. The absence of genetic resistance to malaria in Amerindians, the lack of any local-adapted species of malaria in New World monkeys, the dependence of yellow fever transmission upon a specialised African mosquito vector (*Aedes aegypti*) and historical accounts of early Spanish explorations that made no mention of fever confirm the prior absence of these diseases in the Americas. Particularly destructive epidemics of malaria occurred in the Brazil Amazon region.

During the eighteenth and early nineteenth centuries, European explorations in the Australasia-Pacific region spread Old World infectious diseases to the native populations of that region. The story was becoming familiar. The Australian Aborigines, New Zealand Maori and countless Pacific island populations were decimated by infectious disease epidemics. The impact was most severe when their land was taken by European settlers, which increased the indigenous population's vulnerability by disrupting the economic base, food supply and social-support structures.[33] The native Hawaiian population declined from 300,000 to 37,000 within 80 years of Captain James Cook's first arrival there in 1778. The 1789 epidemic of smallpox in Australian Aborigines around Sydney Harbour, and its subsequent spread into the hinterland, may have been the single greatest shock ever dealt to these indigenous people by the European invasion. The continuing micro-biological rout is well illustrated by records of deadly epidemics of European diseases breaking out among the Aborigines of south-west Australia between 1830 and 1894. They comprised: typhus (twice), whooping cough (twice), influenza (four times), chickenpox, smallpox (three times), measles (twice) and typhoid.[34]

Meanwhile, during the early nineteenth century, the activities of the British military in India mobilised cholera for the first time beyond its traditional home in the Ganges valley, causing epidemics throughout the adjoining Central and West Asian regions. However, India had participated several thousand years earlier in the great Eurasian pooling of infectious diseases, such as smallpox, measles and influenza. Hence, the British colonialists held few infectious disease surprises for that country.

Today's world: the Fourth Transition?

These three historical transitions were processes of equilibration: the first between humans, animal and pest species; the latter two between regional and then transoceanic populations. Throughout these times infectious diseases were the main cause of death, interspersed with recurrent famines. Infectious diseases receded in Western countries throughout the later nineteenth and most of the twentieth centuries. However, as discussed earlier, the trend-lines have faltered in recent decades. In 1996, the annual WHO Health Report stated:

Until relatively recently, the long struggle for control over infectious diseases seemed almost over . . . Far from being over, the struggle to control infectious diseases has become increasingly difficult. Diseases that seemed to be subdued, such as tuberculosis and malaria, are fighting back with renewed ferocity. Some, such as cholera and yellow fever, are striking in regions once thought safe from them. Other infections are now so resistant to drugs that they are virtually untreatable.[35]

Hyperbole aside, *something* unusual does seem to be happening to patterns of infectious disease. As populations become interconnected economically, culturally and physically, the mixing of people, animals and microbes from all geographical areas intensifies. Long-distance travel and trade facilitates the geographical redistribution of pests and pathogens. This has been well illustrated in recent years by the HIV pandemic, the worldwide dispersal of rat-borne hantaviruses and the introduction of the eggs of the Asian tiger mosquito, *Aedes albopictus* (a vector for yellow fever and dengue) into South America, North America and Africa in ship-borne cargoes of used car tyres. Rapid urbanisation is expanding the traditional role of cities as gateways for infections. Population movement between rural areas into cities is opening new vistas of possibility to otherwise marginal microbes. Against this background perhaps it is not surprising that, in the preceding quarter-century, the following infectious diseases or their pathogens have been newly identified:

1999 Nipah virus
1997 H5N1 flu virus (avian influenza)
      Variant Creutzfeld–Jakob Disease (human 'mad cow disease')
      Australian bat lyssavirus
1995 Human herpes virus 8 (Kaposi sarcoma virus)
1994 Sabia virus (Brazil)
      Hendra virus

1993 Hantavirus pulmonary syndrome (Sin Nombre virus)
1992 *Vibrio cholerae 0139*
1991 Guanarito virus (Venezuela)
1989 Hepatitis C
1988 Hepatitis E
     Human herpes virus 6
1983 Human immunodeficiency virus (HIV)
1982 *Escherichia coli O157:H7*
     Lyme borreliosis
     HTLV-2 virus
1980 Human T-lymphotrophic virus
1977 *Campylobacter jejuni*
1976 *Cyptosporidium parvum*
     Legionnaires' disease
     Ebola virus (Central Africa)

The relaxation of traditional cultural norms is yielding newer, freer, patterns of human behaviour, including sexual activities and illicit drug use. The transmission of over a dozen dangerous types of infection is thereby facilitated. Modern medical manoeuvres, including blood transfusion and organ transplantation, are creating new ecological opportunities for viruses to pass from person to person. An estimated 4 million Americans are now infected with hepatitis C virus, silently disseminated by blood transfusion prior to the early 1990s. Other hospitalisation practices have opened up new habitats for various bacteria, such as the *Proteus* and *Pseudomonas* genuses. Over the past half century antibiotics have been used widely and often unwisely, including for livestock and agricultural purposes (approximately half of the antibiotics made in the United States are fed to livestock to enhance growth). Around half the antibiotics prescribed for humans have little or no benefit since they are ineffective against viral diseases. This over-use and frequent misuse of antibiotics has nurtured the rise of drug-resistant organisms.

Infectious disease patterns are also being affected by the intensification of food production and processing methods. The still-evolving story about variant Creutzfeld–Jakob Disease (human 'mad cow disease') in Britain has underscored the health risks of subordinating ecological sense to economic pressures in meat production. Less exotically, the reported rates of food poisoning have increased markedly in Western countries during the past two decades, and almost doubled in the United Kingdom during the 1990s. Several outbreaks of the potentially lethal toxin-producing *E. coli 0157* in North

America and Europe in the mid-1990s originated in contaminated beef imported from infected cattle in Latin America. Large development projects, particularly dams, irrigation schemes and road construction, often potentiate the spread of vector-borne infectious diseases such as malaria, dengue fever and schistosomiasis.

Meanwhile, casting a longer shadow over the future prospects for infectious diseases are the incipient changes in the world's climate, the continued loss of ecosystem-stabilising biodiversity, and the entrenchment of poverty in a market-dominated world. These will all act to maintain and extend the risks from infectious diseases. We are rapidly changing the ecological complexion of life on Earth. We are destabilising ecosystems, disturbing nature's checks and balances, in ways that classically favour the proliferation of small opportunistic species (the so-called *r* species – see chapter 7). This includes the microbes.

LYME DISEASE illustrates the interplay of historical, human, environmental and other ecological influences. This disease was first identified in 1976 in the northeastern United States where it is now a prominent public health problem. The disease is caused by a spirochaete (a spiral-shaped bacterium), *Borrelia burgdorferi*, transmitted by infected Ixodid ticks. Lyme disease also occurs within Europe and across temperate Asia, where it is transmitted via other sub-species of *Ixodes ricinus* ticks.[36] The tick has a complex three-stage life-cycle, and parasitises various mammalian species, especially rodents and deer. Transmission of the spirochaete is influenced by climate because temperature and rainfall affect the geographic range of the intermediate host mammals and the speed of maturation of the immature (larval-nymphal) tick. During its nymph stage, the tick in northeast United States is infected by feeding on spirochaete-infected white-footed mice. The tick also feeds on other small mammals, most of which do *not* carry the spirochaete. Hence, in depleted local ecosystems in which the tick-nymphs may be obliged to feed on infected mice, the proportion of infected ticks is much greater than when the ecosystem has a diversity of vertebrate food sources for ticks.

Human interventions in the landscape – the elimination of wolves as predators of deer, the regrowth of woodland in disused farmland, the extension of suburbia and its golf courses into that woodland, and the warmer temperatures of recent decades – all influence the ecology of the disease and, hence, the likelihood of human infection. The deer population in parts of northeastern United States increased 20-fold during the twentieth century.

There is a longer evolutionary dimension to this disease. The various Borrelian spirochaete species occur in a globalised mosaic across Europe, Asia and North America. Molecular genetic studies indicate that these different bacterial species evolved within separate ecosystems. Palaeo-archaeological analysis suggests that this was because of the ecologically disruptive effects of the advance and retreat of ice-age glaciations during the past million years or so. By creating isolated vertebrate reservoir habitats for the tick, distinct local species of both tick and spirochaete then coevolved. Subsequent genetic mixing of the spirochaete species has occurred, as vertebrate hosts and their ticks have intermingled, particularly under the recent influence of humans. This mixing process has been greatly amplified by the cycles of borreliosis in migratory seabirds. Lyme disease thus exemplifies well how complex ecological changes, with or without human contribution, can cause an infectious disease to 'emerge'.[36]

The widening scope of 'infectious' diseases

There is yet more to this story. As molecular biological research methods advance, and as our assumptions about the causes of cancer, heart disease and neurological disorders become more accommodating, so we see evidence that infectious agents may contribute to the causation of many of these 'non-infectious' diseases.

Schistosomiasis infection has been recognised as a cause of urinary bladder cancer since Rudolf Virchow's astute observations in North Africa in the late nineteenth century. However, only during the last third of the twentieth century was a mainstream role for infectious agents in human cancer revealed. We now know that viruses are directly involved in the causation of cancers of the liver, the uterine cervix and various lymphomas. Worldwide, an estimated three-quarters of all cases of cervical cancer, the most common cancer in women, are due to the human papilloma virus. The several cancer-inducing strains of this virus (particularly HPV-16 and HPV-18) are spread between sexual partners as a sexually transmitted disease.

This recent recognition of the role of infectious agents in human cancer reminds us of the power of prevailing paradigms in science. The theory of chemical carcinogenesis dominated cancer research for much of the second half of the twentieth century. This theory held that DNA mutations caused by reactive chemical molecules were the primary cause of abnormal cellular proliferation. Infectious agents did not fit this theory well. Indeed, in the early twentieth century the idea that infectious agents could cause cancer was actively disdained. This disdain reflected the dominance of the Germ Theory, which prescribed that: (i) every case of a particular (infectious) disease must be demonstrably associated with a particular infective agent; (ii) the agent must be identified in pure laboratory culture; and (iii) it must then induce the same disease when administered to another individual. Since cancer biology did not comply with these 'rules' it did not satisfy scientific standards. Hence, the important finding by Peyton Rous, in 1911, of a transmissible agent (a virus) that caused cancer in chickens was dismissed for half a century. It was, said his critics, irrelevant because chickens were too-distant relatives of humans. Only when the role of infectious agents in cancer became a respectable idea, in the 1960s, did Rous win a Nobel Prize for that early finding.[37]

Today we view this topic differently (but still not necessarily correctly!). We have learnt recently of the efficient molecular mechanisms that repair the continuing damage to our DNA. These have been extremely well-honed by evolutionary pressures, leaving little chance for any particular environmental exposure to produce the several specific mutations required to induce cancer. Hence, it is a reasonable proposition that many 'carcinogens' act by increasing cell proliferation via stimulatory or deregulatory mechanisms. This, in turn, would increase the opportunity for random mutations to occur and for any resultant abnormal cell to multiply into a cancer. The stimulus to cell proliferation can occur via chronic inflammation due to infectious agents such as *Schistosoma haematobium* in the urinary bladder, viral hepatitis in the liver, and *Helicobacter pylori* in the lower stomach and duodenum. Cell proliferation can occur if viruses such as the near-ubiquitous Epstein-Barr virus are released from the host body's normal immunological controls, allowing the virus to induce a proliferation of lymphoid cells which results in a lymphoma. The human papilloma virus can block the cell-stabilising action of certain proteins, thereby causing abnormal proliferative behaviour in the epithelial cells lining the cervix. Worldwide, an estimated 20% of all cancers are due to infection. There are presumably various infective agents that cause other cancers in ways we do not yet know about.

The evidence that infectious agents are somehow involved in the causation of coronary heart disease is recent, and contentious. For half a century we have assumed that this disease entails an essentially biochemical-physical causal process: raised blood pressure damages the inner lining of the coronary arteries, high levels of cholesterol in blood lead to deposition of fatty material at those vulnerable sites, and smoking enhances that deposition process while also increasing the tendency of the blood to clot. However, that configuration of causes is now under siege from several quarters. One such idea is that infective agents may somehow activate the inflammatory process within the atheromatous lesion.

What is the evidence? From reports of over a dozen studies there appears to be about a one sixth increase in risk of coronary heart disease associated with prior infection with the *Helicobacter pylori* bacterium. This microbe is known to release inflammation-inducing chemical cytokines. These, it is argued, might stimulate the activity of macrophages, the body's freelance scavenger cells, at the site of the atheromatous lesion in the coronary artery. Other studies have shown that DNA from the common bacterium *Chlamydia pneumoniae* is present in fatty deposits in the lining of the coronary arteries, but is not present in healthy segments of the artery. But does the bacterium arrive before or after the lesion forms? Several experimental studies have shown that giving antibiotics to patients with heart disease reduces both disease progression and the occurrence of heart attacks. Meanwhile, other experimental studies have found no relationship. Further, if the effect is real and significant why did the timing of the downturn in heart disease mortality in various Western countries differ by more than two decades? Given this inconclusive evidence, larger controlled trials are now getting underway. In the meantime, a further related possibility, supported by experimental studies in mice, is that early-life infections may programme the individual's immune system to produce excessive numbers of macrophages throughout life, and these scavenger cells would enhance the deposition of blood cholesterol in atheromatous lesions. We have not yet heard the last on this complex topic.

During the 1980s and 1990s a high incidence of the neurological Creutzfeld-Jakob disease (CJD) occurred in individuals injected with growth hormone that had been extracted from the pituitary gland of cadaver brains. This made it clear that CJD has an infective basis. We may yet find many more viruses lurking in the human brain – where, in effect, they are beyond the radar screen of the host immune system. The Borna virus may be such an example. This virus is named after a town in Germany where, a century ago, 2,000 cavalry horses were killed by a virus that caused disorders of coordination and behaviour. Virologists have recently found a strain of the virus in the blood of patients with clinical depression or obsessive-compulsive disorders, while other researchers have detected viral markers in patients with depression or schizophrenia, particularly during acute episodes.[38] While controversial, these findings point to the possible role of viruses in human mood disorders.

Finally, the pattern of exposure to infectious agents in childhood can perturb the human immune system in two ways: by influencing its developmental pathway, and by initiating autoimmune disorders. Modern living entails a more hygienic childhood, with the elimination or deferral of childhood infections that have long influenced the development of the young immune system. Most dramatically, this led to the rise of polio in developed countries in the 1950s because children were no longer exposed to the polio virus in early childhood, when the infection is normally harmless. More subtly, this increase in hygiene, along with fewer siblings, has reduced the intensity of childhood exposure to a range of infectious agents, including the many commensal bacteria that, historically, colonised the infant gut. This significant shift in human ecology affects the early-life programming of the immune system, inclining it towards a more 'atopic' (allergic) pattern of response – and this may help explain the recent widespread rise of childhood asthma and hay fever. Likewise, the progressive elimination of bowel parasites such as roundworms, whipworms and pinworms (parasites which coevolved with hominids over several million years) may have contributed to the rise in inflammatory bowel diseases, including Crohn's disease and ulcerative colitis, in Western populations over the past half century.

Infectious agents can also influence the occurrence of autoimmune disorders, in which the immune system erroneously attacks normal body tissues. A basic evolutionary device of parasitic microorganisms is to acquire an outer protein surface that resembles that of the host's tissue. This 'molecular mimicry' provides camouflage against attack by the host immune system, since proteins recognised by the host immune system as 'self' are not normally attacked. Occasionally the immune system gets it wrong, and attacks both the microorganism and the part of 'self' that it resembles. It is likely that insulin-dependent diabetes (which usually begins in childhood), multiple sclerosis and rheumatoid arthritis all involve this type of viral infection-triggered mechanism.

Conclusion

The earliest kingdom of life comprised the *Archaeabacteria*. Today, several billion years later, bacteria remain part of the foundation of life. They decompose organic matter, recycle nutrients and build other molecules. To succeed in life's struggle, all species great and small must secure their life-support supplies. The succession of human demographic, cultural and behavioural changes over tens of thousands of years has provided many new opportunities for microbes.

Today, further opportunities are being afforded to microorganisms by human-induced social-environmental changes on an ever-larger, even global, scale. They include:

• Generalised social changes (world-wide urbanisation, intravenous drug abuse, changing sexual practices).
• Demographic changes (increased and accelerated human mobility, increases in refugee populations).
• Medical care (infections in hospitals and nursing homes) and medical technology (blood transfusion, organ transplantation, re-used syringes for antibiotic injections – a problem in low-income countries – contamination of vaccines, and the increasing incidence of antibiotic resistance in pathogens).
• Economic and commercial trends (intensive food production, extended irrigation, liberalised trading patterns).
• Climatic changes (regional and global).
• Ecosystem disturbance (deforestation, eutrophication of waterways, reduction in predators of disease vector organisms).

We humans are inextricably bound up with the natural world, a world of competition and symbiosis between organisms great and small. During the long history of humankind there have been several major, distinct, transitions in our ecological relationships with wider nature. These transitions have profoundly changed the patterns of infectious disease and, in part because of this, have often altered the course of history.

Today, we may be living through yet another major transition in our evolving relationship with the Fourth Horseman. As the scale of social-demographic change and of human impact on the ecosphere escalates, so the probabilities of infectious diseases, both new and resurgent, increase. The world, as ever, is full of microbes jostling for supplies of nutrients, energy and molecular building blocks. The right microbe in the right place can extend, re-start or found a dynasty. It has happened many times before, and will continue to do so.

5

The Third Horseman: food, farming and famines

The biblical Third Horseman of the Apocalypse, Famine, rides a black horse. Humankind has had long familiarity with that horseman. The Bible recounts how Joseph, leader of the enslaved Israelites in Middle Kingdom Egypt, foresaw for Pharaoh the seven years of drought and famine, symbolised in Pharoah's dream as seven lean cattle. Egypt was ever hostage to the annual rhythms of the Nile and the flood-borne silt that fertilised the fields of the river plain. Indeed, the Old Kingdom, ruled by godlike Pharoahs and adorned with pyramids, had collapsed around 2200 BC because of climatic vicissitudes that caused prolonged droughts, reductions in river flow and serious famine. The same regional drought contributed to the collapse of the Akkadian Empire in Mesopotamia and the Harrapan civilisation of the Indus Valley. A thousand years later, the rulers of Egypt's Middle Kingdom were more alert to the need to manage flood control and conserve agricultural resources, and less disposed to think of themselves as infallible gods on Earth. Even so, there was little practical advice that Joseph could give Pharaoh, other than to store the surplus corn from the seven good years. There was no other way to lessen the impending climatic disaster.

The more usual historical situation has been that famine has struck unbuffered populations, with few food reserves. As in all of nature, human populations tend to increase in size to the limit of the local environment's 'carrying capacity'. Historically, food availability has been the fundamental constraint on human population size. Over time, humans have found ways to expand that carrying capacity. Australia's Aborigines, for example, used controlled fire over tens of thousands of years to remodel the landscape. This 'firestick farming' eliminated pine forests and cleared away the undergrowth, leaving an open woodland of eucalyptus trees in which animal life could flourish, eating the young shoots, leaves and grasses, and in which those animals were more easily hunted. Although the environmental impact was limited in magnitude, and spread over a long time, many species of plants and large mammals were made extinct.[1]

As human numbers have increased, and as agriculture has replaced foraging and hunting, humankind's ways of expanding the carrying capacity of local environments have tended to become less sustainable. Hence the many historical examples of local ecological declines causing the collapse of societies – such as those of Mesopotamia, the Indus Valley, the Mayans, the Anasazi, the West Vikings and the Easter Islanders. The awful fratricide in Rwanda in 1994 is said by some commentators to have reflected the land pressures, and food shortages, in a rapidly growing population of 8 million reliant on an environmental carrying capacity able to support an estimated 6 million.

There are some elusive concepts here. The phrase 'carrying capacity' needs careful consideration – particularly in relation to nature's wild card species, *Homo sapiens*. Arguments over food production statistics, over the definitions of hunger, malnutrition, starvation and famine, and over the provocative term 'demographic entrapment'[2] have also enlivened the debate. Looming large in the debate is the view of the Reverend Thomas Malthus.

Thomas Malthus: mouths versus meals

Thomas Malthus, an English cleric and pioneering political economist, made the famously grim prediction in his essay on population, first published in 1798, that gains in food production could not keep up with natural population increase.[3] He referred to 'the constant tendency in all animated life to increase beyond the nourishment prepared for it' – and to the inevitability of 'positive checks' (starvation and deaths) occurring when mouths outnumbered food. His views influenced Charles Darwin who, in his description of organisms struggling to survive, envisaged that natural selection would display 'the doctrine of Malthus applied in most cases with ten-fold force'. Malthus' views have subsequently been variously contested or supported by other economists. Two prominent economists writing particularly in the 1980s, Ester Boserup of Denmark and Julian Simon of the United States, promoted the argument that humans are themselves a 'resource' – the more humans, the more likely it is that invention and innovation will flow.[4] (In Simon's case, the argument was based on rather flimsy historical evidence.) In contrast, economists familiar with ecological realities recognise that there are fundamental limits to the planet's capacity; that it is essentially a closed system within which continuing and sustainable increases in food production cannot be assumed.[5]

Malthus was one of the first thinkers to foresee that humans were likely to overstep the mark with their burgeoning population numbers. Two hundred years ago, when he wrote of the perennial struggle between population and food supplies, Europe was undergoing very rapid population increase. Linear growth in food production, said Malthus, would always be outpaced by the exponential growth in human numbers. Malthus was contesting the celebrated optimism of his compatriot William Godwin, who foresaw limitless cornucopian possibilities for humans as the culmination of their glorious historical struggle. This optimism had been purveyed also by the Marquis de Condorcet, a liberal French aristocrat who believed in the perfectability of human society and a future of shared abundance. (Despite holding these views the marquis lost his life in the aftermath of the French Revolution, although he was fleet-footed enough to avoid the horror of the guillotine.)

It was Malthus' misfortune to have statistics only up to 1798; but not beyond! In fact, the steep rise in the price of food in the latter half of the eighteenth century, running approximately parallel to the increase in population numbers, flattened out in the early nineteenth century. Malthus was writing in the wake of the French Revolution, which induced apprehensions among social élites elsewhere in Europe. In the two decades before that uprising, population growth had outstripped food production and the price of wheat and bread had approximately doubled. The economist Robert Fogel estimates that, in the late eighteenth century, the poorest 20% of the populations of England and France subsisted on diets so deficient in energy that they were effectively unable to do labouring work. Hence the high prevalence of beggars in those ancient regimes.[6] And hence the occurrence of food riots in France, as prelude to revolution. Then, in the nineteenth century, European agricultural methods modernised, mechanisation increased, chemical fertilisers were introduced, and yields improved. Later in the nineteenth century, there was increased importation into Europe of refrigerated meat and other foods from Australia, New Zealand, South America and elsewhere. For the privileged populations of Europe these nineteenth-century improvements in the amount and quality of food contributed greatly to gains in health and life expectancy (discussed further in chapter 7).

Malthus' argument is, in effect, about exceeding carrying capacity: there are more people than there is food to feed them. The story of Easter Island, in chapter 1, is a vivid example. The term 'carrying capacity' has been somewhat misunderstood in relation to human populations. Unlike other species, human societies typically intervene substantially in the environment in order to increase its carrying capacity. Further, local human populations usually connect with one another by trade, thus acquiring external subsidisation which further modifies the notion of carrying capacity.[7] Hence, argue some environmental economists, any particular estimate of human carrying capacity is of limited meaning, particularly because we cannot know the consequences of both human innovation and biological evolution. Indeed, we may do better to turn the equation around and ask how much damage can be absorbed before the exploited ecosystem 'flips' from one equilibrium state to another.

It is important also to clarify the notion of a Malthusian subsistence crisis. Maurice King describes such situations as 'demographic entrapment'.[8] These are situations in which local, economically disconnected populations, beset by excessive numbers, cannot feed themselves. Resolution can only be achieved by fratricide, starvation, out-migration or food aid. Such a population can survive, in the short term, by depleting their stocks of material, energy and biotic resources. Complex local crises of this kind appear to have occurred in Rwanda and Somalia in the 1990s, and may yet occur in Malawi, Burundi and parts of South Asia where populations are increasing, land pressures are mounting and environmental conditions are declining.[9] The modern hope, however, is that in a better informed and connected world, international cooperation and aid can avert or ameliorate local disasters.

Local subsistence crises, however, have long been part of the human story. We now appreciate that their explanation in agrarian-based societies entails more than Malthus' simple supply-and-demand arithmetic. The key word that requires exploration is 'demand'. The eminent Amartya Sen has shown that it is 'entitlement' that socially determines an individual's access to food, whether by growing, bartering or buying it.[10] In Bengal, India, more people died in 1943 in a 'famine' in which there was actually more food available than in 1941 when no famine deaths occurred. In 1943, the starving rural poor died in front of well-stocked, but well-guarded, food shops in Calcutta. Similarly, in the late 1840s potato famine in Ireland, discussed below, corn was still being exported to England. Entitlement is what converts a person's biological need into a socially effective demand. We are thus reminded that food shortages and famines, as frank food scarcity with resultant starvation and substantially increased mortality, are a reflection of *both* carrying capacity and political economy.

Famines, climate and societal crises in history

Famines typically follow periods of climatic extremes that cause crop failures and livestock deaths. Plagues of locusts and rodents and outbreaks of fungal diseases – both of which, ironically, often follow good rains and abundant green growth – are another cause. Food shortages also result from degradation of the soil. This largely explained the collapse of the Sumerian civilisation in Mesopotamia, 4,000 years ago. Similarly, excessive pastoral grazing is thought to have facilitated the recent desertification in parts of Africa's western Sahel. Finally, two of the other Horsemen – War and Conquest – have been a recurring cause of famine. We need look no further than the siege of Leningrad and the 1944 Dutch Hunger Winter famine of World War II. Fifteen years later, the ill-judged agricultural policies of Maoist China caused a massive famine in 1959–60 when an estimated 15–20 million people died of starvation.

Climatic effects occur on two very different timescales. Long-term changes in climatic conditions can alter the boundaries and viability of a society. The people of the African Sahel have long lived with this reality as the southern fringe of the Sahara Desert advances and retreats several times a century, partly in response to climatic cycles of the great southwest monsoon that brings moist air from the southern Atlantic. In chapter 1 we examined the mysterious demise of the Viking settlements in Greenland in the fourteenth and fifteenth centuries as temperatures began to fall. Their food production declined, food importation became difficult as sea-ice extended, and the unfriendly native Inuit population in Greenland pressed southwards as the climate deteriorated.

Climatic fluctuations can also disrupt food supplies on a much shorter timescale, leading to famine, deaths and social unrest. Indeed, acute famines have long been characteristic of pre-industrial agricultural societies everywhere. The climate is less irregular in Europe and North America than in most other regions of the world, particularly tropical and subtropical regions. Floods in China and famines in India have been notorious killers over the centuries.[11] In China, where the centralised bureaucracy dating from the Han Dynasty of 2,000 years ago kept detailed records and where vegetables and rice have long provided nearly all of the caloric intake by the toiling peasantry, famines occurred in one or more provinces in over 90% of the years between 108 BC and 1910 AD.

Great famines have occurred once or twice every century in India over the past 1,000 years. Smaller famines have occurred more often, usually in association with the weakening of the monsoon system induced by El Niño events. India has long lived and died by the monsoon, the great annual happening that brings in moist air from the adjoining ocean. For 8–9 months there is little rain, the land is dry, the sun is harsh, and the mood of 100 million farmers, initially resigned, eventually becomes apprehensive. When the great southwest monsoon rolls in from the Indian Ocean in early summer, sky and land turn to water, life is rejuvenated, and crops grow. The southeast monsoon feeds Sri Lanka, Bengal India and Bangladesh. El Niño events, originating in the Pacific region, disrupt the monsoon cycle – occasionally severely. In the great Indian famines, hundreds of thousands, sometimes millions, of deaths have occurred. The famines of 1344–45, when even royalty starved, and those of 1631 and of 1791, were all spectacular disasters. The last great peacetime famine in India occurred in 1899,[12] following hard on the heels of a moderately severe famine in 1896–99. The total death toll probably exceeded four million.[13] Those years of the late 1890s entailed strong El Niño events, when droughts occurred throughout Southeast Asia and brought heartbreak to Australian farmers.

EUROPE, TOO, has long been afflicted by famines. Over many centuries diets were marginal and the mass of people survived on a monotonous intake of vegetables, grain gruel and bread. As late as 1870, two-thirds of the French diet consisted of bread and potatoes. Yields of animal foods were low. Cows then, compared to a modern cow, yielded about half the carcass meat and produced one-third the volume of milk. Meat and fish were dietary luxuries. During those centuries, average daily intake was less than 2,000 calories, falling to around 1800 in the poorer regions of Europe. This permanent state of dietary insufficiency led to widespread malnutrition, susceptibility to infectious disease, and low life expectancy. The superimposed famines culled the populations, often drastically. In Finland, for example, the famine of 1696–97 killed one third of the population. France experienced 26 famines that affected the whole country in the eleventh century, 16 such famines in the eighteenth century, and many others in between.

A particularly dramatic example in Europe was the great mediaeval famine of 1315–17. Climatic conditions deteriorated over much of that decade, and the cold and soggy conditions caused widespread crop failures, food price rises, hunger and death. Social unrest increased, robberies multiplied and bands of desperate peasants swarmed over the countryside. Reports of cannibalism abounded from Ireland to the Baltic. Animal diseases proliferated, contributing to the die-off of over half the sheep and oxen in Europe. This tumultuous event, and the Black Death which followed thirty years later, is thought by some historians to have contributed to the weakening and dissolution of feudalism in Europe.

Europe subsequently experienced 400 years of colder weather during the Little Ice Age, between approximately 1450 and 1850 (see Figure 5.1). The later

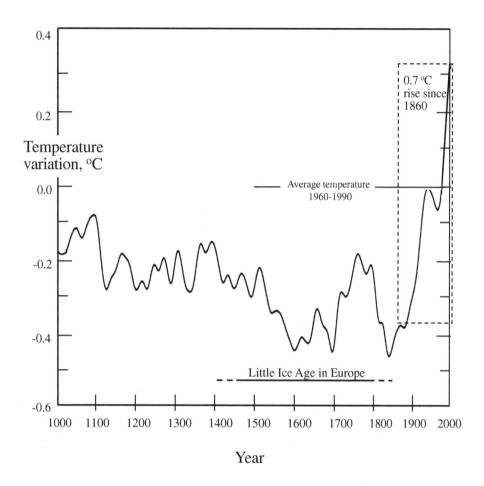

Figure 5.1 A composite, smoothed, graph of estimated northern hemisphere temperature over the past 1,000 years. Prior to 1860, the temperature is estimated from tree-rings and sedimentary isotope profiles. Since then there have been instrumental records. Climatic trends and cycles have long been a major force in regional food production, nutrition, health and survival. The rapid temperature increase in the past century is partly due to human-induced changes in the atmosphere.

The most recent authoritative assessment, by climate scientists within the UN system's Intergovernmental Panel on Climate Change, is that most of the world's temperature increase since 1975 has been due to the human population's emissions of greenhouse gases. The particular pattern of warming during the past quarter-century is as would be expected from a change in greenhouse gas concentrations – and is unlike that caused by volcanic activity, industrial aerosol accumulation or increased solar activity.

decades of the sixteenth century were a time of increasing cold, as this period approached its nadir. This cooling coincided with a much-enlarged European population, which had recovered from the Black Death and was testing the limits of the post-feudal agricultural system.[14] By the 1590s, the growing season had contracted by several weeks and the altitude at which crops could be grown had declined by 200 metres. A succession of four bad harvests in 1594–97 resulted in the desperate eating of cats and dogs – and, reportedly, humans. In Orslosa, western Sweden, the parish register of the late 1590s recorded the local experience thus:

The soil was sick for three years, so that it could bear no harvest. After these inflictions it happened that even those who had good farms turned their young people away, and many even their own children, because they were not able to watch the misery of them starving to death in the homes of their mothers and fathers. Aferwards the parents left their house and home going whither they were able, till they lay dead of hunger and starvation. . . . At times these and other inflictions came and also the bloody flux [dysentery] which put people in such a plight that countless died of it.[14]

An extra chilling occurred in 1601 – perhaps the coldest year of the past thousand years in Europe – when a massive volcanic eruption in the Peruvian Andes cast a pall over the world's skies. Further, solar sunspot activity weakened during much of the seventeenth century (the so-called Maunder Minimum period). As mentioned in chapter 4, this Europe-wide downturn in food production in the first half of the seventeenth century led to widespread political instability, hunger, infectious disease and death. Similar episodes of famine, disease and death occurred in Europe in the late seventeenth and early eighteenth centuries during intensified cold weather. Great famines occurred in France in 1693 and 1709. However, famine began to recede during the eighteenth century as agricultural practices began to modernise. New crops, acquired through trade and conquest, were introduced into Europe, including potatotes, corn and buckwheat. Animal husbandry improved. Indeed, the increased supplies of cattle fodder (alfalfa and turnips) due to mechanised agriculture not only increased the availability of meat and milk; it also helped suppress human malaria, since the anopheline mosquitoes prefer their blood-meals from (non-infectable) cattle rather than from humans.

As populations expanded, there were further food stresses. In the 1780s, in France, the urban food riots, including the dramatic market-women's march on Versailles in October 1789, heightened the mood of pre-revolutionary anger. Meanwhile, world climate patterns were perturbed by an unusually extreme El Niño event that occurred in 1789–91. This climatic convulsion brought severe drought to eastern Australia and its hapless new British colonists and convicts (who, unluckily, had arrived in Sydney Cove in 1788), and to India, Ethiopia, southern Africa and Mexico.[13] The last severe famine to affect the whole of Europe came in 1816–17. Though exacerbated by the Napoleonic wars, the underlying cause was the extraordinary 'year without summer' in 1815 due to the global atmospheric clouding caused by the massive volcanic eruption of Tambora in Indonesia. Crop failure was widespread, food riots broke out across most of Europe in 1816 and 1817, infectious disease epidemics increased and death rates rose.

The Irish potato famine

The last major European famine occurred in Ireland in the 1840s. The climate in Europe had deteriorated during the 1830s, perhaps exacerbated by volcanic eruptions earlier that decade. This was the decade when the early gains in life expectancy that had occurred in England during the late eighteenth and early nineteenth centuries were set back. Simultaneously, famines and heightened death rates occurred in Norway in 1836 and 1838 as that country struggled through a succession of seven bad harvest years. Meanwhile Europe was about to experience a new type of famine, in an introduced crop that had only become widespread in the preceding century: the potato.

The Spanish conquistadors brought the potato back to Europe from the Peruvian Andes in the 1500s, as a minor novelty. There were various official denunications of this irregularly shaped tuber: it was a cause of leprosy, it was the Devil's food, it posed risks to the wellbeing and health of domestic servants.[14] For 200 years the potato was widely rejected, although welcomed as a delicacy by a discerning minority. In Ireland, however, it became clear during the eighteenth century that a plot of land sown with potatoes would feed twice as many people as a plot sown with cereal. Further, subterranean potatoes were less vulnerable to the vicissitudes of climate and airborne pests than were wheat and barley. The word got around, and soon there was state support for growing potatoes in other European countries. The potato had 'arrived', and became a major contributor to the improving food supplies in Europe.

The potato was also a major contributor to the tripling of Ireland's population within the space of a century. By the 1840s, with a congested population of around 8.5 million in Ireland, around 650,000 landless labourers were living in squalid and destitute conditions. The pressure to produce food from tiny plots of land led to even further reliance on the potato such that potato farming accounted for 40% of the total crop area in Ireland, and constituted the dominant food of the poorer half of the population. Potatoes were not yet well adapted to the wet climate of northwest Europe, and were prone to outbreaks of disease. By the 1830s, poor potato harvests were becoming common in Ireland. Then catastrophe occurred, when a fungal disease (*Phytophthera infestans*) causing potato blight wiped out the crops in Ireland – partially in 1845 and totally in 1846. One million Irish died and another million promptly emigrated. The potato blight had been introduced initially into Belgium, from America, several years earlier. Then in mid-1845, after unusually cold and wet weather, the disease spread virulently through north-west Europe, England and Ireland. Being less industrialised and riven with poverty and rural oppression, the Irish population was much more vulnerable to the potato crop failure.

The Irish catastrophe was heightened by the British government's repeal of its own Corn Law in 1846. This allowed the import of grain into England to relieve shortages due to the concurrent bad harvests there. Not only was the impoverished Irish peasantry too poor and powerless to buy imported grain, but Irish grain was now being forcibly exported to England. Of the estimated 1 million Irish deaths from the potato famine, many were directly due to starvation and many were due to the outbreaks of infectious diseases, especially typhus, that accompanied the famine. The Third and Fourth Horsemen, as they had done so often before, rode together. This time, however, they were unusually closely aligned. The cause of the famine was itself an infection. Indeed, the Irish potato famine gave a boost to the contentious theory of contagion, being explored at that very time in relation to human diseases such as cholera and puerperal fever. Several eminent European plant scientists speculated that the fungal blight was the cause, not consequence, of crop failure. Louis Pasteur's seminal ideas of the 1860s were thus being prefigured.

The history of foraging and farming: palaeolithic origins

The preceding review of food, farming and famines over the past two millennia refers to merely the latest episode in a much longer narrative. Finding and producing food has been central to the whole saga of human survival and cultural evolution. Plants, with their solar-panels leaves, capture energy from the sun and, via photosynthesis, use it to build complicated carbon-based molecules. Animals eat the plants to procure both the prepackaged solar energy and the nutrient building blocks. Humans eat both plants and animals, the latter as an efficient source of preprocessed high-quality nutrients. We thus dine at nature's high table.

The menu however, has changed radically over time. We will pick up the story from the account of the Pleistocene legacy explored in chapter 2.

THE PALAEOLITHIC hunter-gatherer diet played a pivotal role in human biological evolution. Some simple arithmetic makes the point. If we assume that the modern human species has existed for around 150,000 years, and that agriculture began around 10,000 years ago, then *Homo sapiens* has been exclusively a hunter-gatherer for well over 90% of its existence. In the absence of very strongly selective survival pressures – such as elicited the anti-malaria sickle-cell trait – the human genotype is unlikely to have changed much since the very recent onset of agriculture. The several diet-related exceptions discussed in chapter 3 entailed an increasing metabolic tolerance of lactose, gluten and total carbohydrate in proto-European farming and dairying populations. Otherwise, we can assume that the general pattern of human nutrient needs and biological responses is as it was inherited from our hunter-gatherer forebears. (This, as we shall see in later chapters, does not preclude the possibility that other dietary adaptations, today, will enhance health and survival in older age – an issue that could only have had marginal relevance in the natural selection stakes of the Pleistocene.)

The first thing to note about the hunter-gatherer diet is that foraging and hunting for food is a year-round commitment. It is difficult to store fresh foods and so, in hand-to-mouth style, food is divided up and eaten. Local seasonal migration, shared memory and basic technology ensure a variety of food sources throughout the year. Typically, there is great diversity of foods, and often considerable seasonal variation.[15] Australian Aborigines make use of a total of around 200 different animals, birds, fish and crustaceans and almost 100 different plant species. The San and Kung! peoples of the southern African Kalahari desert region consume more than 150 plant and 100 animal species. With that dietary diversity, micronutrient deficiencies are very unlikely. Nevertheless, there are good and bad seasons; there are occasional droughts and famines.

The second thing to note is the profile of major nutrients (Figure 5.2). By comparison with the agrarian diet, the hunter-gatherer diet is high in meat, similar in complex carbohydrates, low in simple carbohydrates, low in sodium, and high in vitamin C (ascorbate) and calcium. As we saw in chapter 2, meat

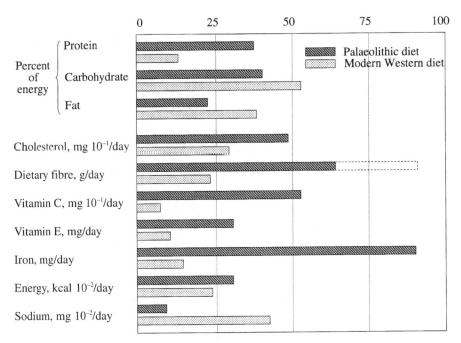

Figure 5.2 Comparison of the nutrient profile of the palaeolithic hunter-gatherer diet (estimated from multiple sources) and the modern Western diet.

typically accounted for 30–40%, and often more, of total food energy. However, meat from wild grazing animals differs greatly in its energy and nutrient content from the meat from domesticated, selectively bred, animals. The meat of domesticated animals is much more energy-dense because it has 20–40% fat content – approximately ten times more than in wild herbivores. Further, the type of fat is different. Most of the fat in domesticated animals is depot fat, and is fully saturated, whereas a high proportion of the fat in meat from wild animals is polyunsaturated fat. As we saw in chapter 2, much of this is 'omega 3' (n-3) long-chain polyunsaturated fatty acids – best known today as health-enhancing 'fish oil'.[16]

Fats serve both structural and energy-storage functions. Fatty acids have a central chain of carbon atoms to which hydrogen atoms are attached by energy-containing chemical bonds. While plant fatty acids are mostly 14 to 18 carbon atoms long, animal fatty acids have 20 or 22 carbon atoms. If the number of attached hydrogen atoms is maximal, then the fatty acid is 'saturated'. The fatty acids in plants, being shorter and unsaturated and therefore of greater molecular mobility, are predominantly oils ('vegetable oils'). Warm-blooded animals, however, use fat both structurally in cell membranes and as an energy store in depot fat. The flexible unsaturated fats meet the structural need, while the less flexible and more energy-dense saturated fats are used for storage.

In contrast to warm-blooded animals, fish and other marine creatures need a storage fat that will remain soft at cold temperatures. This, conveniently, enables cold-water fish to move their tails and fins. (The difference between refrigerated butter and margarine illustrates the point.) The long-chain 'fish oils' are therefore unsaturated. Since this non-saturation occurs first at the carbon atom three places from the end of the chain, these oils are referred to as n-3 (or 'omega 3') fatty acids. Plants contain predominantly n-6 fatty acids, but many (such as soybeans, walnuts and rapeseed) also contain some n-3 fatty acids. Algae which form the base of the marine food web are especially rich in n-3 fatty acids, as therefore are the fish that eat the algae.

Human diets vary greatly in the ratio of n-6 to n-3 fatty acids. Approximately, those ratios are: Westerners = 9:1; Japanese = 3:1; Inuit (eskimoes) = 1:1; other hunter-gatherers = 1:1. Several recent archaeological studies indicate that aquatic foods were more prominent in the palaeolithic human diet, especially during the past 100,000 years, than was previously thought. Human groups were never far from waterways or coasts, and much migration is likely to have occurred along rivers and around coastlines.[17] The many vast middens of shellfish and archaeological clusters of fish bones, on all continents, attest to those human groups having had a substantial intake of aquatic foods. Excavation of the huge cave at the mouth of Klasies River on the coast of South Africa show seafood-rich layers from around 100,000 years ago. Therefore, over most of human hunter-gatherer existence, diets must have had a significant component of unsaturated (n-3) fatty acids – from game animals, fish, other seafood, seeds and nuts. It would not be surprising, therefore, if human biology were evolutionarily well attuned to these n-3 fatty acids. This may account for their many apparently beneficial effects upon the cardiovascular system, including a lowering of blood pressure, a raising of the blood HDL-cholesterol (the 'good' cholesterol) level, a reduction in blood clotting tendency, and an increased resilience of heart muscle against oxygen deprivation.[16] The n-3 fatty acids also suppress the synthesis of saturated fats in the liver. Many epidemiological studies have now shown that dietary supplementation of n-3-rich foods reduces the occurrence and recurrence of heart attacks.

The n-3 fatty acids also have a suppressive effect on the immune system. This is because the n-3 family of fatty acids are precursors to eicosanoid cytokines (inter-cellular chemical messengers) that are mostly anti-inflammatory, whereas the n-6 fatty acids are precursors to the pro-inflammatory cytokines released by white blood cells during the body's immune response. Hence the recommendation of n-3 fish oils for the alleviation of arthritis. What might this imply about the immune defences of n-3-consuming Pleistocene humans and their susceptibility to infectious disease? Probably little, since as we saw in chapter 4 relatively few endemic bacterial infections circulated in ancestral hunter-gatherer bands, and their larger protozoal and helminthic parasites mostly evaded the immune system anyway.[18]

The story of the palaeolithic diet is being gradually pieced together by science, against considerable odds. Archaeological evidence and physical evidence from teeth and bones provides limited information about the conditions of life and health of palaeolithic hunter-gatherers. Isotopic analyses of elements in bones indicate the extent to which meat, sea-food and plant-foods were eaten. The other approach is to extrapolate from surviving hunter-gatherers. It is evident from hunter-gatherers that, although food must be sought continuously, it does not require more than a few hours of effort per day on average. Studies of traditional hunter-gatherer children have shown them to be generally free of nutritional deficiencies, to be healthy, although leaner and of smaller stature than modern Western children, and to have few diarrhoeal or other infections. This, of course, is what one would expect for representatives of a species that has survived successfully with this way of life for almost a quarter-million years.

The origins of agriculture – and of health inequalities

In the several thousand years immediately following the last ice age, there were hectic temperature swings that lasted from decades to several hundred years. Palaeoclimatic studies indicate that temperatures in Britain around 14,000 years ago surged briefly upwards by 7–8 °C within a century – and then, 2,000 years later, fell and then rose again by around 5 °C within the space of centuries (the so-called Younger Dryas event). These massive climatic fluctuations must have created havoc with the environmental and ecological resources upon which human groups depended. Previously well-fed settlements along the Nile Valley disappeared as the river flood-plains contracted and plant foods and fish dwindled. This extreme climatic instability, as Earth shifted from ice age to interglacial, ushered in the Holocene period, and the first stirrings of agriculture. Those early impulses to deliberately cultivate cereal grasses and to herd animals arose in response to a mix of new opportunities and the struggle to maintain food supplies in a changing landscape.[19]

Those few centres that embarked independently on agriculture, as Jared Diamond has persuasively argued, were especially favoured by the range of plant and animal species on hand.[20] Archaeologists think that there were five or six main independent centres of agriculture.[21] The oldest was in the Fertile Crescent of the Middle East, emerging around 10,000 years ago. This was the primary centre from which farming spread northwest, throughout Europe, over the ensuing 5,000 years. The late palaeolithic hunter-gatherers in this area were favoured by the presence of various wild grasses ancestral to wheat, barley and rye. Profuse natural stands of these grasses yielded abundant edible seeds. With selective harvesting of the larger seeds and some fortuitous hybridisation between species, larger-grained wheat would have emerged readily. Further, being annuals, and growing from seeds, these grain plants would have been readily domesticated.[20] The Fertile Crescent also had wild lentils, chick-peas, several types of cultivatable fruits (figs, grapes and olives), herdable populations of animals (the progenitors of today's cattle, sheep, goats and pigs), and a seasonal 'Mediterranean' type of climate. This, for prospective human civilisation, was a Garden of Eden. It opened a way of life in which various simpler hunter-gatherer innocences would be lost.

The next of the primary agricultural centres, chronologically, was in Papua New Guinea. Here the garden-based horticulture of bananas and taro (but no cereals) began around 9,000 years ago. This was followed by northern China (the Yang Shao people, cultivating millet) and by Southeast Asia (the original home of rice), each beginning around 8,000 years ago. Then came Central America and Peru, each around 7,000 years ago, with their distinct indigenous crops: primarily maize, beans and potatoes, along with tomatoes, avocadoes and peppers.

The subsequent emerging centres may have been secondary. The Indus Valley civilisation arose around 6,000 years ago, as did Egypt. Agricultural centres in eastern Africa date from around 5,000 years ago. The archaeological and genetic evidence indicates that domesticated plants, animals and human agrarian genes diffused into those centres from the original Middle Eastern centre.[20] Rice, too, spread from its Southeast Asian origin to southern China, and then, around 4,000 years ago, to Indonesia, Sri Lanka and southern India. Rice cultivation was introduced into Japan and the Philippines, via Korea, within the past 2,000–3,000 years. The colonisers of the Pacific islands originated from that East Asian coast several thousand years ago, as rice farming was becoming established. They took various gardening and farming skills with them, along with yams, taro, breadfruit and chickens, supplemented with locally available coconuts, fish and turtles.

Meanwhile, the Australian Aborigines, other Asian aboriginal groups, and various Amerindian groups in the Arctic (the Aleut-Eskimos and Na-Denes), the northern temperate region, the tropical jungles and the southern reaches of South America had essentially no contact with agriculture. The Pima Indians in the southwest United States depended on an economy of foraging and hunting, supplemented with some agriculture over the past 2,000 years.

THE HISTORY of settled living since the advent of agriculture around 10,000 years ago indicates that we are better at producing than sharing. Poverty and food insecurity have been the lot of the majority of humankind in most settled societies over the ages. The fossil record indicates nutritional disparities between an elite minority and the subordinate peasant majority. In hunter-gatherer societies, in contrast, food tends to be procured and consumed locally, via sharing, since there is little opportunity for preservation and storage.

Comparison of skeletons indicates that adult agrarians were significantly shorter than their immediate hunter-gatherer predecessors.[22] Studies in the greater Eastern Mediterranean region have compared bones from late palaeolithic hunter-gatherers from around 15,000 to 11,000 years ago with those of various early agrarian communities in western Turkey, Greece, the Balkans, the Middle East and north Africa during the neolithic ages and bronze age from around 10,000 to 4000 years ago.[23] As climate and environment changed and as the early tentative cultivation of cereal grasses evolved over several thousand years, human stature decreased by 4–6 centimetres. Over the ensuing 5,000 years, a further 7–8 centimetres of stunting occurred, such that by the early bronze age, around 4,500 years ago, agrarian humans were 12 centimetres shorter than their genetically similar hunter-gatherer ancestors. Interestingly, modern Western populations are only just now regaining that ancestral palaeolithic stature, having gained around 7 centimetres in the last two better-fed centuries.

The evidence of physical stunting during the difficult centuries of learning to farm, of struggling with new endemic infections that sapped nutrients and energy, and of managing hierarchical social systems is widely accompanied by evidence of malnutrition. Skeletal remains typically show evidence of iron deficiency anaemia (especially the tell-tale porotic hyperostosis, an abnormal sponge-like thickening, of skull bone) and of impaired, often arrested, physical growth (with characteristic anomalies in long bones and tooth enamel).[24]

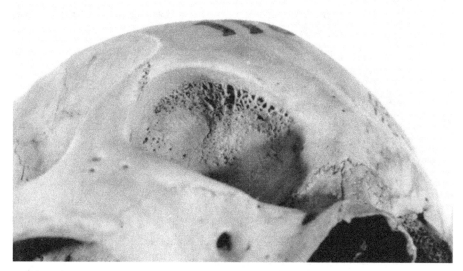

Figure 5.3 Porotic hyperostosis – thinning of the bone – in the right eye socket of a fossil skull (viewed from below, nose cavity on lower right). This condition provides evidence of iron deficiency anaemia, and is used by palaeontologists to assess the level of nutritional stress in populations.

Studies at Dickson Mounds in the Illinois region of the United States indicate that there was an increasing level of biological stress, over four centuries from the tenth to the fourteenth century AD, as the Indian population evolved quite rapidly from hunter-gatherer to mixed economy, to settled agriculture based on maize cultivation.[25] The bones indicate a lowering of life expectancy in adults from an average of 29 to 23 years, a 10% shortening of adult long bones, a tripling in the prevalence of porotic hyperostosis (Figure 5.3), and a doubling in the prevalence of infections, of growth disturbances and of degenerative lesions of joints and backbone. (The researchers, however, caution against generalisation from this study, since any single local population could have been unusually vulnerable to exploitation within a larger regional system of newly expanding agricultural production and trading.)

In agricultural societies hunger is often not equally shared. The fossil evidence from many early neolithic farming communities shows an unequal distribution of the 'hunger lines' (Harris lines) on long bones.[19] Studies in both northern Nubia (now Sudan) and northern Chile have revealed clear differences in stature and nutritional status between the elite and the peasants. In the Chilean Maitas-Chirabaya agrarian culture, the privileged priestly shamans were taller and had fewer bone lesions.[26] It is evident that social inequalities in health have existed for as many millennia as have stratified agriculture-based societies.

WE CAN FINISH this part of the story by looking at the more recent evidence of the relationships between nutrition, infection and growth, and their associated social inequalities in health. There is a close but complex relationship between nutritional state and infectious disease. Thomas McKeown, mentioned in later chapters, has propounded the argument that the improved nutritional status of the population of England and Wales was the key reason for the downturn in deaths from infectious diseases in the nineteenth century. His assumption, widely shared, is that well-nourished individuals are, almost always, less susceptible to serious infectious disease. Evidence that nutritional status inversely affects the severity of infectious disease comes from comparing case fatality rates in children in the United States and Central America infected by the same strain of measles virus in the 1960s, before the advent of vaccination programmes. Death rates from measles were a hundred-fold greater in the Central American children, who were smaller and lighter than the North American children. The corollary of this relationship is that repeated infection in childhood impairs physical growth. Research in Guatemalan highland villages shows that, in low-income populations with high rates of childhood infection, infant growth in the first year of life is 30% less than in their North American counterparts. Records of growth in individual children show a close relationship between infectious disease episodes and growth deficits.[27]

The classic view is that infection and malnutrition constitute a mutually reinforcing 'synergistic package'.[28] However, there is disagreement among scientists. Indeed there is some evidence that a moderately (but not severely) malnourished individual may have a slight biological advantage in forestalling clinical infectious disease. After all, a microorganism requires many of the same nutrients that are essential to the host's biology.[29]

The historical record of the average height of working-class children in England sheds, indirectly, some more light on this complex topic. First, over time, their average height has remained consistently and significantly less than that of upper-class children. Second, the major gains became evident from around 1860. Working-class children aged 15 gained around 10 centimetres during 1800–50, after which there was a spectacular gain of another 15 centimetres or so to 1960. This fits with other evidence that from the middle of the nineteenth century there was an increase in food availability, and a receding of childhood infectious diseases, within the working-class masses of urban-industrial England. Intriguingly, 100 years later, to the decade, Buckingham Palace found that there was a surge in the number of royal telegrams to be sent to English centenarians. The harvest of health gains in the better-fed generations born in the 1850s and onwards was becoming evident in the burgeoning number of Happy Hundredth Birthday telegrams required from the late 1950s onwards.

IN MANY ENVIRONMENTS there are local deficiencies of particular nutrients that impair child growth and development and adult biological function. Many mountainous and arid regions lack iodine, a critical trace element for brain development and normal metabolic functioning. Farming populations, often eating monotonous diets, are vulnerable to micronutrient deficiencies. Rural Middle Eastern populations have long been prone to zinc deficiency because of the high content of zinc-binding fibre (phytate) in local wheat flour. This deficiency adversely affects child growth and sexual maturation. Biological evolution is less able to contrive metabolic adaptations for deficiencies of essential micronutrients (such as iodine, selenium, iron and vitamins) than to contrive basic fuel-switching adaptations such as that which enables Inuit Eskimos to survive on low carbohydrate intakes.

Iodine deficiency remains a widespread problem, seriously affecting several hundred million people. Approximately one-sixth of humankind lives in regions with insufficient iodine in the local diet.[30] This element is needed by the thyroid gland (in the front of the neck) to produce thyroid hormone, which is central to much of fetal development and to metabolic normality post-natally. In iodine deficiency areas goitre is widespread, due to compensatory swelling of the iodine-starved thyroid gland. In the mid-1990s, an estimated half-billion people were affected by goitre. Goitrous women, when pregnant, may deprive the fetus of thyroid hormone and thereby impair the development of the brain and nervous system. The iodine-deprived offspring suffer from a range of iodine-deficiency disorders: mental retardation, spasticity, deafness and physical stunting. Iodine deficiency is an ancient affliction of human populations living on iodine-poor soils, especially in highland regions from which the iodine has been washed away by millennia of rainfall. There is ample historical record of the occurrence of goitre and associated disabilities.[30] A Buddha frieze from southern India of 1,500 years ago shows a goitrous individual playing a large drum in the community procession, apparently protected by his deafness. Woodcuts of battles between late mediaeval warring fiefdoms in the Swiss Alps, where goitre existed until the twentieth century, show the victors slitting the enlarged goitrous necks of the vanquished.

Several experiences in India in recent decades illustrate how nutritional hazards from natural sources have coincidentally improved or become worse following human interventions in the environment. Both pellagra (niacin deficiency due to amino acid imbalance) and lathyrism (exposure to a neurotoxin in lathyrus cereal seeds) were alleviated in the 1980s by economically driven changes in India's production of alternative cereal grains. Wheat and, to a lesser extent, rice substantially displaced pulses and jowar. Meanwhile, goitre and intellectual stunting due to dietary iodine deficiency increased their geographic range, as did skeletal fluorosis. The former occurred because both the spread of irrigation and the expansion of sugar-cane production depleted soil iodine levels. The latter resulted from the use of dams and tubewells that increased the content of bioactive fluoride in drinking water.

Food production, land degradation and health

Since sunlight is the source of virtually all food energy on Earth, our food supply is primarily limited by the efficiency of photosynthesis in plants in the human food chain. On average, a natural wilderness environment supports approximately one hunter-gatherer per 10 square kilometres, and provides a seasonally varying mix of plant and animal foods. This low-intensity figure contrasts with that of traditional farming which supports up to 50 people per square kilometre, depending on the richness of soil and water resources. In fertile river plains this figure approaches 100 people per square kilometre, or one person per hectare (a hectare being one hundredth of a square kilometre – about the size of a baseball ground). With more intensified farming methods, even more people can be supported, at least temporarily. Indeed, in the modern world, with widespread intensive farming practices, the global average is now three persons per hectare of arable land. That is, the world's approximately 1.6 billion hectares of arable land, which currently yield about 2.2

billion tonnes of cereal grains, support 6 billion people. There are a further 3 billion hectares of pastoral land upon which livestock grazes.[2,3]

Ever since human societies began replacing the low-impact hunter-gatherer life with that of farming and pastoralism there has been a need to find and clear fertile land. The expansion of populations and the rise of ancient civilisations depended crucially on the extension of labour-intensive agriculture, capable of yielding a food surplus to feed the urban elites and workers. The thousand-fold increase in human numbers since the advent of early agriculture has necessitated the clearing of forest and woodland on all continents. Between the tenth and fifteenth centuries in Europe, approximately three-quarters of natural lowland forest was cleared. Likewise, there has been rapid and extensive clearance of lowland forest in Australia over the past two centuries. The process continues today in many parts of the world, most spectacularly in the Amazon basin, central and west Africa, Southeast Asia and parts of Siberia.

From the world's arable land, approximately one-sixth of which is now artificially irrigated, comes the plant food that makes up the majority of the human diet. Two-thirds of our dietary energy comes from cereal grains, predominantly wheat, rice and maize (corn). During the 1980s and 1990s, the combination of erosion, desiccation and nutrient exhaustion, plus irrigation-induced water-logging and salination, rendered unproductive about one-fifteenth of the world's readily arable farmland. Much more land was seriously damaged. In Australia, for example, the spreading salination of denuded farmland is becoming a serious national problem. As population size increases, as regional climates alter in response to global climatic changes, and as biodiversity loss increases the probability that pests and diseases will afflict food crops and livestock, there will be further stresses on the world's food-producing systems.

The world's per-person production of cereals seems to have faltered a little since the mid-1980s. The reasons for this are unclear and contentious.[31] However, it is well recognised that the celebrated successes of the 'Green Revolution' of the 1960s to the 1980s depended on laboratory-bred high-yield cereal grains, fertilisers, groundwater and arable soils. In retrospect, those productivity gains appear to have depended substantially upon the expenditure of ecological 'capital', especially via damage to topsoil and depletion of groundwater. In India, for example, an estimated 6% of cropland was taken out of production because of waterlogging, salinity and alkilinity that occurred during the 1970s and 1980s.[32] The International Food Policy Research Institute has concluded that the Green Revolution, while achieving widespread caloric success, exacerbated maternal anaemia and childhood deficiencies in iron, zinc and beta-carotene, because the higher-yielding strains of wheat and rice, while replete with more energy-rich macronutrients, contain relatively lesser amounts of micronutrients.

Around one-quarter of total animal protein consumed by humans comes from the sea. Indeed, in many countries, such as the Philippines, Bangladesh and the Pacific islands, fish is the main source of animal protein. The annual global catch of seafood, which rose rapidly during the 1960s to 1980s to around 100 million tonnes, has increased little over the past decade. Most of the world's great ocean fisheries are being exploited at or beyond their limit. Several are now in serious decline, as the annual catch drops. The great Grand Banks cod fishery, off Newfoundland, appears to have collapsed permanently since the urgent moratorium of the early 1990s. The North Sea cod fishery is going the same way. The annual catch has declined by 90% over the past two decades because of over-fishing. Furthermore, scientists think that cod spawning may have been impaired by the gradual rise in water temperature that has accompanied the recent global warming.

THERE IS CONTINUING debate about the capacity of the growing world population to continue to feed itself. The profile of the contemporary situation is summarised in Table 5.1. Overall, as world population has doubled from 3 to 6 billion since the 1950s, the per-person production of food has marginally increased. As is often pointed out, this statistic is only an average. The real challenge is to achieve an equitable distribution of the world's food, in order to alleviate the continued malnutrition, and sometimes starvation, that affects one-sixth of the world population. Approximately 830 million people, particularly women and children, are underfed to the extent that their health or their physical capacity is impaired.[35] In young children malnutrition increases the risk of stunted development or of succumbing to diarrhoeal disease or respiratory infections. Alongside this continued hunger and malnutrition, obesity rates are increasing in urban populations everywhere. This is a world in which many Americans, in particular, are desperate to find weight-reducing drugs or to eat designer foods that, by whatever unaesthetic mechanism,[36] reduce the intestinal absorption of fat.

Given the dimensions of the task of feeding a growing world population, it is likely that neither world poverty alleviation nor the voluntary sharing of food will be sufficient to eliminate hunger and malnutrition. The problem will

Table 5.1. Profile of world food production, distribution and consumption

- The proportion of hungry and malnourished people in the world is slowly declining. However, in absolute terms, there remain an estimated 830,000 undernourished people – 95% of them in developing countries.[33] Meanwhile obesity is increasing in urban populations everywhere.
- Per-person food production has increased over the past 4 decades. 'Green Revolution' gains were achieved via intensive inputs of energy and chemicals, and at the expense of soil and water resources. Around one-third of all arable land was significantly degraded over that period.[34]
- Per-person grain production has plateaued since the mid-1980s. The reasons are not clear, and have been partly economic. Selectively bred high-yielding strains may yet provide another round of yield gains, but extra fertiliser and water will be needed.
- The annual harvest from wild fisheries has plateaued at around 90 million tonnes per year. Many fisheries are overexploited. Aquaculture, growing fast, now accounts for approximately one-quarter of the world's total fish and shell-fish production.
- The promise of genetically modified food species, while potentially great, is currently offset by uncertainties about genetic, nutritional and ecological consequences. The genetic engineering of food species should be a cooperative public–private partnership, with agreed environmental, social and public health objectives.

persist at some level for decades. Therefore – and despite the evidence that the world's per-person grain yields peaked in 1985 (at around 380 kilogrammes per person) and have trended downwards since (to around 360 kilogrammes per person in the late 1990s) – the immediate need is to increase the global harvest. If this can be done by increasing labour-intensive agriculture within developing countries, then rural wages will increase and so will 'food entitlements'. However, those production gains must also be achieved by ecologically sustainable means.

Although world food production managed to outpace population growth over most of the past half-century, those successes were achieved partly by depleting natural environmental resources; that is, by borrowing against the future. So, what types of diet will be ecologically sustainable in future? What is the balance of gains and losses due to intensive agriculture and livestock production, both to the environment and human health? And what types of diet will be acceptable in a world in which consumer expectations in urbanising lower-income countries are rapidly changing towards the meat-enriched, highly processed, freight-intensive diets that have been typical of high-income countries? There is an irony in this situation. As lower-income countries aspire to diets richer in animal foods and less dependent on plant staples, diets in high-income countries are evolving towards those of the Mediterranean and non-Western cultures – with more fruit and vegetables, more whole-grain foods and less animal fats.

There are some other environmental dilemmas here. For example, transport is energy-intensive; and fruits and vegetables have high water content and are therefore much heavier to transport, per unit nutrient, than are cereal grains and lentils. And yet, increasingly, the epidemiological evidence shows that diets high in fresh fruit and vegetables lower the risks of many major types of cancers, heart disease, diabetes and other diseases.[37] The eventual answer to this particular tension will lie in developing transport that is powered by renewable energy sources, in encouraging the consumption of locally grown plant foods and, where appropriate, genetically adapting non-local species of fruits and vegetables to facilitate their local production.

In considering future options for feeding the world we must keep the criterion of population health to the fore. To this end we should note that: (i) the types of diet eaten by our agrarian and, particularly, our hunter-gatherer predecessors provide a template for thinking in evolutionary terms about human biology and its dietary needs; (ii) the health gains that have accrued in Western societies over the past 150 years have in part reflected improvements in food transport, refrigeration and distribution systems, and the associated increase in seasonal importation of fresh fruits and vegetables; and (iii) the diets in some high-income countries today, such as those of the Mediterranean region and Japan, appear to confer widespread health benefits. From the diversity of historical and contemporary experience we can learn much about how diets affect population health.

Future prospects: security and sustainability?

The experts are divided on the outlook for feeding the world in the coming decades. World population will reach an estimated 9 billion by 2050 and, if economic development (including the elimination of hunger) proceeds in low-income countries, then the total demand for food will increase approximately threefold. Meeting this demand is likely to prove a tall order, especially in view of the recent slowing of gains in total terrestrial and marine food production. Nevertheless, anticipating biotechnological advances and gains in the efficiency of production, and noting the continuing decline in the market price of cereal grains, most international agencies foresee future food production matching increased population and rising demand at the global level over the next two to three decades.

Fish farming, which has grown at over 10% annually during the past decade, is of considerable potential.[38] Within a decade it may overtake world beef production, which has plateaued at around 55 million tonnes per year. Indeed, in response to environmental pressures, we may be about to make a basic shift in the human diet: fish ponds offer great advantage over cattle feed-lots in a protein-hungry world of land and water scarcity. As we will see in chapter 6, feedlot beef production requires enormous inputs of water, grain and fossil fuel energy. China, with 3,000 years experience, leads the way with aquaculture: its ponds, lakes and rice paddies currently account for two-thirds of the world's annual aquacultural yield of approximately 35 million tonnes. However, aquaculture is prone to problems of infection and pollution and it entails some particular ecological difficulties. Salmon and shrimp, currently each accounting for around 1 million tonnes per year, are especially problematic. Salmon are carnivorous and their production therefore intensifies environmental pressures – they require 5 tonnes of fishmeal per tonne of salmon produced. In Norway, the waste produced by salmon farming approximates the sewage output of that country's 4 million people. Salmon stocks, selectively bred for fast growth, are prone to lice and viral infections, despite heavy chemical treatment of their water. Their escape and inter-breeding with wild salmon may impair the latter's survival capacity. Shrimp farming, especially around Asian coastlines, has widely destroyed mangrove forests and polluted coastal waters. Further, since most farmed shrimp is for export to higher-income populations, its production does not directly alleviate local food shortages.

At the regional level, meanwhile, food shortages persist. The prospect over the coming decades is for worsening food security in sub-Saharan Africa and only marginal improvement in South Asia.[31] On current trends, by 2025 Africa will be able to feed only around 40% of its population, likely by then to total about 1 billion. Africa's soils are relatively thin and infertile, and poverty and population size have precluded both restoration of those soils with fertilisers and organic matter and any respite from production pressures. Over the past three decades the per capita yields of food in Africa have declined by about one-tenth, whereas in the world at large they have increased by about one-tenth.

Most of the world's gains in food production have been due to the use of improved high-yielding variants of rice, wheat and maize (corn) in combination with great increases in synthetic fertiliser and pesticides. The rate of recruitment of new land has slowed; there is little good land not already in use (with some exceptions in South America). The Food and Agricultural Organization anticipates, optimistically, an increase in irrigated land by 5–10% over the coming decades. Yet much of that 'increase' will merely replace abandoned, salinated, irrigated land. Further, the increasing awareness of the ecological and social costs of dam-building and irrigation may limit that option, as must the fact that freshwater supplies are dwindling.

Food yields, especially of agricultural crops, are also likely to be affected by human-induced global warming, entailing warmer temperatures, changes in growing seasons, altered patterns of precipitation, and (in many rain-dependent regions) reduced soil moisture. Such climatic changes may not all be adverse. Regions currently with a temperate or cold climate might undergo increased yields in response to increased temperature. However, many mid-continental and semi-arid regions would be vulnerable to crop failures caused by increases in warming and soil drying. Irrigation-dependent agriculture would be vulnerable to reduced rainfall, exacerbated by heightened evaporative losses. We will consider this topic further in chapter 10.

MANY SCIENTISTS THINK that because of soil erosion, depleted aquifers and the already high levels of fertiliser use (except in Africa, where chemical fertiliser cannot be afforded), a continuing Green Revolution is not possible. We must, instead, find ways of improving yields that leave the natural resource base intact, including biological methods of pest and weed control, adequate crop rotation, and mixing of crops with forestry and livestock. We must also find ways to make food more accessible and affordable for all people. This proposition, seemingly banal, highlights a fundamental tension: most of the emergent new yield-increasing techniques, grounded in genetic engineering, are best suited to the world's flat lands with good soils, plenty of water, and effective commercial and governmental infrastructures. In other words, these techniques are better suited to temperate First World regions than to the often food-insecure, agriculturally marginal regions in developing countries.

The conventional options for boosting plant-food production would include pressing more land into service, extending irrigation, increasing fertiliser use severalfold in Asia and at least twentyfold in Africa. However, limits are being reached on various environmental and biological fronts. Therefore, higher priority must be given to sustainable methods. Meanwhile, there are hopes for newly engineered high-yielding plant varieties. The various specialist international agricultural research centres hold out hope for a new designer breed of rice with 25% higher yields, of a potato that is resistant to tropical bacterial disease and is much faster-growing, and of drought-resistant maize. There is, however, often a mismatch between technical developments in crop production and the circumstances of poor Third World rural populations. If new developments are not tailored more to those populations, via dialogue between scientists, extension workers and local farmers, the rich–poor gap will continue to widen and widespread malnutrition will persist. Particular attention must be paid to the age-old problem of postharvest loss. An estimated 20–50% of maize (corn) and cassava (manioc) in Africa is lost in this way, whereas losses for similar staples in Europe (e.g., wheat and potatoes) are less than 1%. Opportunities to reduce losses include improved scientific understanding of indigenous crops and their handling and greater insight into the socioeconomic context in which new technologies might be applied.

Livestock production must optimise the use of plant-food energy. Plant and animal production do not necessarily compete with each other: ruminants such as cows and sheep *can* graze on land that otherwise would not be useful for growing crops. However, grazing animals often have heavy impacts on the environment, resulting in soil erosion, competition with indigenous animal species, and the eutrophication and microbiological contamination of waterways. The routine use of antibiotics in animal feed as growth promoters induces antibiotic-resistant bacteria within livestock that then pass to meat-eating humans. The problem is worldwide. In Kenya, for example, most farmers now use a wide range of over-the-counter antibiotics for growth promotion, prophylaxis and treatment of farm animals. One survey there showed that three-quarters of healthy chickens carried tetracycline-resistant *Escherichia coli* and around one-quarter carried *E. coli* that was resistant to ampicillin and gentamicin. Another such problem arises from the widespread use of chicken manure from battery farms as an inexpensive source of protein-rich feed for cattle and hogs in the United States. Aesthetics aside, this carries an obvious risk of transmission of salmonella, *E. coli* and campylobacter bacteria – all increasingly antibiotic-resistant – from chickens to four-legged mammals and then to two-legged mammals.

There is, of course, great promise in the genetic modification of food species, particularly in adapting them to the available environment. However, there are also unresolved worries about potential adverse ecological and health consequences. As discussed in the next chapter, we face a major challenge in directing this ingenious biotechnology to socially beneficial ends.

Conclusion

We began this chapter with a review of how history's Third Horseman, famine, has left a trail of misery and early death along his trail. All food derives from the natural world and is therefore subject to both the constraints of ecological systems and the vicissitudes of weather, pests and diseases. Obtaining food has been a central task in all human societies – a task that eventually led our anxious ancestors towards the agrarian diet. The evolution of both human biology and of human society has been intimately shaped by the types and amounts of food available.

For most of human agrarian history the balance between population demands and food supplies has displayed the precarious arithmetic that underlies potential Malthusian subsistence crises. Climatic variations have played a central role as both immediate and longer-term determinant of food production. Life in today's rich countries – a tiny and historically unusual part of the total human experience – can easily mislead us about the security of food supplies. Today, as the scale of the world-feeding enterprise mounts, and as consumer preferences for animal-based foods grow in urbanising populations, so too does our reliance upon environmentally damaging modes of food production.

Meanwhile, we have not noticeably improved our ability to share; approximately one in seven persons in the world are significantly malnourished, alongside increasing obesity in overfed, underactive, urban populations. If we are to feed the expanding human population during this coming century adequately, safely and equitably, then we should strive to:

- Constrain world population growth.
- Develop ecologically sustainable methods of food production.
- Encourage consumption of fresh fruit and vegetables, thereby reducing consumption of energy and materials-intensive processed foods and animal foods.
- Achieve greater equity in world trade; encourage economic development that allows for local production of dietary staples as opposed to emphasising export crops; and seek fairer and more efficient food distribution systems.

We may already have pushed the world's food-producing systems to, or sometimes beyond, their limits – both on land and at sea. In view of the ongoing increase in world population, and the rise in consumer expectations, we will need to triple world food production by around 2050. Without remarkable new technical breakthroughs, and new ways of ensuring ecological sustainability, such increases may not be achievable. The emergence of global environmental changes is adding further stresses to food producing systems. The twenty-first century may yet provide the first global test of the ideas of Thomas Malthus who foresaw, 200 years ago, an intrinsic mismatch between the growth trajectories of human populations and food production.

6

The industrial era: the Fifth Horseman?

Over the broad sweep of history, changes in environment, in human ecology and in contacts between civilisations have largely determined the tides of infectious diseases and the changing nutritional fortunes of populations. For several thousand years, disease and death have been dominated by the biblical Four Horsemen – war, conquest, famine and pestilence. Within the European region over recent centuries, the gradual 'domestication' of epidemic infections and the attainment of famine-free food supplies laid the foundations for a healthier living environment. This broadly coincided with the onset of industrialisation. Two thousand years ago the fevered mind of St John the Divine, with his vivid vision of the horsemen as agents of divine wrath,[1] could not have foreseen human society's eventual industrialisation and its many health consequences. Is industrialisation the Fifth Horseman? (Or, with some poetic licence, is it a variant of the First Horseman, Conquest – the conquest of nature?)

There have been great material benefits and social advances associated with industrialisation, beginning in England in the late eighteenth century. Via the accrual of wealth, the processes of social modernisation and the development of specific public health and medical interventions, the industrial era has contributed enormously to the gains in life expectancy in economically developed countries over the past two centuries. However, industrialisation has also caused much environmental blight and ecological damage and, consequently, has created various risks to health. Over the past half century these negative aspects have become a focus of public concern and formal research in rich countries. Today, we have a clearer idea of the immediate health gains and losses associated with this stage of human socioeconomic development. We have also begun to see that, globally, the aggregate weight of industrial activity and material consumption is beginning to overload Earth's life-support systems.[2]

The industrial revolution emerged in late eighteenth-century England, with the development of machine tools such as the steam engine, the spinning jenny and new metallurgical processes. Our nineteenth-century predecessors then embarked on the path of industrialisation, powered by fossil fuel combustion,

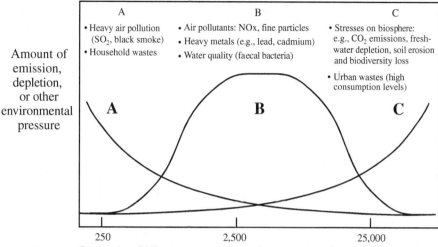

Figure 6.1 Schematic view of three historical 'waves' of different categories of environmental hazards, reflecting how increasing wealth affects society's management of environmental problems. Graph A represents the typically early reduction of traditional, manifest and usually localised environmental hazards. Graph B represents conventional industrial pollutants that impinge on whole communities or regions, and which have now been generally controlled in high-income countries. Graph C represents the newer, larger-scale category for which solutions have not yet been found, and which are continuing to increase.

in a spirit of post-Enlightenment optimism. In practice, whether driven by the creative energy and profiteering of capitalism or, in the twentieth century, by the clumsy, ideologically competitive, urges of communism, the early phases of industrialisation caused great environmental damage. Further, industrial workplaces in mines, factories and sweat-shops have brought new hazards, causing physical injuries, lung diseases, assorted cancers, blighted fertility and reproduction, and the psychological stresses of depersonalised, machine-paced work. In recent decades, wealthy countries have constrained the environmental excesses of industrial activity by reducing air pollution, applying stricter standards to liquid and solid effluent, regulating agricultural chemicals, monitoring radiation hazards, enforcing food safety standards, and so on.

This evolution of human impact upon the environment over the past several centuries, and of society's level of understanding and response, is summarised in Figure 6.1. Three successive 'waves' of environmental hazard are shown: the traditional hazards (graph A), the hazards of industrialisation (B), and those of the late-industrial stage (C). Graph A refers to long-standing environmental hazards that families and local communities can remedy, such as unsafe housing, lack of sanitation, contaminated drinking water and smoky emissions (from domestic coal burning and local factories). They tend to be ameliorated early in the process of economic development. Graph B refers to larger-scale environmental problems such as the industrial and automotive emissions that cause high levels of gaseous air pollutants (sulphur dioxide and nitrogen oxides) and the contamination of drinking water and food with organic chemicals and heavy metals. In Western societies, those exposures have been progressively brought under control over the past three to four decades. Such intervention becomes possible with the accrual of scientific understanding, new technologies and sufficient wealth. The political will derives from public pressures and 'consumer sovereignty' in the market place (whereby consumers perceive directly beneficial trade-offs from environmental amelioration).

Graph C refers to larger-scale forms of environmental degradation and change, the adverse impacts of which are usually displaced in both space and time. These include the release of acidic gases which convert, over distance, into 'acid rain', the accumulation of urban wastes in distant massive dumps, the build-up of greenhouse gases in the atmosphere, the depletion of stratospheric ozone and the loss of biodiversity. There are several impediments to curtailing this third category: the processes and their consequent hazards are harder to understand; the costs of remediation may be large; and the trade-off benefits may be less apparent – and less real at the time and place of intervention. The difference between graphs B and C is illustrated by air pollutants in Sydney, Australia. Between 1970 and 1990 the per-person emissions of carbon monoxide, the nitrogen oxides, sulphur dioxide and particulates all fell (the last two by approximately fivefold), whereas the greenhouse gas, carbon dioxide, rose by almost one quarter.[3]

The orderly diagrammatic sequencing of these three categories is not meant to imply that every society follows exactly this path. These phases overlap in time, and they do so particularly for the socioeconomically disadvantaged subpopulations. The urban poor in Delhi or Mexico City face all three categories of environmental hazards. For example, they are exposed to unsafe drinking water, urban air pollution and (soon, if not now) the intensification of heatwaves due to global climate change.

In addition to this historical sequencing, we can view our environmental incursions in terms of basic ecology and thermodynamics.[4] As industrialisation has proceeded, our use of energy and materials has increased. The size of our ecological footprint has thus increased; we walk with a much heavier tread. This is not just a simple 'physical' impact; it also entails an increasing disordering of the natural environment. Our actions, after all, are subject to the all-important second law of thermodynamics. According to this law continuous inputs of energy are required to create and maintain 'order', against the intrinsic tendency of the material world to lose that order, to become entropic. This law applies across systems and at all levels. For example, it applies to our individual bodies, to whole ecosystems, and to the human-made economy. Organic life and industrial activity each entail a struggle against the natural tendency for order to be lost and for energy to be degraded to heat. Living organisms therefore must take in nutrients and chemical energy to maintain themselves as ordered, internally differentiated entities, and in so doing they export wastes and heat to their environment. Similarly, human economic activity creates ordered entities from raw natural materials and energy. That is, via the processes of extraction and manufacturing we impart order to our industrial products, while exporting entropy into the environment in the form of heat, disseminated pollutants and the disruption of nature.

We should note one more thing. Many of the wastes generated by our industrial metabolism play no useful role in nature. In this our species is unique. Along with the large mass of 'natural' wastes that we produce – sewage, animal dung, food wastes, carbon dioxide, dirt-tailings, fibre (wood, cotton textiles, etc.) and so on – we also produce wastes that the biosphere cannot recycle and, increasingly, cannot absorb. Various of our non-natural wastes are toxic to living organisms. These include the heavy metals (such as lead, cadmium and mercury) that we have mobilised and various of the synthetic persistent organic chemicals that have now been disseminated worldwide via atmospheric and marine convection. Some of these illustrate, again, Graph C in Figure 6.1. As human numbers and economic activities escalate, so various limits in the biosphere's sources and sinks are now being exceeded at the global level.[5] This is a first in human history, and we will return to it in chapter 10.

Historical perceptions of environmental hazards

The health consequences of the transition from hunter-gatherer to village agrarian were mostly those of newly acquired infections from livestock and rodents, which then circulated person-to-person or via rodents and insects.

The risks of infectious disease were amplified by the growth of towns, the extension of irrigation and the growth of trade. As technologies evolved and as specialised craft skills arose, exposures to new physical and chemical hazards gradually emerged. Lead exposure, for example, dates back to around 5000 years ago on the Anatolian plateau in south-eastern Turkey where the metal was first smelted and used. By Roman times, lead exposure had become a serious occupational, environmental and domestic exposure. As we shall see, it may eventually have dulled the wits of Roman senators.

Urban air pollution from coal-burning became a nuisance, and a matter of official concern, in the thirteenth century in England. By the mid-seventeenth century, the diarist John Evelyn was driven to fulminate against the 'hellish and dismal cloud of Sea-coale' that smothered London: 'an impure and thick Mist, accompanied with a fuliginous and filthy vapour, which renders them obnoxious to a thousand inconveniences, corrupting the Lungs, and disordering the entire habit of their Bodies; so that Catharrs, Phthisicks, Coughs and Consumptions rage more in this one City, than in the whole Earth besides'.[6]

Meanwhile, as small-scale manufacturing and commerce grew in revitalised post-Renaissance Europe, Ramazzini in Italy began cataloguing the major physical and chemical health hazards in the workplace. In 1775, the English surgeon Percival Pott noted the unusually high incidence of cancer of the scrotum in chimney sweeps and correctly attributed it to the soot that accumulated in the unwashed skin folds. All of this was a long prelude to the much vaster proliferation of human-made environmental hazards that accompanied the industrial revolution from the late eighteenth century onwards.

AS HUMAN ECOLOGY and its environmental interfaces and impacts have changed over the centuries, so have the ways in which people interpret the hazards they encounter. In Western society up until late in the eighteenth century, older ideas about disease and calamity arising as God's judgement on the human condition prevailed. This idea was of ancient lineage. The Christian Bible's Old Testament reports that God frequently embarked on bouts of smiting the wicked, the idolatrous, the non-believers and the enemies of the Israelites in general.

More generally, the weight of religious authority and the inertia of folklore has fostered a generally passive and fatalistic approach to environmental adversity. Indeed in most primitive cultures such external forces were construed as supernatural or as some kind of magic. In the eastern highlands of Papua New Guinea, the mysterious neurological disease kuru – confined to the Fore tribe, and still a puzzle to Western science in mid-twentieth century – was understood within the afflicted communities to be the work of sorcerers. It was the result of a malicious act of retribution. This bizarre 'laughing death' affected the brain and central nervous system of children and of adult women, but not adult men. Hence, for the male tribal elders it was evident that the sorcery was directed at their families. (In the 1960s, scientists showed that the disease was caused by a 'slow virus', apparently transmitted to women and children during funereal preparations of the body of the affected dead, and perhaps ritually consuming portions of brain – referred to as ritual cannibalism.)

While early popular Western culture was essentially fatalistic and god-fearing, there were coexistent formal views grounded in philosophy and science. The classical Greeks were the first to attempt a rational analysis of how aspects of the environment affected human biology and health. Theirs was a cosmos made up of opposites: heat and cold, wet and dry, solid and liquid. The tangible world was made up of earth, air, fire and water. And human function and mood reflected the balance of bodily humours: blood, black bile, yellow bile, and phlegm. Greek philosophers therefore had many degrees of freedom in their explanations of disease. The pre-Socratic philosophers, such as Alcmaeon of Croton, sought an environmental explanation. Disease, he wrote, occurs sometimes 'from an external cause such as excess or deficiency of food . . . certain water, or a particular site, or fatigue, or similar reasons'.[7] For its time, this was a radical and visionary statement. It anticipated the famous ideas of Hippocrates and followers, from around 400 BC, recorded in *Airs, Water and Places*. In that great opus Hippocrates writes that physicians should have 'due regard to the seasons of the year, and the diseases which they produce, and to the states of the wind peculiar to each country and the qualities of its waters'. He exhorts them to take note of 'the waters which people use, whether they be marshy and soft, or hard and running from elevated and rocky situations, and then if saltish and unfit for cooking', and to observe 'the localities of towns, and of the surrounding country, whether they are low or high, hot or cold, wet or dry . . . and of the diet and regimen of the inhabitants'.[8]

The ancient Greek philosophers thus had some interest in ecological processes and relationships. The Hippocratic view that human health and disease were strongly affected by the external environment remained influential in medicine and public health until the rise of the germ theory with its specific microbiological explanation of disease. Even so, the Hippocratic frame of reference was confined to local environments and local ecosystems. The biosphere's larger-scale life-supporting processes were generally beyond that earlier field of vision. Indeed they went largely unremarked during the 2,000 years between Hippocrates' time and the origins of the industrial revolution. During those centuries, the world's populations were much smaller than today's and they had much lower environmental impact. Besides, before the Copernican revolution in Western science there was no understanding of Earth as a bounded system.

Natural environmental influences, of the kind that Hippocrates drew attention to, remain relevant today. They include extremes of weather, seasonal and latitudinal variations in solar ultraviolet irradiation, locally circulating infectious agents, and local micronutrient deficiencies that reflect soil composition. For example, there are regions of exposure to dietary selenium deficiency in China and elsewhere, that cause oft-fatal Keshan disease of the heart muscle in young adults and Kashin-Beck disease of the bones and joints in older persons.[9] This relationship between local geochemistry and human biology is a basic aspect of our ecological dependency on the natural world. As such it warrants a brief exploration here.

THE HUMAN SPECIES has dispersed more widely around the world than has any other large animal species. We now inhabit all non-polar regions of the world. Given that each species evolved originally within a restricted habitat range, such migration into unfamiliar environments is a risky venture. In particular, the chemical composition of soil and water, along with climate, varies greatly around the world. Humans, however, are buffered by culture. They trade food, goods and artefacts. They can detoxify and fortify processed foods. In this way, the natural hazards of a widely varying geochemical environment are diminished or side-stepped. Given sufficient time, a regional population may also acquire, through genetic evolution, some specific metabolic defences against ingested hazards.[10]

In poor agrarian settings, however, humans often live in an intimate, largely unbuffered, relationship with the local soil and water. One-sixth of the world population lives on ancient, leached and often mountainous soils where they are at consequent risk of iodine deficiency and its several serious health disorders, as was discussed in chapter 5. An estimated 350 million persons worldwide suffer from severe iron deficiency; around 60% of reproductive-aged women in India have iron deficiency anaemia. And, as noted above, there are pockets of selenium-deficient soil in East and Southeast Asia.

These local natural exposures are, today, often supplemented by the consequences of mining, forest-burning, and the spread of industrial and transport effluent. Hence, for example, the toxic food-borne exposures to cadmium from mine-tailings and landfill that have afflicted Japan and parts of Poland over the past half-century, resulting in kidney damage and, sometimes, severe bone damage. Or, more recently, the hazard posed by mercury in the river ecosystems of the Amazon, downstream to unruly hordes of inexperienced gold prospectors who use mercury compounds to precipitate the gold.

OVER THE PAST several decades, the main category of 'environmental' concern for epidemiologists and general public has been local human-made contamination of the environment within the industrial-urban setting. In popular understanding, prototypical environmental health problems include the organic mercury disaster of Minamata Bay, Japan, in 1956, the Great London Smog of 1952, and, subsequently, the chemical disasters of Seveso (Italy, 1976) and Bhopal (India, 1984).[11] Then, in 1986, the nuclear reactor disaster in Chernobyl, Ukraine, occurred. In industrialised countries research and environmental management has been directed predominantly to the plethora of chemical contaminants entering air, water, soil and food, along with various physical hazards such as ionising radiation, non-ionising radiation, urban noise and road trauma. As technologies evolve and as levels of consumption rise, the list of candidate hazards seems endless: in the late 1990s we began to worry about the cancer hazard of electromagnetic radiation from mobile phones and about the risk to the fetus from chlorinated organic chemicals occurring in chlorine-treated water supplies.

In low-income countries environmental exposures are more mixed, reflecting the 'old' and the 'new'. Microbiological hazards, especially in drinking water, remain widespread in rural populations and in urban slums: approximately 40% of the world's population still lack safe drinking water and 60% lack sanitation. Domestic air pollution levels are often high, especially where biomass fuels or coal are used for heating and cooking. These exposures cause high rates of infant and child mortality from diarrhoeal diseases and acute respiratory infections. Meanwhile, as industries proliferate, as chemical-intensive agriculture spreads, and as cities fill with motor vehicles, so various additional physical, airborne, water-borne and food-borne exposures occur in these developing country cities. Further, the rapid pace of industrialisation in these countries and the lax environmental and occupational health standards have often resulted in hazardous practices and exposures. In some cases, Western industries have simply moved their discontinued manufacturing practices 'offshore'.[12] More generally, the combination of population pressures and economic intensification is placing increasing stresses on local environ-ments, including agroecosystems, aquifers and coastal waters.

That, then, is an overview of how beliefs, attitudes and social priorities in relation to environmental health problems have evolved over the centuries. How has the actual practice of environmental management and public health protection evolved?

Environmental management: evolving priorities and practices

The foundations of modern empirical science were laid in Western Europe during the seventeenth and eighteenth centuries. Francis Bacon in seven-teenth-century England, rejecting the rationalism and occasional sophistry of classical Aristotelian science, argued for scientific enquiry based upon empiri-cal observation and comparison. Descartes advocated a reductionist approach to studying the external world, as a machine-like entity amenable to disaggre-gation. Later that century Newton elucidated the laws of physical motion, light and gravity. With the ensuing growth of the Enlightenment, the rise of induc-tive logic and a more utilitarian application of scientific knowledge, there emerged a more 'activist' approach to exploiting and managing the environ-ment. This interventionist philosophy nurtured the 'social hygiene' movement in Europe, originating in France in the late seventeenth century.[13] This move-ment aimed to cleanse the environment and lessen its pathogenicity and its epidemic-promoting capacity. Major social expenditures were required for these ambitious projects, ranging from the draining of marshes, the removal of urban refuse and the improvement of roadways. Governments were per-suaded, sometimes grudgingly, that such investments would improve the health of workforces and increase the amount of arable land – leading to gains in productivity and taxes.

After the convulsion of the French Revolution at the end of the eighteenth century, more humane and egalitarian social ideologies emerged in Europe. In the early decades of the nineteenth century it was recognised that a popula-tion's health was affected by the social and physical environment, and that the resultant infectious diseases often swept through the social ranks. The condi-tions of life and work were notorious in early and mid-nineteenth-century urbanising England. This was the age of the industrial miseries of Dickens' *Hard Times*, and of William Blake's 'dark satanic mills'. In 1845, Friedrich Engels described Manchester's factory-working masses as 'pale, lank, narrow-chested, hollow-eyed ghosts' afflicted with ricketts and scrofula, and subject to early death from consumption (tuberculosis), typhus and scarlet fever.[14] His basic epidemiological research revealed that, within the industrial quarter of the city, the death rates were twice as high in the worst houses in the worst streets as in the best houses in the best streets. Around 1840, life expectancy in England's industrial centres ranged from 25 years in labourers to 55 in the gentry.

Following the crisis of urban-industrial blight and a bleak decade of social unrest and increased mortality in the 1830s in Britain, the Sanitary Idea emerged. Edwin Chadwick, the erstwhile but frustrated enforcer of the Poor Law and its punitive workhouse requirements, was the moving force. He was appalled at the filthy living conditions of the working class and was convinced that their persistent illness and susceptibility to disease kept them impoverished – and a financial burden on society. Chadwick's sanitary reforms of the 1840s were, temporarily, linked with larger ideas of urban sustainability, including the recycling of sewage and in the fertilising of adjoining soils and attaining local self-sufficiency in food production. His ideas about the benefits of sanitation, garbage disposal and housing improvements were grounded in assumptions about the disease-inducing role of miasmas, those foul telluric emanations that arose via decay in dank, squalid, urban environments.

Four decades before the germ theory, miasmas were a compelling idea. Friedrich Engels in 1845 wrote:

All putrefying vegetable and animal substances give off gases decidely injurious to health, and if these gases have no free way of escape, they inevitably poison the atmosphere. The filth and stagnant pools of the working people's quarters in the great cities have, therefore, the worst effect upon the public health, because they produce precisely those gases which engender disease; so, too, the exhalations from contaminated streams.[15]

In the same year Charles Darwin, in his chronicle *The Voyage of the Beagle*, wrote: 'In all unhealthy countries the greatest risk is run by sleeping on the shore. Is this owing to the state of the body during sleep, or to a greater abundance of miasma at such times?'

Meanwhile, the alternative, minority, view was that of the contagionists, who believed that particular agents of disease could be transmitted between persons. The studies of Ignaz Semmelweiss in Viennese lying-in hospitals in the 1840s, showing that puerperal ('child-bed') fever was preventable by clinician handwashing, and those of John Snow in London in the 1850s implicating sewage-contaminated domestic drinking water in the causation of cholera pointed clearly to the role of infectious agents. Nevertheless, the struggle between ideas continued for several more decades. The miasma idea was embraced by Florence Nightingale during the Crimean War, in the 1850s. Seeking to reform hospital sanitation, and contemptuous of contagionist ideas, she wrote: 'There are no specific diseases.' The task, she said, was to eliminate the malevolent disease-inducing conditions by infusing the hospitals with pure air. The subsequent enthusiasm for 'garden cities' in England was partly inspired by the prospect of minimising unhealthy miasmas. It also reflected an emerging belief in the possibilities for enlightened collective action in urban planning and in the management of nature. In this it challenged the values of the prevailing *laissez-faire* ethic in mid-nineteenth-century England.

As the industrial revolution proceeded in Western countries, widespread environmental hazards of a non-microbial kind arose. The heavy metal, lead, is illustrative. The great increase in the mobilisation of lead in Europe and North America during the industrial revolution is shown in Figure 6.2. (So too is the brief but acute spike in lead usage, dissemination and human exposures during the Classical Greek and, in particular, Roman eras.) Lead became a dramatic occupational health hazard in late nineteenth-century England, particularly in pottery glazing factories, where lead poisoning was common. Workers suffered from muscle paralysis and wasting, colic, high blood pressure, kidney failure and oft-fatal strokes. Reproductive failure afflicted women employees. Meanwhile, lead began to accumulate in the general urban environment from industrial, domestic and traffic exhaust sources, and posed an increasing, often insidious, hazard to the health of children and adults.

Late in the nineteenth century, a radical shift in causal concepts occurred. Miasmatic theories of environmental disease causation were replaced by the highly specific ideas of the germ theory. Microbes were now deemed to be the primary cause of disease. This powerful new germ theory, along with new theories of cell biology, the specific agents of heredity and micronutrient ('vitamine') deficiencies, refocused the health sciences on the idea of specific agents causing specific diseases in individuals. Ideas of shared environmental exposures and their risks to the health of communities receded; the ecological perspective that had prevailed earlier in the century was eclipsed. This shift was reinforced by the identification of particular health problems caused by specific occupational exposures. Many newly synthesised organic chemicals were becoming commercially useful as dyes, solvents, pharmaceuticals and pesticides. In Germany in the 1890s, scientists observed that occupational exposures to aniline and related dyestuffs were causing an epidemic of bladder

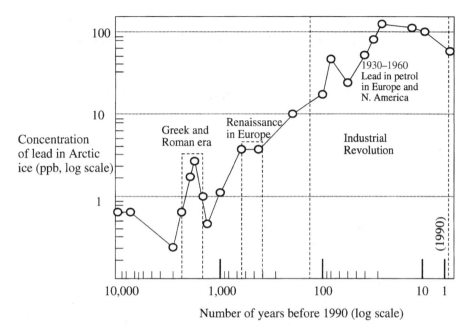

Figure 6.2 Increases in concentration of lead in Greenland ice-cores over the past 10,000 years (shown on a logarithmic scale). The vertical scale, also logarithmic, indicates that the greatest absolute increase, from around 10 to 100 parts per billion, occurred with industrialisation. In recent decades various persistent organic pollutants have, like lead, also disseminated world-wide and accumulated in polar regions.

cancer in factory workers. Similarly, the synthetic pesticides, which often contained arsenic, were beginning to afflict agricultural workers.

The notion of specific environmental, microbiological and nutritional agents as the cause of each particular disease had thus become dominant by the end of the nineteenth century. This was a triumph of reductionism in science. The proclaimed role of toxins, germs and micronutrients foreshadowed the dominant themes of much of twentieth-century health research. Here were the foundations of the 'biomedical model' which shaped a great deal of the clinical and epidemiological research of the twentieth century. It was now the details of the foreground rather than the larger constructs in the background that commanded attention.

In addition to the panoply of new chemical environmental exposures, there were some new physical hazards too. Following the pioneering efforts of Daimler and Benz in Germany in the 1880s, internal combustion engine motor cars were coming into use in Europe. This invention would not only play a central role in shaping the evolution of twentieth-century cities; it would also confer a range of benefits and detriments to human health. In 1896, a novel and shocking event occurred in England: Mrs Bridget O'Driscoll was run over and killed by a motor car. At the subsequent inquest the coroner expressed the solemn hope that such a death would never occur on the roads again.

Environmental health hazards in the modern world

The spread of industry and motorised transport systems in the early part of the twentieth century hugely increased the inventory of human-made environmental chemical exposures. Petroleum products were becoming more widespread, spurred on by the advent of the internal combustion engine. From the 1920s, lead compounds were added to petrol to enhance the performance of car engines. During the 1930s various chlorinated organic chemicals were synthesised. These were unusually stable and persistent chemicals. They included DDT, a potent pesticide able to suppress mosquito populations in malaria-infested areas, and first manufactured commercially during World War I. Among these newly discovered chlorinated organic chemicals were the versatile and seemingly inert chlorofluorocarbons (CFCs), used particularly in refrigeration. However, as we shall see in chapter 10, the CFCs underwent a remarkable and unexpected character change once they had drifted upwards into the extreme cold of the stratosphere.

Following World War II the proliferation of new technologies, industries and wealth in Western countries intensified the building of highways, the reshaping of landscapes, the extension of oil exploration and of mining ventures, and the consequent degradation of environments by modern rich societies. The consolidated communist world embarked on an intensive industrialisation that was seriously negligent of environmental protection. Meanwhile, Europe's empires, freed from the colonial yoke, joined the ordained procession to the promised land of democratic government, industrialisation, trade, consumption and wealth. Textbook-style economic development was there for the asking – a linear staged process, clearly prescribed by the World Bank, the International Monetary Fund (IMF) and their controlling Western interests. This Development Project was intended to achieve a convergent procession of modernising industrialising nation-states.[16]

During the 1950s and 1960s, however, evidence of environmental deterioration and adverse health effects began to accumulate in industrialised countries.

Urban air pollution episodes had become more serious. The famous London Smog of December 1952 killed an estimated 4,000 persons over the course of a frightful week when street-signs could not be read from more than five paces and buses could only proceed with a torch-bearing conductor walking in front. The least-endangered citizens were those living near, or working in, horse stables where the pungent ammonia from horse urine neutralised the acidity of the sulphurous smog. In Japan in 1956, the infamous Minamata disaster occurred when the industrial discharge of mercury wastes from a plastics factory entered the local coastal fishing grounds, poisoning those who ate the fish. Bizarre uncoordinated behaviours were reported in seabirds and cats. Among humans, hundreds of cases of brain and neurological damage occurred over the ensuing decade. Even so, the link to environmental mercury exposure was only accepted following a similar disaster in Niigata Japan, in 1965.

Rachel Carson, in 1962, alarmed Americans when she wrote of a 'silent spring' devoid of birds, the victims of the insidious bioaccumulation of persistent chlorinated pesticides in nature.[17] These chemicals, she argued, impaired the oxidative enzymes that were crucial to the cells' production of energy. Biological functioning, including DNA replication, was thus damaged. Non-human species and whole ecosystems were being adversely affected. Her particular concern was with the indiscriminate use of 'the miracle insecticide' DDT in agriculture, forestry, malaria control and recreational amenity programmes. She documented how, in Clear Lake in California where DDT was used to get rid of nuisance gnats, it was concentrated up the food chain, from 0.02 ppm in the water, to 5 ppm in algae, to several hundred ppm in fish, up to several thousand ppm in fish-eating carnivores. Overall, this was a 100,000-fold bioamplification. We were on notice, said Carson, that such chemicals could have effects that would ripple through the natural world, eventually impinging on human biology and wellbeing. This was a radical shift in how people perceived environmental pollution: a recognition of the systemic ecological disruptions that could result; an understanding that humans could inadvertently poison the natural world. This was the type of thinking which, as we saw in chapter 1, made the science of ecology 'subversive' – a challenge to the cosy assumptions of the military-industrial complex during the Cold War decades.

These emerging environmental health concerns culminated in the groundbreaking UN Conference on the Human Environment, in Stockholm in 1972. There was a new and palpable sense of unease. Humankind, people said, was seriously fouling its nest. *The Ecologist* magazine published *Blueprint for*

Survival and The Club of Rome published *The Limits to Growth*.[18] In response to the accruing evidence and the groundswell of public concern, the UN Environment Programme was established, new national environmental agencies were created, and new national laws were enacted to control the quality of air and water.

The advent of acid rain as an international issue, in both Europe and North America, showed clearly that environmental health hazards were transcending landscapes, crossing boundaries and becoming larger in scale. Today that problem is spreading as China's massive coal-fired industrialisation releases acidic gases to drift eastwards over Japan. Acid rain results from the long-distance atmospheric movement of aerosols of sulphur and nitrogen oxides, usually drifting from west to east. It acidifies waterways and damages soils, crops and forests.[19] The acidification of soil mobilises heavy metals and aluminium into waterways and this may pose a risk to human consumers. The greater problem is likely to be the long-term leaching of calcium and magnesium from soil. These minerals are essential for plant growth. Acid rain may thus impair human food supplies, both from local crops and freshwater fisheries.

During the last third of the twentieth century, technologies and consumer expectations were evolving in tandem. Of the tens of thousands of modern synthetic organic chemicals in current use in the United States, most have not yet undergone adequate toxicity testing. Nevertheless, over 1,000 are either known or presumed to be hazardous to humans – although most of these pose negligible risk at their usual environmental concentration. As new chemicals proliferate, overburdened regulatory systems must, like the Red Queen, run hard just to maintain position. Meanwhile, in much of the Soviet bloc during those years, corruption, inefficiency and state propaganda compounded the profligate environmental contamination and destruction by intensive industrialisation and irrigated agriculture.

Spanners in the metabolic works

Men are naturally most impressed by diseases which have obvious manifestations, yet some of their worst enemies creep on them unobtrusively. (René Dubos)[20]

In the 1980s, concerns about the direct toxicity of environmental chemical exposures were supplemented by heightened suspicions that cumulative exposures to various non-biodegradable chlorinated hydrocarbon chemicals, such as DDT and the polychlorinated biphenyls (PCBs), could disrupt the workings of the reproductive system, the immune system and the neurological system.[21] Consonant with Rachel Carson's earlier concerns, particular attention was paid to the question of environmental 'endocrine disruptors' – chemical exposures that have hormone-like actions and which might therefore disrupt fertility and reproduction. Indeed, there is persuasive evidence from various animal species that such effects do occur.[22] Nevertheless, the notion that such exposures have caused the apparent decline in male sperm count (except in Finland!) over the past half-century remains controversial.[23] It has been reported that thousands of men working in Costa Rican banana plantations in the 1970s and who were exposed to the nematicide dibromochloropropane (long after it was banned in the United States) suffered from reduced fertility.[24]

In 1950, scientists reported that DDT had a hormone-like effect when injected into young male chickens. The birds grew up to look and act like hens. This remarkable observation was largely ignored. In this it was like many in science that do not accord with orthodoxy (from earlier chapters, recall Gregor Mendel, Peyton Rous and Raymond Dart). Forty years later, Theo Colborn, an American biologist working for an environmental organisation, unearthed the report of that finding while examining ecological disturbances in the Great Lakes caused by industrial chemical pollution. She connected this earlier experimental finding with the puzzling observation that female herring gulls around the lakes were sharing nests that contained double-sized clutches of unfertilised eggs. It transpired that male birds had lost interest in mating, pairing and child-rearing. Related findings of abnormal genital development in male alligators exposed to pesticides in the Florida waterways and sexual ambiguities in chemically contaminated fish indicated that such chemicals have a general 'endocrine-disrupting' effect. Despite the current lack of clear evidence in humans, Colborn and colleagues point out that the sex hormones affected by 'endocrine disruption' have been highly conserved through aeons of vertebrate evolution.[25] Thus, the hormones that direct the metamorphosis of tadpole to frog are the same chemical molecules as those that control human sexual development. Therefore, goes the argument, chemical exposures that can malform frogs may well harm human reproduction.

Over forty chemical compounds had, by 2000, been deemed to be endocrine disruptors. Many belong to the 'persistent organic pollutant' (POP) category, able to persist in the environment for decades and, having high lipid solubility, undergo bioaccumulation in biological tissues. They comprise various chlorinated hydrocarbon pesticides (DDT, chlordane, heptachlor, aldrin, dieldrin and endrin), industrial chemicals such as the PCBs and dioxin, and various chemicals used in plastics. Indeed, those POPs that are semi-volatile undergo a type of 'distillation' in the atmosphere, being passed from lower latitude to higher latitude via a process of serial concentration across adjoining compartments ('cells') of the lower atmosphere.[26] For this reason, scientists have recently found unexpectedly high concentrations of some of these chemicals in the Arctic region in fish, seals, polar bears, Inuit and Faroe Islanders. For example, very high levels of dioxins in wildlife in the Canadian arctic have recently been traced to industrial sources in the United States and southern Canada. This global spread has recently prompted the international community to take action to restrict the further use of these chemicals. This, in turn has highlighted a moral and practical dilemma – the trade-off between protecting the health of current populations with useful chemicals and avoiding long-term damage to ecological systems and species that may be important to the health of future generations. A spirited debate has centred on DDT, which is still a major asset in the control of mosquito populations that spread malaria, dengue fever and other diseases. If DDT use were confined to essential public health purposes, and not used in profligate fashion in agriculture and forestry, then a tolerable balance between meeting the needs of the present and future generations could be achieved.[27]

What of the risks to the development and functioning of brain and immune system? Laboratory studies of animals suggest, for example, that exposure to PCBs prenatally or via breast milk can interfere with the production of thyroid hormone and therefore with the growth and maturation of the young mammalian brain. Indeed, some epidemiological studies have found supporting evidence of an adverse impact of prenatal exposure to PCBs or dioxin on brain function in young children.[28] Environmentally induced impairment of immune system functioning could be expected to increase susceptibility to infections and cancers and, perhaps, to affect the occurrence of auto-immune diseases. In recent decades there have been widespread, unexplained, rises in non-Hodgkin's lymphoma, brain cancer, kidney cancer and multiple myeloma. Might these increases, in part, have been due to the immune-suppressive effect of exposures to environmental chemicals? After all, immune-suppressed organ transplantation patients and AIDS patients incur considerably increased risks of various cancers, especially the lymphomas. An array of evidence indicates that the human immune system is indeed affected by many external exposures and stresses, including various chemicals, solar ultraviolet radiation, exogenous oestrogens, cigarette smoking and psychosocial stress.

Uncertainties aside, we now realise that certain environmental chemical exposures can cause sub-clinical disturbance of the endocrine system, the central nervous sytem and the immune system. Such effects fall outside the conventional framework of 'environmental health', with its focus on the risk of specific diseases such as cancer, respiratory damage and birth defects. This is therefore a technically difficult research topic. The biological effects of exposure to chemicals that affect organ system function, while potentially widespread in the population, are likely to be subtle. Further, the mix of chemical exposures keeps changing, as industrial technologies evolve. The use of DDT, demonised by the environmental movement, has been widely curtailed in wealthy countries since around 1970. This is reflected in the approximately tenfold reduction in levels of DDT in breast milk in all continents since that time.[29] Meanwhile, chemical exposures to some other POPs are becoming globally pervasive.

Hazard avoidance or habitat maintenance?

There are many examples of environmental health hazards that could be considered under this heading. The important point to note is that there is an ecological dimension to many of these environmental health problems.[30] The task, in addition to characterising the immediate hazard to human biology, is to understand the extent to which the problem has arisen both because of the scale of human intervention in the environment and because of the oft-complex sequence of resultant impacts on natural biophysical systems.

Each of the problems discussed below entails the overloading of local environments by human pressures and demands. Hazards then arise either directly from noxious exposures or less directly from the disruption of some normal environmental processes, with consequent risks to the health of local communities or whole populations. The adverse exposures must, of course, be recognised and specifically countered. However, there are wider lessons to be learned if similar environmental hazards are to be avoided in future.

Arsenic in groundwater: the Bangladesh disaster

The concentration of various elements varies naturally in groundwater supplies. Localised areas in southwest India have long experienced problems of bone-damaging 'skeletal fluorosis' because of the naturally high fluoride levels in drinking water. In countries such as Taiwan and Argentina, the high levels of arsenic in drinking water have been recognised since around mid-century as a serious health hazard. High levels also exist in Chile, Inner Mongolia, parts of the United States, Hungary, Thailand and China. More recently, the exposure has assumed epic proportions in Bangladesh and neighbouring West Bengal, where tens of millions of people in recent decades have been drinking heavily arsenic-contaminated water obtained via tubewells. The number that have experienced toxic effects, especially skin lesions, probably number in the hundreds of thousands. Allan Smith and colleagues from Berkeley University, who have done much of the recent fieldwork research on this topic, describe it as the greatest episode of mass poisoning in history.[31]

The prolonged consumption of arsenic causes a succession of toxic effects, typically appearing five to ten years after first exposure. Early manifestations include thickening and pigmentation of the skin. This may be followed by dysfunction of kidneys and liver, heart and blood vessel disorders, and, perhaps, by damage to peripheral nerves that can lead to gangrene of feet and fingers. There is also a substantial increase in the incidence of cancers of the skin, lung, bladder and kidney.[26] Indeed arsenic appears to be the most widespread cancer hazard in drinking water in the world. In Chile, for example, 5–10% of all adult deaths have been attributed to arsenic-induced cancers.

West Bengal shares with Bangladesh a subterranean geology with arsenic-rich sediments. Much of the villagers' drinking water now comes from the several million tubewells sunk over the past two decades to provide a safe alternative to drinking faecally contaminated surface water. The irony is obvious: a new public health problem has occurred inadvertently in the course of avoiding an old public health problem. Many of the tubewells yield water with arsenic concentrations 10–50 times higher than the WHO guideline (0.01 mg/litre). For example, in the village of Samta, in Jessore District on the boundary between Bangladesh and West Bengal, approximately 90% of the 265 tubewells were found to have arsenic concentrations greater than 0.05 mg/litre.

It is not clear how to solve this problem – or whether it can be fully solved. One partial solution, where possible, is to drill the tubewells deeper, in conjunction with rapid field testing able to identify arsenic contamination. Meanwhile, the use of arsenic-contaminated water should be restricted to washing only, while using boiled surface water for cooking or drinking. That, of course, requires ready availability of both surface water and firewood – in local environments that are already burdened beyond their carrying capacity. In such situations risks to health are inevitable.

Environmental degradation in the Soviet Union

Dump sites or high-temperature incinerators for hazardous wastes are a source of great public anxiety and controversy. Despite this public concern, the documented health impacts of hazardous waste sites in developed countries have mostly been slight – and considerably less than more mundane forms of air and water pollution. It is interesting, therefore, to speculate on why hazardous wastes attract disproportionate public attention. In part it reflects moral outrage. It also reflects a natural mammalian tendency to treat 'waste' suspiciously, an in-built 'disgust' reaction with obvious evolutionary advantages. It is for this reason that tempting rats to consume poisoned bait is difficult.

Hazardous wastes have assumed a spectacular scale in the former Soviet Union, where vast environmental damage resulted from the industrial, agricultural, military and weapons-manufacturing activities. In some respects this may correspond to the environmental calamities that afflicted Western countries in the early stages of their industrialisation. In other respects, though, it is the grim legacy of decades of production-driven environmental pollution by industry, compounded by the authoritarian prohibition of environmentalism.

The Russian environmental catastrophe has involved much more than radioactive wastes. It includes pesticides, leaking oil pipelines, toxic wastes, chemical weapons and rocket fuel. The aerial spraying of agricultural pesticides over the cotton crops in the Aral Sea basin resulted in soil concentrations of pesticides that often exceeded the official safe levels by several hundred times. Regrettably, the unreliable nature of health statistics records in the Soviet Union has frustrated attempts by epidemiologists to assess the risks to health posed by these environmental disasters. Meanwhile, there remain mountains of solid wastes such as the several billion tonnes of toxic wastes stored precariously in Ukraine. There are, reportedly, thousands of tonnes of highly toxic liquid rocket fuels in depots scattered around Russia and tens of thousands of tonnes of stored chemical weapons, most of it ecologically lethal organo-phosphorus compounds with no ready means of disposal.

The environmental contamination caused by the Soviet Union's production of plutonium for nuclear weapons was extraordinarily high. For example, the Mayak nuclear complex in the southern Urals, established in the 1950s, leaked an estimated five times more radioactive isotopes (strontium-90 and caesium-137) into the environment than had all of the world's atmospheric nuclear tests plus the Chernobyl and Sellafield episodes combined. Beyond the immediate hazard posed to regional residents, via contaminated food and drinking water, there is the serious prospect of these nuclear wastes reaching the Arctic Ocean and spreading more widely via the marine food chain.

Does rapid industrialisation in China portend similar environmental hazards to ecosystems and to human health? Current levels of urban air pollution might well suggest that it does. The smoky sulphurous air pollution, from massive burning of coal, has reduced crop yields in northeast China by around one-third. China has experienced other widespread environmental damage from industrial wastes and agricultural chemicals over the past several decades, including extensive contamination of aquifers by chromium and other wastes. In a more open and interconnected post-Cold War world, however, there is a better chance of earlier rectification of this type of environmental problem in China.

Urban air pollution

Air is our most acute survival need. Humans can go for weeks without food, for days without water, but only for minutes without oxygenated air. Further, the atmosphere is one of the world's great 'commons'. Old ideas about miasmas, and recent debates about acid rain, motor vehicle exhaust gases and environmental tobacco smoke all remind us that, on varying scales, we share and depend upon common access to the atmosphere. It is a 'global public health good'.[32] Yet, out of political necessity, in order to ensure international progress on the abatement of global climate change, we have embarked on establishing an international market in permits to pollute the lower atmosphere with greenhouse gases (especially carbon dioxide). While this affirms the 'polluter pays' principle, it opens up the possibility of wealthy countries or corporations acquiring control over a disproportionate share of the lower atmosphere.

Urban air pollution has, over the past several decades, become a worldwide public health problem. Various studies in North America and Europe implicate short-term fluctuations in air pollution in daily variations in death rates and hospital admissions. Of more significance, several long-term follow-up studies of populations exposed at different levels of air pollution implicate fine particulates in raising the death rate, especially from heart and respiratory diseases.[33] Air pollution also plays an exacerbating, but not initiating, role in childhood asthma.

All of today's car-congested cities, rich and poor, share the modern airborne blight of exhaust emissions: fine particulates, nitrogen oxides and photochemical oxidants (including ozone that forms in the lower atmosphere from precursor pollutants). But for cities in developing countries, the problem is compounded. As they expand rapidly in size – often without the cushion of time and wealth accumulation that would allow planned and managed growth – so air pollution levels rise in response not just to the growth in motorised urban transport, but to increases in industrialisation, open domestic fires in slum housing and the burning of garbage. Today's large cities in East Asia, South Asia, and Latin America have the sorts of levels of smoky particulates, sulphur dioxide and acidity that were banished from most Western countries by the 1970s. Air pollution levels in New Delhi are now so bad in winter that many incoming domestic flights are cancelled. Over the past two decades the number of cars in Delhi has increased at an average of 12% per year, while population has increased by 4% per year.

China has great problems of urban air pollution with particulates and sulphur dioxide. Beijing and Shanghai are now among the world's most air-polluted cities. The World Bank has recently assessed that morbidity and mortality in China will increase steeply over the coming two decades. On current industrialisation trends, increases in air pollution will result in an estimated fourfold increase in premature deaths from this exposure (currently around 20,000 per year), chronic bronchitis cases and bouts of respiratory symptoms.[34] The main source of pollution in China is the industrial use of coal, with its relatively high sulphur content, supplemented by increasing emissions from domestic cooking and heating fuels as poor urban settlements expand.

These figures sound compelling enough. Yet, surprisingly, of all the deaths in the world attributable to air pollution, only one-tenth are due to external environmental exposures.[35] By far the greatest aggregate burden of disease and premature death from air pollution is due to traditional heavy exposures to indoor air pollution in Third World rural and urban slum settings. The exposure results from the inefficient and unventilated use of low-grade cooking fuel, including various types of biomass – wood, dung and crop residues. The concentration of respirable particulate matter is typically 1,000 times greater than in external urban air; carbon monoxide concentrations may be 100 times greater. This domestic exposure blights the respiratory health of women and children particularly, contributing an estimated half of the annual toll of 4 million childhood deaths from acute respiratory infection. There is also epidemiological evidence that it increases the risks of tuberculosis, cataracts of the eye and lung cancer.[36] It is, *par excellence*, a consequence of defective human ecology – the reliance on low-grade energy sources and inefficient technologies within traditional low-income housing, perpetuated by low levels of income, education and knowledge transfer. The serious hazards of indoor air pollution thus reflect the circumstances and way-of-life of whole rural communities and urban sub-populations. It is the type of hazard that was dealt with at a community level in the early decades of the industrial revolution in Western society.

The human species is not alone in being adversely affected by urban-industrial air pollutants. Sulphur dioxide and the nitrogen oxides increase the susceptibility of plants to both fungi and insects. Before the airborne grime of nineteenth-century industrialisation, gardening books in England made no mention of aphids. Many controlled experiments have confirmed that the intensity of aphid attack on plants increases as the concentration of sulphur dioxide in air rises.[37]

Environmental lead and health

Lead, one of the heavy metals, was first smelted around 5000 BC in the Anatolian plateau, and may have been the first of the metals to be smelted. Various leaden beads, trinkets and tumblers have been discovered in eastern Mediterranean, Mesopotamian and Egyptian sites. Lead water pipes were used in Ur, the main city of Mesopotamia, around 3000 BC. Leaded bronze work has been dated to around 2000 BC in Thailand. The use of lead had increased greatly by the age of Classical Greece. This is evident in the geological record in Greenland ice-cores (Figure 6.2). Even more spectacular was the release of lead into the environment during the expansion of the Roman Empire, with its massive lead mines in Greece, Gaul and England. During the European Dark Ages, lead usage sagged to pre-Rome levels, before being rehabilitated in the Renaissance.

The Romans were the original high-volume 'plumbers'. They lined their aqueducts and cisterns with sheets of this versatile metal, plumbum; they rolled it into pipes for their domestic water pipes. In the excavations on the imperious Palatine Hill, adjoining the Forum in Rome, you can see the lead water-pipes in the house of Lyvia (wife of Caesar Augustus and scheming mother of Tiberius). Although Emperor Augustus had prohibited using lead for water pipes, there is little historical evidence that Romans obeyed this law. Clearly Augustus' wife was above the law.

Lead was central to the Romans' lives. They used it for plumbing, roofing, kitchen utensils, coins, children's toys, coffin linings, net sinkers, amulets, pottery glazes, cosmetics, and, eventually, as a sweetener (lead arsenate) of wine. One particularly hazardous use was in lead-lined cauldrons used for boiling down fruit juices in order to produce a concentrated sweetener. Simulation of this process according to extant recipes yields lead concentrations in syrup thousands of times greater than modern drinking water standards. The historian S.C. Gilfillan sparked considerable debate, in 1965, by proposing that the decline in the numbers of Roman aristocracy after around 60 AD might have been due to selective lead poisoning of the upper classes.[38] He reasoned that this would have impaired fertility. Indeed, the prohibition of wine consumption by reproductive-age Roman women was lifted at about that time. Others have suggested that the increasingly bizarre behaviour of many Roman rulers in the latter half of that century (Caligula appointed his horse to the Senate) may have been due to neurological damage by lead ingestion. Overall, the Romans increased the release of lead into the environment by a factor of ten, as is evident in the Arctic ice record (see Figure 6.2).

Historical speculations aside, it is certainly true that over the centuries there have been many poisonings from lead-contaminated food and alcoholic drinks. These include: the 'colic of Poitou' in France in the 1570s associated with wine making; the seventeenth-century epidemic of 'dry gripes' in eastern American colonies using lead-tubing devices to distil rum; the eighteenth-century epidemic of 'dry bellyache' in the West Indies plantation slaves due to the concentration of sugar-cane juice in lead-lined cauldrons and its subsequent use to make rum; the 'colica pictonum' in Holland in the eighteenth century caused by drinking lead-contaminated rainwater collected from leaden roofs; the poisoning of British imbibers of imported Portugese port wine made with brandy from lead-lined stills; and the 'colic of Devonshire' in cider consumers in the eighteenth century due to local use of lead-banded millstones to crush apples. In early industrial Europe and America, chronic domestic lead exposure and poisoning often arose from lead-containing kitchen utensils, storage containers and expensive prestigious pewter-ware that often contained more than 20% lead. That part of the story continues today: within the past decade there has been a report of lead contamination of sherry and port from the high-lead crystal decanters in England's stately homes. Shades of Roman senators?

Environmental lead exposure has accrued over time in many of the world's cities from lead water pipes, delapidated lead-based house-paint, lead smelting, cottage industries (e.g., battery breaking) and the use of leaded petrol for motor vehicles. Epidemiological studies over the past quarter-century have shown that environmental lead exposure impairs the development of young children's intelligence. The best estimates come from studies that have followed young children from birth in several Western urban populations with a typical range of blood lead concentration of 5–30 microgrammes/decilitre. Children whose blood lead concentrations during early childhood differ by around 10 microgrammes/decilitre – typically the difference between the top one-fifth and bottom one-fifth of children in an urban population – display an average difference of 2–3 points in IQ (the standard measure of intelligence, with an expected population mean of 100).[39] A downwards shift of 2–3 points of IQ in a population of children approximately doubles the number of them below the critical IQ value of 70, requiring remedial education.

In today's cities, most of the lead in air comes from leaded gasoline. Lead, as tetra-ethyl lead, was first added to petrol to improve its performance (its 'octane rating') in the 1920s. By the late 1960s the scientific evidence of various, often subtle, adverse health effects from lead, plus the fact that body burdens in the United States had increases 100-fold over the century, led to moves to abolish lead in petrol. Over the subsequent quarter-century, blood lead concentrations in the American population declined by over three-quarters. Meanwhile, leaded petrol is still standard in the developing world. Exposures in young children from industrial and petrol-derived lead exposure have been edging up in cities such as Bangkok, Jakarta and Sao Paulo. In Mexico City, 4 million cars pump 32 tonnes of lead into the air each day. In Dhaka, Bangladesh, the airborne lead concentration is very high, and the mean blood lead concentration in a large sample of rickshaw-pullers was 53 microgrammes/decilitre – five times higher than the acceptable limit in high-income countries. The lead content of petrol sold in Africa is the highest in the world and is associated with high lead concentrations in atmosphere, dust and soils. In recent surveys, over 90% of the children in the Cape Province, South Africa, had blood lead levels over 10 microgrammes/decilitre.[39] Although the world is gradually converting to the use of non-leaded petrol, childhood lead poisoning will remain a serious problem in many low-income countries as urbanisation, poorly controlled industrialisation and car usage grow.

Radon: the domestication of a hazard

In its earlier years Earth was a slow-burn nuclear reactor. When the four innermost, solid, planets of our solar system coalesced from cosmic dust, much of their core material was uranium – unlike the sun, which formed by coalescence of hydrogen gas. Uranium and other heavy elements are formed by the nuclear fusion of lighter elements in stars when, as brilliant supernovae, they finally explode and shower the interstellar void with heavy elemental dust. The subsequent radioactive decay of this uranium, plus thorium and potassium, has generated Earth's internal heat.[40] This causes convection currents in Earth's mantle layers, causing the tectonic movement of continents, along with earthquakes and volcanic eruptions.

One intermediate product in this chain of radioactive decay is the gas, radon, which seeps slowly through Earth's crust, escaping into the atmosphere. Humans, particularly as cave-dwellers, have therefore always breathed traces of radon and its gaseous radioactive decay products, called 'radon daughters'. Today, however, many of us inhale much larger amounts of this radioactive emanation because we live inside houses and work in buildings. Epidemiological studies have established that these inhaled radioactive gases are a cause of lung cancer. This is most obvious in studies of uranium miners, who over many years are typically exposed to a high cumulative dose of these gases. From some of the studies of miners, where individual exposures have been quite low, and from Swedish, British and North American studies of persons living in houses with above-average levels of radon gas, it emerges that there is an increased risk of lung cancer at those lower, more typical, levels of exposure. Estimates in the United States suggest that around 5% of all lung cancers are due to this domestic exposure.

This has come as something of a modern surprise. After all, houses are a major defining characteristic of post-hunter-gatherer life. They represent settled living; they represent physical security. Yet now we find that houses in many parts of the world, especially in colder climates where they are sealed against the external weather, actually serve as trapment chambers for radon and its daughter products. Well, we can reassure ourselves that there is clear positive net health benefit of good housing. But we must also remind ourselves, again, that most changes in human ecology have consequences for health.

Environmental and social impacts of modern food production

Homo sapiens has been foraging for food for 200,000 years, farming it for 10,000 years, and industrially processing it for just 100 years. Much of the contemporary health-related concerns about food in modern urban consumer societies relates to eating too much. In all societies there are concerns to avoid micronutrient deficiencies, minimise exposure to toxic contaminants, and avoid food-poisoning and diarrhoeal disease. For one-seventh of the world population, total daily food supplies are inadequate, causing hunger and malnutrition.

As the world industrialises and as trade becomes global, the international food industry is also making larger footprints. First, its energy-intensive chemical-dependent methods place stresses on productive land. Second, it creates economically efficient but ecologically vulnerable monocultures, as it diminishes the diversity of traditional strains of crops. The Andean farmers of Peru have several hundred types of potato, whereas US farmers get by with three types. In South Asia, there are several thousand types of rice acquired by crossbreeding over several thousand years, but in a world dominated by agro-industry and genetically modified rice that could change dramatically. Third, large-scale export-oriented food production often displaces longstanding sustainable patterns of land-use. Farmland in the Punjab in northwest India, for example, incurred substantial damage from the Green Revolution.

Agrarianism, by definition, puts pressure on the land in order to increase the yield of edible food. In simple, traditional, societies this can be done sustainably by the use of fallowing, crop rotation, and the direct return of nutrients via animal and human excreta. This has long been so in China, where today 22% of the world population must be fed by 7% of the world's arable land. Fortunately for China, smallhold farming over several thousand years has largely maintained the cycle of nutrient extraction and return, via manuring, fertilising and avoidance of erosion. Nevertheless, the increase in population pressures in China over the past half-century has caused increased damage to land and substantial depletion of groundwater in some regions. In general, as urban super-structures evolve, agrarian-based societies tend to break the ancient cycle of hunter-gather ecology wherein nutrients are returned to the soil. As villages became towns, excreta were disposed of in and around settlements or in nearby rivers.

Once agrarian production became established, regular food surpluses were produced. Food thus became a tradeable commodity. Human societies have traded food throughout recorded history, especially rare or exotic foods – whether spices entering Renaissance Europe or salt and iodine-rich coastal foods reaching up the mountain slopes in Papua New Guinea and South America. At the height of the Roman Empire, 1,000 tons of wheat were imported daily to Rome from North Africa. This, in the Roman world, was international trade at its near maximum. Providing Bread and Circuses for an urban population of approximately 1 million was a constant struggle. Many tonnes of imported elephants, bears, lions and Christians were also required.

During the 1930s, energy-intensive agriculture developed strongly in the industrialised world. The world food system that subsequently emerged immediately after World War II – dominated by Western, particularly US, interests and their beholden international institutions of finance and trade – fostered an increasing standardisation of food production. Consumption of wheat and, subsequently, meat was promoted in urban populations everywhere. During the 1950s and 1960s, cheap food for the Third World's urban industrial populations was a prerequisite for their economic development. This nicely coincided with vast US food surpluses, useable for both commercial and political ends. The net effect of this economic regime, with subsidised food imports from the United States, resulted in the contraction of local food production in many developing countries, leaving them dependent on food imports. Their local agricultural base was sometimes further eroded by the restructuring actions of international agribusiness. For example, Mexico – which had been an early Green Revolution 'success' – became food-insufficient in the 1970s as its agricultural food base was diverted into livestock production and export crops.

The economically volatile 1970s, followed by the collapse of various commodity prices and the resultant Third World debt crisis in the 1980s, unleashed new forces of globalisation in production and trade. Nation-states were adrift on a turbulent and swollen ocean of deregulated capital. The Green Revolution, which had produced some spectacular gains in agricultural yields during the 1960s and 1970s, began to lose momentum as marginal yield gains declined, soils lost fertility, and in some countries rural poverty increased. National economies, including their agricultural sectors, were increasingly subjected to the imposition of restructuring by the World Bank and IMF. Subsistence production of staple foods, by small farmers, was thereby replaced by the more intensive agro-industrial model of food production. Under this model, food is produced for export to redeem national debts; it thus becomes a commodity rather than a locally produced source of nutrition. Under the structural adjustment programme negotiated with Zimbabwe in 1991, and which entailed extension of plantation agriculture for export crop production, child nutrition and growth was impaired and infant mortality rates increased markedly.[41]

The global reorganisation of the production, distribution and marketing of food has opened up commercial opportunities for niche marketing (fresh fruit and vegetables, exotic tropical fruits, fragrant coffee beans, etc.) to First World markets and to Third World urban elites. Today, the world's 100 largest transnational agribusiness companies produce about one-quarter of the world's food, predominantly export grains and export luxury foods (e.g. vegetables from Mexico during the US winter, orange juice concentrate from Brazil and peanuts from Senegal). Much of this intensified, export-led, food production is environmentally damaging. In particular, 40% of all corn and coarse grain produced in the world is fed to livestock (in the United States the figure is nearly 70%). To produce one unit of food energy as beef, pork or poultry requires an input of, respectively, eight, four, or two units of grain-food energy. It is not surprising that birds are the most efficient converters of grain since that is part of their natural diet; cattle, however, have evolved to graze on grass.[42] Feed-lot production of beef cattle also requires huge inputs of water, chemicals and electrical energy, and generates extensive nitrogenous wastes and the greenhouse gas, methane. Meanwhile, two-thirds of all arable land in Central America has been converted to pasture for producing export beef for hamburgers and processed meats. Little of the wealth generated by the export of these commodified foods from low-income countries filters back to the poorer, food-insecure segments of those populations.

In Britain, the amount of fossil fuel energy required to produce, process and distribute the average person's annual food intake is about six times greater than the energy content of the food itself. To many hunter-gatherer groups this would be flagrant deficit budgeting, incompatible with survival.[43] Indeed, in the natural selection stakes an aspiring species must be able to achieve sufficient food-energy credit – that is, energy consumed minus energy spent finding it – to sustain reproductive activities. Agrarian and industrial humans, however, have harnessed various sources of extra-somatic energy to the task of food production. Today, we spend fossil fuel energy in producing fertiliser and pesticides; in ploughing, sowing, irrigating and harvesting; in processing and packaging food; in transporting it, often long distances, to market; in commercial and domestic storage; and in disposing of containers, wrapping and food scraps.

Modern industrial food production thus entails the substantial conversion of fossil fuel energy into food energy, with extra energy inputs from the sun and trace element inputs from the soil. Globally, approximately one quarter of the excess emissions of human-made greenhouse gases that accumulate in the atmosphere each year derives from food production, processing and consumption.

Genetically modified foods

The genetic modification (GM) of food entails the deliberate and specific manipulation of an organism's genome in order to modify aspects of its biology, such as nutrient composition, resistance to pests and herbicides, tolerance of adverse growing conditions, and durability of the edible product. This is an ingenious technological achievement. Molecular biology has matured to the extent that we can edit nature's genetic code, including by inserting, *en effet*, words from a foreign language: genetic modification often entails the insertion of genes into food plant species from unrelated species.

In some respects this human-made genetic intervention is equivalent to the processes of random mutation that occur in nature as plants reproduce themselves and of the trial-and-error hybridisation used in traditional cross-breeding by agriculturalists. All three entail a haphazard element in that, depending on where the genetic change occurs within the genome, the function of other existing genes within the host genome may be altered. However, in three respects the GM technology is different. First, the genetic change is specific, planned and deliberately sought – and the desired result may be obtained more rapidly. Otherwise it makes no difference whether a gene has been introduced via classical cross-breeding or through *Agrobacterium*-mediated DNA transfer. Second, the introduced genes can come from any species of plant, animal or microbe – i.e., the procedure can be *transgenic*. It is this aspect that has been a particular source of public concern and scientific uncertainty: in transcending the barriers between distant species, might some surprising changes be induced in the functioning of the altered host genome? One possibility is that potential toxins or allergens could be produced via the transgenic gene itself. Or such compounds might arise inadvertently via other changes in plant chemistry caused by the action of inserted gene switches and gene promoters, or from the accidentally altered functioning of host organism genes. Third, the technology requires the use of marker genes to confirm the successful insertion of the index gene. Those marker genes may confer properties such as antibiotic resistance which could inadvertently be taken up by the genome of gut bacteria – for example, in livestock being fed GM plants. Although scientists consider such gene flow unlikely, it poses a theoretical risk to humans who might subsequently ingest those antibiotic-resistant bacteria.

In principle, we should hope that the genetic engineering of food species will increase world food production. Further, it should do so in ways that lessen pressures on the environment by, for example, reducing the amount of insecticide required. Indeed, one attractive aspect of genetic modification is that we may be able to 'fit' the plant or animal to the available piece of environment, rather than having to modify the environment (by irrigation, fertilisation or pesticide use) to suit the plant or animal. The nutritional quality of foods could also be improved. For example, rice can be engineered to produce vitamin A by inserting the daffodil gene that makes yellow carotenoids (the precursors to vitamin A), thereby helping counter a great nutritional problem that afflicts around 400 million people. Nevertheless, we should be aware that the vitamin A deficiency problem is largely a human-made problem in the first place. The diminished diversity of plant foods in our agrarian ecology, versus forager ecology, and the increasing simplification of agrarian diets as various green leafy vegetables have been reclassified as 'weeds' that impede the production of monoculture staples have resulted in various micronutrient deficiencies. Further, as discussed in chapter 5, the higher-yielding Green Revolution cereal grains are now recognised to have been proportionally deficient in several essential trace elements and vitamins.

A more sobering consideration is that, whereas the expression of herbicide resistance, insecticidal activity or salt tolerance may be under the control of single genes, the photosynthetic capacity of the plant is influenced by many genes. It is a polygenic trait, and may not – at least soon – be amenable to genetic modification. Commenting on the prospect of modifying photosynthesis, the Australian plant scientist Lloyd Evans concludes: 'Having been subject to intense natural selection for 3.8 billion years or so, yet having maintained an extremely slow rate of evolution . . . the improvement of its efficiency by genetic engineering constitutes a supreme challenge, and a little molecular modesty may be in order.'[44]

The greater worry over GM foods, at least theoretically, is in the ecological realm. Here uncertainties persist. What are we to make of early studies showing that pollen from GM plants expressing the *Bt* insecticide gene is toxic to Monarch butterflies, or that ladybirds feeding on aphids on insect-resistant maize are less able to reproduce? Might the newly inserted genes in crop species accidently become feral and spread into wider nature? Could 'super-weeds', resistant to herbicides, result? Whereas society can dismantle unwanted industrial machinery, mobilised genes cannot be recalled. It is the very nature of genes as compulsive self-replicators to seek wider circulation within the living world.[45] There have been many examples in recent years of how human disturbances of natural ecosystems have had unexpected adverse impacts, including facilitating infectious diseases. Similar chains of ecological detriment could follow the inadvertent spread of transgenic organisms or hybrids into natural ecosystems.

Finally, if there is now to be a gene-based 'green evolution' can we carry it out in a socially enlightened and ethical fashion? Market incentives encourage the types of genetic modifications that appeal to the economic interests of farmers and the preferences of affluent consumers in high-income countries. Hence there is commercial profit in producing pesticide-resistant maize or long-life tomatoes for Western markets. In contrast, the production of vitamin A-enriched rice to be grown in the backblocks of Asia will require the support of international agencies and charitable foundations. We must seek a way of handling this type of molecular biotechnology so as to balance the legitimate interests of venture capital with the needs and rights of underfed populations everywhere, and with the achievement of ecological sustainability. Activist organisations pressing for land reform in the Philippines have pointed out that even a ten-fold increase in yield in transgenic cereal grains would have little social benefit. Tenant farmers would still have to hand over virtually all of the product to the landowner.

Conclusion

The industrialisation of erstwhile agricultural-mercantilist human societies during the nineteenth and twentieth centuries has transformed many aspects of the human habitat. It has also contributed centrally to the great gains in material security and longevity, most evident in the industrial countries. Cities have grown rapidly, factories have proliferated, electrification and communications systems have arisen, and motorised transport systems have come to dominate urban landscapes and to spread their asphalt tentacles throughout the land. As populations have increased, as wealth has accrued, and as consumerism has emerged as a late twentieth-century way-of-life, so our aggregate environmental impact has increased. The various forms of environmental pollution, degradation and impoverishment pose a spectrum of risks – toxicological, microbiological and ecological – to human population health. Characteristically, these risks bear on whole communities, sometimes whole populations. Some of them, such as intensive food production methods and the dissemination of persistent, bioaccumulating organic pollutants, act by weakening ecosystems and diminishing the environment's carrying capacity.

As we shall see in chapter 10, the problem of humankind's increasingly large foot-prints has led us into frank ecological deficit budgeting, and on a global scale. Meeting the needs of the current total world population, with its high levels of consumption and waste generation, now depends substantially on depleting global stocks of resources and on overloading environmental 'sinks'.[46] Industrialisation has thus greatly increased the intensity and scale of our environmental impact, and radically altered many aspects of human ecology. These larger-scale risks to health will be explored in the final chapters. First, though, let us consider the changing demography of humankind, the ways in which modern consumerism heightens various disease risks, and the consequences for human wellbeing and health of urbanisation and its restructured social relations.

7

Longer lives and lower birth rates

Humankind has just lived through a demographically phenomenal century. During the twentieth century the following four things happened: human numbers increased almost fourfold, the proportion of people living in cities increased fivefold from approximately 10% to 50%, world average life expectancy doubled and, during the second half of the century, birth rates approximately halved. We are now heading towards a world of large, urban and long-lived – indeed, elderly and therefore dementia-prone – populations. The consequences of these various demographic changes for patterns of health and disease have already been great. In future they will be equally great.

In 1999 total human numbers passed 6 billion. Another 750 million will be added during the first decade of the twenty-first century. The global total is likely to reach 8–9 billion by 2050. Beyond that the projections are, of course, less certain. Although most demographers forecast a plateauing at around 9–10 billion later in the twenty-first century, we could yet be surprised by a much higher or lower figure. If it is the latter, one hopes that it will be because of reduced fertility, not increased mortality. Recent experiences in the wake of the socioeconomic collapse in post-communist Russia and the now catastrophic HIV/AIDS epidemic in Africa remind us that increased death rates remain possible.

Our passage through these demographic and social transformations over the past 150 years has entailed changes in contraception, human sexuality and family structures. It has brought social and economic emancipation of women in modernising societies. Recently we have learnt much about the biology of human reproduction, and we have developed many radically new techniques of intervention in those processes. We are less certain about their various social consequences, and how best to manage them. Those consequences include the new sexual freedoms, changes in family dynamics and the rapid 'ageing' of populations – soon to be illustrated *in extremis* by the extraordinary age profile of China's population following a quarter-century of the 'one-child family policy'.[1]

In Western countries, contraception based on 'barrier' devices began to be popularised in the later nineteenth century. Hormonal (oral) contraception became available in the early 1960s, as also did intra-uterine contraceptive devices and sterilising operations on both men and women. Technical control over human fertility thus took a giant step forwards. Contraception was becoming simpler, more democratic (available to all, and more acceptable because it was not linked directly to the coital act) and socially legitimate. In developing countries, the next task was to create the three preconditions for fertility restraint: cultural acceptance; motivation through anticipated benefits to the household; and access to contraception. As India painfully discovered in the 1960s, providing the third component (operative sterilisation) without creating the first two preconditions can be a social and political disaster.

Meanwhile, the problem of unachievable pregnancy also began to recede. Beginning with the 'test-tube embryos' of *in vitro* fertilisation (IVF) in the 1970s, techniques for assisting fertility have proliferated. Surrogate motherhood has now become possible. So too has deferred motherhood, by freezing eggs that are surgically removed in younger adulthood, thus also avoiding the risk of the chromosomally defective eggs characteristic of middle-aged maternity.

As sexual behaviours changed, especially in response to new contraceptive freedoms, so, inevitably, did the incidence of sexually transmitted infections. The ancient scourges of syphilis and gonorrhea increased again in many Western populations during the 1970s and 1980s. These were accompanied by the more insidious bacterial infection, chlamydia, and the often persistent genital herpes virus. Cancer of the cervix, one of the world's leading causes of cancer death in women, was also found to be predominantly an infectious disease, caused by the sexually-transmitted human papilloma virus. Then in the 1980s came a shock. HIV/AIDS appeared unexpectedly and began to spread in epidemic fashion, facilitated by changes in patterns of sexual behaviour and human mobility. The ever-inventive microbial world had played a trump card: here was a virus that actually infected and destroyed the body's first-line defence, the immune system's white blood cells.

The contraceptive, reproductive and other recent changes in human ecology have altered the hormonal and reproductive rhythms of adult womanhood. Women nearly everywhere are deferring their first pregnancy. Western women, especially those with higher education and professional employment, now typically defer having a baby until their late 20s. Since menstruation now begins at around 12 years of age in well-nourished under-exercised girls, their bodies are exposed to an historically aberrant 15 years or more of cyclical hormonal stimulation before the breast tissue-stabilising process of pregnancy occurs. In those same populations, hormone (oestrogen) replacement therapy (HRT) has become commonplace in post-menopausal women. As prolonged survival beyond the age of natural menopause becomes usual, women now have post-reproductive lives that are as long as their reproductive lives. This has no counterpart in other mammalian species. Not surprisingly, these various changes in the reproductive and hormonal life-course of women influence the risks of various diseases – including cardiovascular disease, gallstone disease, several types of cancer and osteoporosis.

Scientists, meanwhile, continue to push back other frontiers. In the late 1990s the cloning of animals such as sheep and pigs was achieved. This cloning of whole organisms is a novel type of reproduction, achieved by direct 'carbon-copy' replication based on the diploid genes of a somatic (body) cell, rather than by nature's luck-of-the-draw recombination of two sets of haploid genes from sperm and egg. Cloning will become a major social and ethical issue early in the twenty-first century as its application extends from livestock and domestic pets towards humans. For clinical medicine the great promise is of 'therapeutic cloning', creating from the somatic cells of ailing individuals genetically identical organs as spare parts.

Genetic screening of the unborn baby – indeed, of the preimplantation embryo during IVF – has also advanced. Next comes the possibility of somatic gene therapy of the fetus or new-born, entailing genetic repairs on targeted body cells. What, then, of the fine line between repairs and 'improvements'? Via the genetic engineering of germline cells, the possibility looms that babies could be made to order: hair colour, height, blood group and, perhaps, intellectual talents. The spectre of neo-eugenics thus arises, this time using direct molecular intervention as opposed to the cruder device of controlled breeding.

The extent and rapidity of these various changes in human birth and death rates, population age-structures, social relations, sexual behaviour and reproductive technology have no precedent. We are living through a remarkable set of demographic, social and health transitions. To get this in perspective, let us look first at how human population size has grown over time.

Human numbers: three great surges in 80,000 years

Over the past 80,000 years humankind has undergone three great increases in population size. We are living through the third, and most spectacular, of these.

A combination of ecological reasoning and anthropological observation indicates that the savannahs of eastern and southern Africa would have supported approximately 50,000 early humans. From around 80,000 years ago, as *Homo sapiens* began dispersing around the world, human numbers began a gradual 100-fold increase, reaching an estimated 5 million by the advent of agriculture. Since that time, a brief 10,000 years ago, human numbers increased another 100-fold, to approximately 500 million by the beginning of the industrial revolution. Those were the first two large-scale surges in human numbers. To call them 'surges' is to use some poetic licence. Those first two increases occupied long time-spans. As the American demographer Joel Cohen states: 'Before the several local inventions of agriculture, local human populations grew at long-term rates just above zero. Where agriculture was invented, local human populations grew ever so slightly faster.'[2] The annual percentage growth rate in world population of the past half-century, of 1.5–2%, has been markedly faster than in those two earlier periods.

Throughout those 80 millennia the size of local populations generally remained within the limits set by the local environment's carrying capacity (as modified by human technology and culture). Local population size often fluctuated, in response to catastrophic ravages by the Four Horsemen. An extreme example is that of Egypt, where population has fluctuated hectically between around 5 million and 30 million over the past 3,000 years. Elsewhere in greater Eurasia, in Western Europe, China and Japan, occasional disasters such as the bubonic plague or extreme famines culled up to half the local population, but the deficit was typically replaced within several decades. Population fluctuations in European and Chinese history relate most strongly to variations in political stability and to climatic change.[3]

Since the eighteenth century, total human numbers have increased another tenfold, to 6 billion. Overall, then, the modern human species has now increased 100,000-fold (i.e., $100 \times 100 \times 10$) since the initial dispersal out of Africa. This third, ongoing, surge has occurred much faster than ever before. It may yet end up by having added an extra 8–10 billion to the pre-industrial half billion. That figure implies that we will have augmented the Earth's (human) carrying capacity by an extraordinary 10-fold to 15-fold over the past two centuries. Can Earth sustain those numbers in the long term? We will return to this topic in chapters 10–12.

Fertility rates are now falling in most parts of the world, albeit at greatly differing rates. The annual population growth rate, which peaked at around 2% per year in the 1980s, declined to 1.3% by the year 2000. The average fertility rate in the world declined from around a total of 5 births per woman in 1950 to 2.6 in 2000. In most of Europe the figure has now declined to below replacement level (approximately 2.1 births per couple). Catholicism notwithstanding, Italy has the lowest fertility rate within Western Europe, at 1.2 births per woman. Japan, too, has moved below the replacement level. At the other extreme, countries such as Yemen, Uganda, Niger, Ethiopia and Afghanistan still have fertility rates of 6–7. The demographic giants, India and China, entered the twenty-first century with total fertility rates of around 3.0 and 1.8, respectively.

Why have these radical trends in population growth, fertility and life expectancy occurred over the past two centuries? The answer lies in understanding the recent great transitions in human ecology.

HUMAN POPULATIONS have undergone several major, inter-related big transformations in their death rates, birth rates and disease profiles over recent centuries. Today's Western countries began the process earlier and are much further down this path than are most of the developing countries. The two best-recognised changes are the demographic transition and the consequent epidemiological transition.[4] Underlying these two transitions has been a protracted transformation in health risks, a 'risk transition', as urban environments, workplaces and ways-of-living have changed.

These several interrelated changes in human living conditions, survival and health status have occurred much more rapidly than did the other two great prehistorical transitions in human ecology: first when early humans became tool-users and meat-eaters, and later when neolithic humans began farming and herding. The complex interplay between gains in material wealth, in social modernisation and in levels of health is a matter of continuing debate between historians, economists, other social scientists and epidemiologists.[5]

On a larger scale, the combination of expanding populations and increased economic activity in the world at large, over the past half-century, has caused the relatively rapid emergence of various types of global environmental disruption. In later chapters I will argue that this turn of events, and the hazards posed to human health, must direct us towards a third, great, transition: the Sustainability Transition.[6]

The demographic transition

Pre-modern human societies have high rates of birth and death. Modern societies have low rates of both. In between lies the process of demographic transition. Typically this entails initially a reduction in the population's death rate[7] – particularly deaths in infancy and childhood – followed later by a reduction in the birth rate. In the intervening period (with a low death rate but a still high birth rate) population size expands. So, initially, does the base of the 'population pyramid' (the population's age structure) as an increasing proportion of children survive the early years (Figure 7.1).

This transition occurs in response to variable combinations of increased food security, sanitary improvement, literacy, social modernisation and other gains in the material and social conditions of living.[8] The conditions of life in Europe began to change radically during the late eighteenth and nineteenth centuries as the industrial revolution got underway, supplemented by the bounty of empire. Death rates began to fall from the 1750s as more new-borns survived childhood. The subsequent decline in fertility that appeared first in France late in the eighteenth century (largely achieved by the use of coitus interruptus) spread through most of Europe in the nineteenth century. A new equilibrium between fertility and mortality was thus established in Western society as high rates of births and deaths were replaced by low rates of both. The lag between the fall in deaths and the fall in births occurs, according to many demographers, because fertility patterns are deeply embedded in the system of cultural norms and therefore change more slowly than mortality-reducing behaviours.

The demographic transition is not a law of nature. Its form and timescale are situation-dependent. In some countries, such as the Netherlands, birth rates remained high long after death rates fell. Indeed, industrialising Europe was able to alleviate the pressures of its expanding populations via large emigrations to America and, less so, to Australia and New Zealand. In China, a gradual slow decline in death rates began as early as the seventeenth century. This has been variously attributed to the introduction of higher-yielding crops from the Americas via Europe, improved agricultural practices, variolation (immunisation) against smallpox, and the introduction of basic family and community hygiene.[9] Elsewhere in the world the demographic transition has generally begun more recently and has followed varied paths, typically proceeding faster in the developing world than it did in Western countries.

In many of those developing countries, however, the transition is not yet complete; hence their populations are expanding. In some countries, particularly in sub-Saharan Africa, the process has stalled, leaving birth rates well above the now-lowered death rates. Here, again, the situation dependence is apparent. On the one hand, over the past half century those poorer countries were able to reduce their infant and child mortality with simple public health

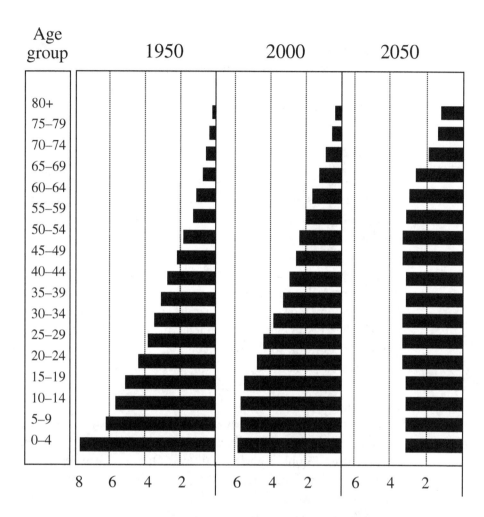

Percentage of total population

Figure 7.1 Transformation of the age distribution of the male population in Southeast Asia region, 1950, 2000 and (projected) 2050. So long as the proportion of individuals aged below 20 is high (as is still the case in 2000), the population will keep on growing as these younger age-ranks reach adulthood and reproduce themselves. The picture is similar for females. After 2050 – if populations become wealthier and healthier – the height of these increasingly narrow-based age 'pyramids' will increase as more individuals survive beyond 85 years. The pyramid will thus tend to become column-shaped and a little taller.

and medical interventions. But, on the other hand, fertility decline in many such countries has been impeded by economic isolation, social conservatism and the retreat of international support as the developed world moved from the normative Development Project of the 1960s and 1970s towards today's global market free-for-all.[10]

The epidemiological transition

As infectious diseases recede and life expectancy lengthens, the demographic transition ushers in the epidemiological transition. Initially, this entails an age-related shift in the profile of diseases. The noncommunicable diseases of later adulthood such as coronary heart disease, stroke, diabetes, arthritis, cancer and dementia thus become more common in longer-living populations. Because gains in life expectancy occurred first in the richer stratum of Western society, coronary heart disease and other noncommunicable diseases emerged early on in that stratum. However, as behaviours such as cigarette smoking and eating high-fat diets became mass phenomena, and eventually more prevalent among the poorer stratum, so the socioeconomic distribution of most of these diseases reversed. The adverse health impacts of socioeconomic disadvantage and associated chronic life stress would have further amplified this inverse gradient between individual wealth and health.[11]

Again, the paths followed by early-developing Western countries and later-developing other countries have generally differed. Many poorer countries have incurred a 'double burden of disease'. One burden arises from the fact that the fruits of economic advance and the modernisation of public health and medical care have bypassed a billion poor people who continue to suffer heavily from infectious diseases.[12] The toll of infectious disease and malnutrition falls particularly upon women and children. Meanwhile, the other burden in these poorer countries is the rise in noncommunicable disease as a consequence of population ageing, urbanisation and altered consumer behaviours. Cardiovascular disease, cancers, diabetes, mental health problems and injuries (especially on the roads) are becoming the leading causes of disability and premature death in most regions of the world.

This retreat of infectious diseases and the rise of adult noncommunicable diseases reflects a succession of changes in the backdrop of risks to health. This process, sometimes referred to as 'the risk transition', has had many facets. As early industrial wealth accrued, as societies became more liberal, as mass production techniques evolved, and as urban wage-earners became consumers, so the conditions, behaviours and exposures of daily life changed. Physical activity at work declined, diets changed, cigarette smoking was promoted and family size decreased. Then, after World War II, physical activity decreased as labour-saving devices proliferated. Hormonal contraception appeared, and patterns of sexuality became freer. The industrial workplace became gradually cleaner and safer. Wealthy Western societies became better able, and more motivated, to control various types of local environmental (especially air) pollution.

The upheavals of the Vietnam War and the struggles for land and livelihood in parts of the rural Third World contributed to the rise of international trafficking in hard drugs. This was reinforced by the growing numbers of alienated and often economically marginalised young adults in harsh inner-urban environments everywhere. The prime profitable markets for the international drug cartels have been in the rich countries. More generally, as social relations in large cities became more fluid, as the sense of community weakened, and as family life became more fragmented, so the risks of isolation and of persistent life stress increased for many people in the later decades of the twentieth century. An interesting twist in all of this is that the reemergence of various infectious diseases in recent decades represents a partial reversal of the epidemiological transition – even as the ageing of populations takes us into a further variant of the epidemiological transition: the age of delayed degenerative diseases.[13]

The remainder of this chapter considers population trends in relation to environmental carrying capacity, looking particularly at trends[14] in life expectancy and in fertility rates, and the evolutionary basis for reproductive and parenting behaviours.

Life expectancy: historical trends

Average life expectancy has doubled since 1900. This figure refers not to the average age of adult death, but to the average expectancy of life *at birth*. Populations with high infant and child mortality have low life expectancy. If three of ten babies survive to age 60 years, and the other seven all die before age 5 years, then the life expectancy at birth for that 'population' will be around 20 years. Thus, the biblical 'three score years and ten' referred to a reasonable upper limit in ancient Israelite populations, not to the average life expectancy. Before and long after Christ's time, life expectancy would have been closer to one score years and ten – 30 years. Today, for the world at large, the figure is well over 60 years – and in some wealthy countries life expectancy now approximates 80 years. These figures were unimaginable before the twentieth century.

Human skeletal remains from prehistoric hunter-gatherer communities indicate that about one quarter of babies died soon after birth.[15] In the poorest agrarian communities, with superimposed risks of 'crowd infections', similar figures have persisted until recent times. Today, infant death rates are much lower, especially in rich countries where the figure is less than 1%. Nevertheless, in the natural world such losses among new-born are widespread. Approximately two-thirds of the offspring of birds, reptiles and small mammals perish in early life.

Among those young humans who survive the hazards of early life there is the possibility of living for another seven, eight, even nine decades. This raises an intriguing question about the potential human life-span. The American demographer Jay Olshansky has estimated that, if cardiovascular diseases, diabetes and cancer could be eliminated, life expectancy in the United States would increase to around 90 years.[16] Will the average life-span in developed countries extend to and beyond 100 years before the end of the twenty-first century? To answer that question we will need to understand better the biological process of ageing – something that is explored further later in the chapter.

A half-century ago the British evolutionary biologist Peter Medawar proposed that the rate of ageing of any particular species is proportional to the force of external mortality.[17] That is, the greater the daily risk of death by physical mishap or predation, the greater the investment of biological resources into producing offspring – and the less the investment in maintaining body tissues for long life. For those animal species that acquired large size, that could evade most predation by taking to the air (birds and flying or gliding mammals), or that evolved physical defences (such as shells or sharp spines), life was less urgent. Natural selection could reasonably invest them with bodily maintenance and repair capacities in the expectation that they would survive long enough to reproduce again in future.[18] Hence birds live longer than mammals of the same body size; bats live longer than other mammals of similar size; and porcupines live longer than their non-spiny rodent cousins. Indeed, humans, long the beneficiaries of culturally reinforced survival strategies, now live several decades longer than do similarly sized chimpanzees and gorillas.

THE LIFE EXPECTANCY of hunter-gatherer humans, and, indeed, through much of agrarian and early urban history, has long corresponded to that in

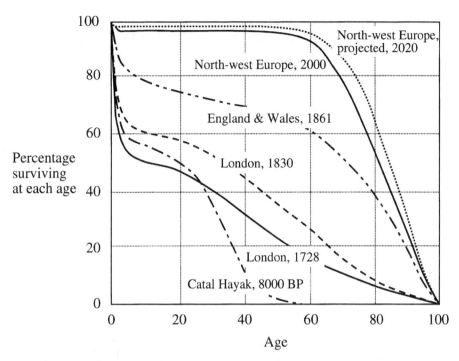

Figure 7.2 Survival curves in human populations over the past 8,000 years. The mortality data for Catal Hayak in southern Turkey are derived from burials around 8000 years ago. Note also the much poorer survival in urban London in 1830 than in England and Wales as a whole in 1861.

other mammals. That is, few individuals survived beyond the end of their reproductive period (Figure 7.2). The somewhat sparse fossil evidence from the late palaeolithic period – probably biased (who qualified for burial?) – indicates that prehistoric hunter-gatherers had a life expectancy of around 20–25 years. Less than one in ten appear to have lived beyond age 40 years.

Fossilised skulls from Greece, from around 6,500 year ago, indicate a small rise in average survival. That era coincides approximately with the establishment of agrarian living in southeast Europe. During the subsequent 3,000 years adult height increased, arthritic damage to bones decreased, teeth were healthier and average life exectancy at birth rose to around 25–30 years. In the Golden Age of Pericles, in the fifth century BC, life expectancy was around 30 years. Subsequent piecemeal evidence from Rome, comprising taxation records (socially selective), military conscription (males only) and tombstones (mostly well-to-do men), indicates a similar life expectancy.

In late medieval England the life expectancy of the general populace was approximately 30 years. Over the next five centuries life expectancies in Europe fluctuated between 25 and 35 years, depending on socioeconomic conditions, military circumstances and the ravages of epidemics such as the Black Death. Life expectancy declined a little during the bitterly cold and politically turbulent seventeenth century (as was shown in Figure 1.2). Interestingly, during these centuries the differences in life expectancy between Europe's rich and poor were small. Studies of life expectancy in European ruling families and in the Geneva aristocracy in the sixteenth and seventeenth centuries reveal figures around 30–35 years.[19] Even well-fed Jesuit monks in sixteenth-century Italy, whose initial selection depended on their being in good health, had a modest life expectancy of around 30 years. It seems that infectious disease mortality within the increasingly crowded urban environment of post-Renaissance Europe must have pressed equally on all classes of persons, irrespective of how full their bellies were at night.

Not until the second half of the eighteenth century did a clear survival advantage for the nobility begin to emerge. In the last decades of France's pre-revolution *ancien régime*, aristocratic life expectancy approached 47 years – ten years better than the general average. The widening rich–poor gap and the worsening food shortages of the 1780s hastened the advent of The Terror and the trimming back of the aristocracy's life expectancy. In Britain, the infant mortality rates began to diverge between nobility and commoners around 1750, in part because of the advent of inoculation against the great killing infection of the time, smallpox. As in France, life expectancy in these two strata of society had diverged by approximately ten years by later in the eighteenth century.[20] In nineteenth-century Britain, the life expectancies of rich and poor began to diverge more obviously as material conditions improved from the 1840s, particularly for the upper and emerging middle classes.[20] The differences in nutrition and child health between England's rich and poor at that time resulted in a difference of approximately 5 inches in height at age 14 between upper-class cadets at Sandhurst and working-class boys. Indeed, the *Dictionary of Statistics* of 1884 recorded that: 'Fellows of the Royal Society on average are 3.9 inches taller and 21 lb heavier than burglars and other convicts.'

During the eighteenth and nineteenth centuries, life expectancy in French and British colonies in North America and Australasia differed little from the parent populations in Europe. This, despite their generally better food supplies and less crowded living conditions. Again, one suspects the levelling power of infectious disease in a world in which infectious agents were now well distributed, courtesy of European colonialism. Gains in life expectancy began to accelerate from mid-nineteenth century in European populations at home and abroad. Average adult heights in British males increased across successive generations during this period, presumably due to reductions in malnutrition and childhood infectious disease. By the 1870s, cholera, smallpox, typhus and tuberculosis had all begun to recede. This was a transformation in the conditions of human life and health. Here were the foundations for attaining, by the end of the twentieth century in Western countries, a life expectancy of almost 80 years.

Modern gains in life expectancy

What accounts for the modern gains in life expectancy in developed countries? This question continues to provoke professional and ideological passion. The three main contending schools emphasise, respectively, society's material advances, specific public health interventions, and the importance of social modernisation via, in particular, gains in literacy, democracy and the strength of civil institutions.

A central figure in this debate has been the social-medical historian Thomas McKeown, writing mainly during the 1960s–70s. Focusing on Britain, McKeown argued that improved nutrition accounted for most of the reduction in infectious disease deaths in the second half of the nineteenth century and early twentieth century.[21] His analyses for the period 1840–1950 show that by the time specific medical interventions such as vaccination and antibiotics were introduced in the twentieth century, mortality from various infectious diseases had already declined by 80–90% from their high rates in mid-nineteenth century. Mortality from tuberculosis, a disease closely associated with poverty, crowding and malnutrition, declined from around 4,000 deaths per million per year in England and Wales in 1850 to around 400 per million by the time antibiotics were introduced in the 1940s. The annual death rate from measles in children dropped from 1,200 per million in the late nineteenth century to about one-tenth of that figure by the mid-1930s, when treatment of life-threatening secondary bacterial infections became possible. Similar trajectories apply to mortality from tetanus and from childhood whooping cough. In contrast, the retreats of smallpox and diphtheria were substantially boosted by the introduction of smallpox vaccination in the 1800s and diphtheria antitoxin in 1895 and immunisation in 1942.

McKeown's is essentially a materialist argument, and thus represents the first of the three contending viewpoints mentioned above. Gains in food production and overall wealth from mid-nineteenth century onwards improved the average levels of nutrition, he argued, and this increased resistance to infectious disease. Since the main declines were in diseases spread by inhalation such as tuberculosis, measles and diphtheria, McKeown reasoned that cleaner water was not the main benefactor. He concluded therefore that improved nutrition must have been important, shoring up bodily defences against all infections. More generally, this thesis has drawn attention to the profound influence of social and economic conditions as prime determinants of the health of populations. It has stimulated a generation of researchers over the past quarter-century.

Researchers espousing the second viewpoint have criticised McKeown's thesis for undervaluing the historical role of deliberate public health interventions – and because of the lack of direct evidence of benefit due to gains in nutrition.[22] Such interventions included the safer drinking water and more hygienic streets that Edwin Chadwick's sanitary engineering achieved in Britain, the improved housing design and ventilation, better midwifery practice, and the increasing use of smallpox vaccination. In France, for example, substantial gains in life expectancy emerged first in Lyon (beginning in 1850s), then Paris (1860s–70s, albeit more protractedly) and then Marseille (around 1890). This occurred in direct association with improved public water supply and sanitation in each of those cities.[23] Similarly, in both England and Sweden, the mortality decline accelerated markedly after 1870, the period when there were widespread municipal advances in water treatment, sanitation and waste removal. However, the fact that non-industrialised Sweden's mortality decline matched that of much wealthier England also testified to the importance of improved literacy, the enhancement of civil institutions and greater social cohesion. That is, it gave support to the third viewpoint, emphasising the central role of social modernisation.

Consonant with that third viewpoint, some of the recent strong gains in life expectancy, including reductions in infectious disease mortality, have been made by countries that have focused on building up stocks of social and human resources, via education, social security provisions and primary health care. This includes Costa Rica, Cuba, China and Sri Lanka. Costa Rica, for example, has a GDP per capita that is one-tenth that of Britain, but has a near-identical life expectancy. Within India, regional declines in mortality have been correlated much more with social modernisation, such as high school attendance rates by girls in rural areas, than with rising incomes. For example, the state of Kerala with high schooling levels and lower incomes has a higher life expectancy than has the Punjab with its higher incomes but lower female educational levels. Such data indicate that the enhancement of social relations, civil institutions and investment in human resources create the conditions for improved population health. Indeed, in recent decades this appears to have been more important in the less developed countries than it was historically in the West.[24] An analysis of gains in life expectancy between 1960 and 1990 in 115 low-income and middle-income countries has attributed 20% of the gain to increased real incomes, 30% to schooling for girls, and the remaining 50% to the generation and use of a range of new knowledge.[25] That is, most of the health gains that flow from economic development reflect increases in stocks of social and human 'capital': roads and schools are built, teachers are trained, electronic communications are improved, and children, especially girls, are educated. Indeed, the education and social autonomy of females is probably the main key to mortality declines, especially in poor societies. When young unmarried girls can assume roles outside the house and when older women can appear freely in public, then girls are more likely to remain at school and mothers are more likely to seek medical care for themselves and their families.[26] We will return in chapter 9 to further consideration of the importance to population health of how a nation spends its wealth.

McKeown's analysis of death rates extended from the 1840s to the 1950s. In fact, life expectancy in England had already increased from around 35 years in the 1740s to 40 years by the late 1840s (see, again, Figure 1.2). The scourge of smallpox had begun a long retreat with the introduction of rudimentary inoculation in the 1740s, followed in the early 1800s by Edward Jenner's cowpox-based vaccination. Typhus, too, had begun receding in the early 1800s. More effective social policies to avert famine followed the food price crisis in Europe in the late eighteenth century.[27] So far, then, social and economic historians have not offered a clear explanation for the gains in life expectancy in England in the 100 years before the 1840s.[28]

In the second half of the twentieth century, clinical-medical interventions began to contribute significantly to gains in longevity in Western societies. Death rates from at least those conditions considered 'amenable' to medical treatment (including tuberculosis, cervical cancer, Hodgkin's disease, stroke, gallstone disease and maternal mortality) fell markedly, compared to a much more static picture for other causes of death. An estimated two-thirds of the seven-year gain in adult life expectancy in the United States since 1950 is attributable to improved medical treatment and care.[29] Even so, we should not apply an overly technical interpretation to these statistics. After all, the recently completed international MONICA study of cardiovascular disease trends and their causes found that seemingly beneficial 'treatment effects' were rather non-specific in their actual biomedical impacts. The research team therefore concluded that much of the significance of improved medical care is that it is *also* an index of a society in which other preventive measures are likely to be undertaken.[30]

Returning to McKeown's 1840–1950 time window, and looking through it from another angle, we can glimpse the underlying dynamics of change in British mortality. Life expectancies and annual death rates are routinely calculated cross-sectionally, by collating the simultaneous experience of the different age-groups within the population. However, by rearranging the data to allow analysis of the longitudinal mortality experience of successive generations, an interesting pattern emerges.[31] Childhood (excluding infant) death rates fell from the 1860s onwards; death rates at ages 45–54 years declined from around 1900, and those at ages 75–84 years declined from around 1930. The important point is that each of these onsets of mortality decline come from the same generation, born around 1850, as it moves through the age ranks and pushes down the death rate at each newly attained age. Apparently some biological advantage acquired by that generation in childhood resonated throughout that generation's lifetime. Intriguingly, infant death rates (i.e., deaths in the first year of life) did not begin to decline until the last two decades of the nineteenth century – that is, about 25 years after the above-mentioned initial downturn in childhood death rates. From what we have learnt recently about the importance of a woman's lifelong health and nutrition as a determinant of the lifelong health of her own children, it looks as if the decline in infant mortality in Britain had to await the arrival of a new, healthy, generation of young mothers, born in the 1850s and having babies in the 1880s and 1890s.

MEANWHILE, WHAT has been the trend in non-fatal disease? The picture here is more mixed and less easy to interpret.[32] During the last third of the twentieth century, while life expectancy in Western populations increased by around seven years the estimated *healthy* life expectancy (i.e., years lived free of disability and chronic illness) has also gained ground. The picture that emerges is generally a positive one. Note, however, the potentially misleading arithmetic: to move from a life expectancy of 75 that includes five unhealthy years of life to one of 80 with seven unhealthy years is to make gains in both life expectancy and healthy life expectancy – even though the duration of unhealthy life becomes two years longer.

Greater life expectancy gains are now being made at older than at younger ages, as the probability of reaching age 80 years increases and as the population of centenarians increases. The earlier assumption, prevalent in the 1980s, was that the human life-span was relatively fixed and that health gains would be made by compressing ('rectangularising') morbidity – that is, by deferring its age of onset – within that otherwise fixed frame.[33] However, a more open-ended vista seems now to be emerging, as both the age of death and the age of onset of disabling chronic disease are being deferred in modern populations. Meanwhile, figures published by the World Health Organization in 2000 indicate, again, the important influence of social and economic context upon patterns of disease and disability. The countries with the longest *healthy* life expectancy were Japan, Australia, France and Sweden (all in the range 73–75 years of healthy life). The United States, despite its wealth and high-tech medical care, was ranked 24th. This was attributed to the heightened impact of diseases of poverty (including among native Americans, rural African Americans and the inner-city poor), to the marked inequality in access to medical care, to the relatively high impact of HIV/AIDS, tobacco and coronary heart disease, and to the consequences of violence and drug abuse.

It is difficult to forecast to what extent chronic disease and disability will contract in future. Cardiovascular disease, which caused around two-fifths of deaths in Western countries several decades ago, is now on a well-established down-trend in those countries. Meanwhile, it is rising in urban populations in developing countries, and it surged upwards during the 1990s in most of the former communist countries – particularly in Ukraine and Russia. There are clear long-term health gains from some modern medical interventions, such as drug treatment of hypertension, insulin replacement in child-onset diabetes mellitus, a widening range of vaccinations, and hip replacement in elderly persons. Even so, the incidence rates of various low-fatality conditions have risen recently in Western populations, including childhood asthma, eating disorders (especially in young women) and mental depression. Meanwhile, in ageing populations, the number of persons with dementia is increasing.

Ageing and the human life-span

The ongoing increase in human life expectancy invites the inevitable question about the limits to longevity. Among scientists, there is a divergence of views.[34] We know that 'ageing' entails a cumulative loss of function in body cells and organs. Molecular and tissue damage accumulates over time, as stresses on the body exceed its repair capacity, and this impairs metabolic function and micro-structure.[35] Studies of DNA in body cells taken from people of varied ages reveal an accumulation of unrepaired genetic damage with increasing age. This accumulation is evident from childhood onwards (and the rise occurs more steeply in smokers than in non-smokers). Nevertheless, the noncommunicable diseases, such as coronary heart disease, chronic bronchitis and osteoarthritis, are not a necessary consequence of growing old. Various traditional hunter-gatherer communities do not develop these diseases at older ages. Therefore, the fact that these diseases occur predominantly at an older age in more developed societies reflects not ageing itself but the long 'incubation' period during which tissue damage and biological malfunction gradually accrue in response to detrimental aspects of our late-industrial way of life.

Why does ageing occur at all? Might it serve the needs of evolution? The principle of natural selection requires that the limited supply of environmental resources induces competition among those individual, genotypically variant, members of a population who are still of reproductive age. That competition would be most efficient if older players had left the field. This argument, however, imputes strategic objectives to natural selection. That is neither necessary nor reasonable. Rather, the basic evolutionary theory of ageing explains senescence as the inevitable result of the competing needs of healthy young adulthood and reproduction versus the continuation of individual survival. Nature, seeking to sustain transmission of the genetic lineage, necessarily invests in the former and neglects the latter – that is, reproductive achievement takes precedence over extension of the post-reproductive lifespan. Ageing is the price of sustaining the genetic line.[36]

There have been many theories about the biology of ageing.[37] Two major theories were propounded in the 1950s. Peter Medawar reasoned that natural selection has acted to defer the time of action of deleterious genetic mutations, preferably until after completion of reproductive life. Although our ancestors were all healthy young adults, and reproductively successful (otherwise we would not be here today), we know from the fossil record that only a few attained old age. That is, nature necessarily selects for healthy young age, and is indifferent to healthy old age. The net effect of this heaping up of late-acting deleterious genes, Medawar argued, was to ensure a healthy young reproductive life, but an increased likelihood of a disease-prone older age.

The alternative view, argued by the evolutionary biologist George Williams, is that genes can be double-edged swords: many alleles are 'pleiotropic', having both beneficial and detrimental effects.[38] Further, to have been positively selected for in the first place, the beneficial effect must have acted well before the detrimental effect. The obvious example, he noted, is that of sickle-cell anaemia which protects young children against dying from malaria, but which causes problems at later ages. A more recently identified example pertains to a genetically based defence against tuberculosis. One of the biological actions of vitamin D, circulating in the bloodstream, is suppression of part of the body's immune system – as it turns out, the part that defends against the tuberculosis bacterium. Within tuberculosis-prone populations, therefore, natural selection is thought to have favoured those individuals with defective cellular receptors for vitamin D since their immune activity is thus unimpaired. However, this genetic mutation of the vitamin D receptor molecule also renders these individuals, in later life, more susceptible to osteoporosis.

Jay Olshansky and colleagues have sought evidence of 'Medawarian' diseases in what they refer to as a late stage of the epidemiological transition: 'the age of delayed degenerative diseases'.[13] If that hypothesis is correct, they say, then strongly genetically determined diseases should tend to appear after about age 30 years – the age by which most reproduction has occurred throughout the long course of human evolution. However, so far there is little supportive evidence for this, other than perhaps for the onset of Parkinson's Disease.

There is cause for some optimism about the future of human ageing. In nature, as we saw earlier in this chapter, there is usually an urgency about the maturation of young creatures and their early reproduction. The evolutionary race goes to those who move quickly and leave the greatest number of descendants. However, for any particular vertebrate species, when the levels of danger and environmental stress are reduced, breeding can proceed at a more leisurely pace and ageing is slowed. Isolated island-dwelling possums, for example, live longer and age more slowly than do their more environmentally pressured mainland cousins. If longevity is an agreed social goal for humans, then the conclusion to be drawn from the possum experience is obvious: a reduction in biologically damaging life-stress would be beneficial.

Old age, dependency and dementia

As the demographic transition has spread around the world, the age structure of the human population has begun to change radically. Between 1950 and 2050 the proportion of persons aged less than 15 years is projected to fall from 35% to 20% while the proportion over 65 years will rise from 5% to over

15%.[39] Further, by 2050, there will be almost 370 million people aged 80 years or over – that is approximately 4% of the population, compared to 1.3% today. Societies everywhere, both developed and developing, thus face major new challenges of shrinking employment, increasing pension liabilities and extended health care in old age.

We are entering an era when that focal point of human biological evolution, the brain, moves once again to centre stage. The human brain is relatively well protected against the stresses and toxins of daily natural life. Unlike the lungs and the gastrointestinal tract it is not exposed to the external environment. Unlike the liver and kidneys it is not involved in detoxification and excretion. It is physically encased, and semi-isolated by the blood–brain barrier. Nevertheless, it seems that in all cultures 'senile dementia' (that is, dementia not attributable to toxicity or manifest vascular disease) rises markedly with increasing age over 60 years. The currently incurable Alzheimer's disease is the most common form. Prevention is as difficult as treatment, since we know very little about the determinants of Alzheimer's disease. Several genes that predispose have been identified, especially for the earlier onset 'familial' type. But, other than the increased risk associated with high blood cholesterol level and arterial atherosclerosis, little is known about the non-genetic risk factors. There is evidence that types and levels of intelligence may play a role, as might continued active 'intellectual' use of the brain. One intriguing retrospective follow-up study of young novitiates in a contemplative order of nuns found that those whose essays (written upon entry into the convent) were richest in texture and ideas were much less likely to develop Alzheimer's disease.

Other studies indicate that dementias may result from an age-related breakdown in the metabolic handling of trace metals, particularly copper, iron, zinc and manganese.[40] These metals are integral components of the several antioxidant defences provided by zinc-dependent enzymes, beta-amyloid protein and prion protein. Human biological evolution has faced a major challenge in devising durable ways of minimising oxidative damage to the brain's finely tuned neuronal networks. Slight age-related changes in the brain's chemistry – of a kind that were never seriously tested by natural selection, with its focus on young adulthood – may well underlie the dysfunction of the cerebral housekeeping molecules in older age.

We humans have found other ways of modulating brain function. These, too, often cause residual damage or frank dementia. Other large mammals are known to chew narcotic leaves or occasionally to imbibe seasonal fermenting fruit juices. Occasional bouts of karaoke thus occur among chimpanzees and elephants. But only *Homo sapiens* has found ways of growing, fermenting, curing and refining psychoactive substances; and of inhaling, ingesting, injecting and inserting. With our large brain, we excel at breaching the very defences with which nature has protected that organ.

FOR WOMEN, longevity means prolongation of post-reproductive survival. This raises an interesting question: the mystery of the human menopause? The dispassionate logic of nature means that in most species there is little time cushion between ceasing reproducing and ceasing living. Indeed, in some species the point is made rather forcefully. The female praying mantis bites off the head of her male partner after copulation. Once mayflies take to the air they can only mate, lay eggs and die – since they have no gut. Something about larger mammals, however, especially primates, has evidently favoured the survival of adults beyond reproductive age. This is particularly so in the human female, for whom the menopause is a distinctive biological transition, not a precursor of impending death.

Menopause also occurs in apes and, perhaps, in pilot whales. However, only in humans does it loom so large, with about one third of the female life-span still to follow it. Menopause marks the transition, in women, from active breeder to mature-age adviser, knowledge repository, supplemental food gatherer and assistant child-carer. In genetic terms, there appears to be a trade-off: an older woman may enhance the propagation of her genes more by assisting the survival of grandchildren than by having more children of her own at an age when the survival prospects of both herself and the baby are diminishing. This 'grandmother hypothesis' about menopause remains controversial among evolutionary biologists.[41] Some support for it comes from recent research in West Africa, revealing that child survival is significantly higher in families in which grandmothers (especially maternal grandmothers) are present.

The human male, who does not have to sustain a pregnancy and lactation in order to reproduce, is not subject to this trade-off. His reproductive capacity persists until older age and then it tapers off.

Fertility rates

Fertility, alongside death rates and life expectancy, is the other major variable in the demographic equation. Fertility, in nature, is essentially a joint function of the health of the breeding stock and the permissiveness of the environment.

Australia's kangaroos, for example, have evolved to be able to suspend the progression of pregnancy temporarily while food is inadequate. Baboons, in times of environmental stress, undergo hormonal changes that prevent pregnancy occurring. Rodents are able to resorb their fetuses if conditions become adverse or threatening. Humans, by comparison, are more persistent, and less situation-dependent, in their reproduction. The buffering effects of social organisation and culture have apparently, through hominid evolution, relaxed some of the environmental strictures on reproduction.

In nature, plant and animal populations display a dynamic equilibrium. Numbers rise and fall in response to fluctuations in food supplies, predators and disease-causing pathogens. These fluctuations are often hectic, and population numbers can surge and crash. There are two polarities in reproductive strategy, which the biologists call the 'r', and the 'K' strategies. As we shall see later in this chapter, those names refer to two contrasting aspects of the equation that describes the 'logistic' graph of typical population growth. Opportunistic, usually small, species that can capitalise on the nutrient bonanzas that arise in disturbed ecosystems follow the 'r' strategy. These species, many of which we regard as pests, weeds and pathogens, reproduce rapidly to exploit the transient opportunity. Algae, locusts, rodents and herring gulls are examples. Larger species, with specialised biological needs and attributes, and which reproduce optimally in stable ecosystems, follow the 'K' strategy. They reproduce at a steady rate, with moderate numbers of surviving offspring. Humans and other primates are 'K' strategists. Indeed, the human species exhibits the most prolonged and intensive 'K'-type parenting because of the immaturity of the human new-born and infant.

Humans are, by nature, slow-breeding large mammals. As with other foraging primates, births in early humans were spaced between periods of pregnancy followed by prolonged breast-feeding. The natural child rearing pattern of frequent suckling has the hormonal consequence of suppressing ovulation. The evidence from surviving hunter-gatherers today indicates a usual total of around five to six live births in a full reproductive life, with approximately four years between births (nine months of pregnancy, about three years of lactation, and some time to next conception). However, once humans changed to agrarian living, weaning could occur a little sooner and extra children meant more hands in the family fields. Fertility rates for completed reproductive lifespans increased to six to eight live births on average. India, early in the twentieth century, with a life expectancy of 20–25 years, had a fertility rate of around 7. Anthropologist Beverley Strassman's detailed study of the women of the traditional agricultural Dogon tribe in Mali, West Africa, in the 1980s revealed an onset of menstruation (menarche) at age 16 years, first birth at age 19, almost two years of lactational suppression of ovulation after each pregnancy, and a fertility rate of 8.6 live births.[42]

As aspects of early modernisation emerged in Western Europe after the Renaissance, social devices to limit child-bearing evolved. During the seventeenth and eighteenth centuries the 'European pattern' of deferred marriage limited family size. Subsequently in Europe's urbanising populations, and with the social and economic dislocations of early industrialisation, family size tended to increase. However, most of that increase was offset by the greater early-life mortality from infectious diseases. In Western society, family size peaked during the nineteenth century when women would often have ten or more children. In Britain, Queen Victoria had nine children. My own maternal grandmother, born of solid Protestant stock in the 1880s in South Australia, was one of 12 children. Two of them died in childhood – one when dropped overboard by a solicitous ship's captain – and two were killed in World War I. It was the evidence of biological and social penalties imposed upon women by this excessive fertility of the late nineteenth century that ultimately activated the various campaigners (mostly women) in Western countries who, often in the face of trenchant official disapproval, advocated contraception and family planning services.

Nature's 'r strategists': the example of turtles

The prodigious egg-laying of many insects, fish, reptiles and amphibians anticipates a heavy attrition among young offspring. It is a classic 'r' strategy. The green turtles that breed widely in the Pacific region have an average life expectancy, at birth, of days rather than years. Very few of the hatchlings reach sexual maturity. Most of the rest perish within hours of hatching.

Each year, the gravid females labour up the sandy beaches of Pacific islands and coast-lines to each lay clutches of several hundred eggs at the vegetation verge. Weeks later, via the finely tuned processes of nature, the hatchlings all emerge together – often on a moon-lit night – and make a floundering dash across the sand, apparently attracted towards the flickering reflections of the water's surface. But many never make it to the water. En route they provide a culinary bonanza to the gulls. Those that reach the water soon become prey to reef-sharks and other marine predators. Within hours most of the hapless hatchlings have been eaten. They thus become part of the great recycling of nutrients along the world's coastlines, as mature breeding turtles bring in their accumulated nutrient stores from a season of foraging in deeper waters that have been enriched, via diverse routes, by nutrient run-off from the land.

Among the young turtles that reach deeper waters, the few eventual survivors then enter what scientists call the 'lost years'. Fragmentary evidence suggests that these pre-adolescent turtles drift for years around the oceans on rafts of vegetation and other debris, feeding on algae and seaweed. Ultimately, by the fifth decade of life, around 1 in every 5,000 of the original hatchlings survives to achieve sexual maturity. Then, for 20 years, the adult females lay about 500 eggs annually, yielding a lifetime total of 10,000. Of these, on average, two will survive to adulthood – one to become a sexually mature female and one a male. So the extravagant 'r strategy' arithmetic of turtle life continues in great slow cycles.

Human fertility then and now

Most animal species breed on a seasonal basis. Although humans are year-round breeders, evidence from hunter-gatherers shows that critical hormonal changes can be triggered by seasonal food supplies. The San people of the Kalahari Desert have a skewed seasonal birth rate, which peaks nine months after food abundance. There is also intriguing evidence, in agrarians, that seasonality of birth can make a difference to health and survival. A study in West Africa, based on birth records from the 1940s, identified a much lower mortality during young and middle adulthood in individuals born in the harvest season compared to those born at other times.[43] The scientists speculated that the nutritional circumstances of early infancy, maybe of fetal life, affected the maturation of the young individual's immune system and hence the level of resistance to infectious disease.

Humans are the one species that can deliberately avoid reproducing. Alongside tool-making, fertility control is a primary defining characteristic of the human species. In addition to various ritualised constraints on sexual intercourse, hunter-gatherer bands, including Inuit, Australian Aborigines and the Amazonian Yanomami, have widely practised infanticide. It is safer than abortion, and it can be applied more selectively in relation to both the viability and sex of the baby. Where infanticide is used, male:female ratios of up to 2:1 have long been common. The Greeks and Romans used various devices, concoctions and behaviours for contraception and abortion. Infanticide, by subjecting infants to environmental 'exposure', was approved of by the Greeks.

Subsequently, the early Christian Church was somewhat antinatalist and tolerant of homosexuality and infanticide. This was changed several centuries later
within the christianised Roman Empire by St Augustine, keen both to popu-
late Heaven and to enlarge the Earthly flock. Neverthless, in mediaeval times
there was widespread infanticide, especially by maternal overlying (which in
England attracted a punishment of three years penance, or two years if it was
deemed unintentional).

In pre-industrial Western Europe, late marriage and celibacy kept fertility at
economically sustainable levels. Various forms of infanticide and abandonment also occurred, especially during 1750–1850 with the crowding and privations of the early industrial revolution.[44] In China, as in Japan and India,
population growth was restrained by a mix of female infanticide and widespread bachelorhood.[45] The most spectacular current example of fertility
control is the 'one-child policy' in China, where the number of births per
woman fell from six to two in the last quarter of the twentieth century.[1] (The
equivalent fertility reduction in Europe took 150 years.) However, state coercion is clearly not a prerequisite: in impoverished Bangladesh the total fertility
rate fell from almost seven in the 1970s to three in 1998 in response to the
effective public provision of contraception. In Latin America, despite official
state disapproval of birth control, fertility rates began to fall in the 1960s and
1970s. However, there is still great diversity, with fertility ranging from below
replacement level in China and some Southeast Asian countries to 6–7 births
per woman in parts of sub-Saharan Africa and West Asia.

Contraception is now becoming a normal practice around the world. The
proportion of women now using contraception is around 30% in Africa, 50% in
South Asia, 70% in Latin America and 80% in East Asia. However, the persistence of poverty and illiteracy in much of the world means that several hundred
million couples still have no access to contraception. The resultant 40–50
million abortions each year in developing countries account for up to a quarter
of overall fertility control in those countries. Half of the abortions are done via
unsafe procedures, resulting in much maternal trauma, infection and death.

HUMANKIND'S RAPIDLY INCREASING control of fertility is radically altering the biological and social consequences of reproduction and sexuality. The
change in the maternal age and number of pregnancies has contributed to
reducing the age-old risks of maternal mortality. These changes in behaviour,
along with use of the contraceptive Pill, have hormonal and metabolic consequences for women that affect the risks of several diseases. Uncoupling sexual

intercourse from conception, and often doing so with the Pill, has resulted in an increased incidence of sexually transmitted diseases (STDs). Those diseases illustrate well the importance of ecological, population-level factors in determining whether an individual becomes infected. A woman who lives in a community with a high prevalence of STDs and extensive sexual networking is at much higher risk of contracting an STD – even if she has only one partner – than a woman living in a low-prevalence community who has multiple partners.

Fertility reduction, by changing family size, influences other aspects of health. As we saw in chapter 4, the reduced incidence of early-life infections in families with fewer children and living in more hygienic households apparently influences the development of the immune system. This, in turn, may increase susceptibility to allergic disorders. As family structure changes, the changes in within-family interactions and socialisation processes influence the formative 'neural sculpting' of the young child's brain, thereby modulating lifelong patterns of physiological response to stressful situations and affecting cognitive abilities (see also chapter 9).

The contraceptive revolution of the twentieth century is a pivotal event in human history, with enormous social and biological repercussions. In response to declining death rates, especially infant mortality, humans had no choice but to reduce birth rates. Inevitably, they found ways to do this. Yet contraception is a basic confrontation with the evolutionary imperative to maximise the transmission of one's genes to the future. Human biological evolution, blind to the future, could not have foreseen the need for contraception. Indeed, if natural selection had focused our instincts upon reproductive success *per se*, and not on physical survival and copulation, then the advent of contraception would have deterred us from most sexual activity. This has *not* happened.[46] Hence, the spread of oral contraception has potentiated the recent increases in sexually transmitted diseases, including HIV/AIDS.

Annulling natural selection?

The transformation of human death rates and birth rates has wrought a quiet revolution at the core of human population biology. In rich countries today, nearly all newborns survive to adulthood and, hence, to reproductive age. Reproductive 'fitness' therefore no longer has much to do with surviving the shoals and rapids of early life. As we saw in chapter 4, there is evidence of a genetic influence on the severity of infectious disease within individuals. We have, however, greatly attenuated the process of natural selection in relation to that genetic variation by largely averting childhood death from infectious disease, malnutrition and other hazards of early life.

That attenuation in selective force over the past two centuries may have caused a one-off shift in the population's genetic profile. By precluding the culling of the immunologically weak, might we have inadvertently altered the incidence rates of some immune-related diseases? For example, over the past several decades in Western societies there has been a widespread, unexplained, increase in Non-Hodgkin's disease, a malignancy that is known to increase markedly in immune-suppressed persons. This could reflect a population shift in the immunological genotype that now survives a childhood that is relatively free of life-threatening microbial challenge. Or it could be due simply to an altered immunological phenotype, with later-life disease consequences, because of the change in pattern of childhood infectious diseases.[47]

Meanwhile, other changes in the overall genetic profile of humankind are occurring because of the different fertility rates between major regional, ethnic or religious populations. Most human genetic variation, however, is *within* populations (i.e., between individuals) rather than between populations. Hence, a change in the relative size of different populations in the world has negligible impact on the overall human genotype.

Future prospects: sustaining 9 billion

Human population growth cannot be reined in at short notice. For the moment, great absolute growth continues, even though the annual percentage increase has been steadily declining for several decades. This reflects the 'flywheel' phenomenon of demographic momentum. Most of the next quarter-century's parents have already been born. This momentum has been evident in the accelerating annual increase in the number of women of child-bearing age in the later decades of the twentieth century, respectively. Although this surge in reproductive-aged women is now slowing, the demographic fly-wheel will almost certainly keep turning for another half century.

The 1960s was a crucial decade in reshaping public opinion and governmental policy in favour of fertility restraint. Today half of the world's population is reproducing at below the replacement level (2.1 babies per couple), heading for an estimated 75% in 2025. Nearly all of the residual growth in world population is now occurring in developing countries. India, which reached 1 billion in 1999, will add a massive half billion by 2050, and may overtake China in the process. Sub-Saharan Africa, too, will swell the world's total. Its high fertility and late demographic transition may yet cause its population to triple from 600 million to almost 2 billion by 2050 – unless the African HIV/AIDS catastrophe escalates.

The task of achieving a socially and environmentally sustainable world supportive of human wellbeing and health is a multi-faceted one. To summarise, the following are the main demographic components of that challenge:[48]

- Virtually all (non-migratory) population growth in the twenty-first century will occur in non-Western countries, particularly in South Asia and Africa where poverty and unemployment are already widespread.
- In Europe, where below-replacement levels of fertility are already widespread, population will decline. By 2050 Europe's share of world population will have almost halved from 12% today to 7%.
- There will be increased economic and environmental pressure for international migration.
- Rapid urbanisation will, by 2030, result in the world's urban population being twice the size of the rural population. (Today, they are approximately equal.)
- The number of people aged over 65 years will approximately triple by 2050. This will greatly increase the demands for health and social security provision.
- In low-income countries, population ageing and the double burden of poverty-associated disease and increasing rates of noncommunicable disease will put great pressures on health care systems and economic resources.
- In high-income countries, ageing will augment the ratio of children and elderly to working-age population. In contrast, demographic change in low-income countries will initially swell the ranks of young unskilled adults, with social consequences that will depend on employment prospects.

Carrying capacity, and population growth patterns

In nature, the characteristics of the local environment limit the population size of each particular species that can be supported. The population size fluctuates around that number as environmental conditions vary over time. For the human species, as we saw in chapter 5, the notion of environmental carrying capacity remains contentious. While ecologists see it as important and meaningful, many economists dismiss it on the grounds of substitutability – if you run out of one resource stock (e.g., oil) then you find another (e.g., uranium). Now, if this were always possible, then 'carrying capacity' would be infinitely expandable, and hence not relevant. In fact, it is not always possible. We cannot substitute for extinguished species, lost topsoil and depleted stratospheric ozone.

Nevertheless, Thomas Malthus' forecast of local subsistence crises arising from excessive human numbers within a food-limited environment seem increasingly unlikely, as localised disasters, in today's interconnected world. Indeed, the famines that have occurred in recent decades – the most serious being the Chinese famine of 1959–61 with around 20 million deaths – have arisen from either economic mismanagement or warfare, and not directly from inadequate food-producing resources. However, local population pressures on dwindling natural resources may have exacerbated some of those conflicts. Bangladesh, already with less than one-tenth of a hectare of cropland on average for each of its 130 million people, will face similar difficulties this century as population size doubles and as the combination of sea-level rise and land subsidence displaces up to one-quarter of that population. India has seen its per-person supply of fresh water drop from 5,500 cubic metres per year in the 1950s to around 1,800 cubic metres now – just over the recognised scarcity threshold of 1,700 cubic metres.[49] By 2050 India's supply is projected to be around 1,400 cubic metres per person per year. This poses basic risks to health via the hazards of unsafe drinking water, poor sanitation, deficient personal hygiene and water shortages for food crops.

Meanwhile, the Malthusian perspective is becoming relevant at a larger scale. We have begun to exceed the carrying capacity of the planet as a whole. So, for humankind at large, what is the world's 'carrying capacity'?[50] Or, rephrased: What would be a comfortable number of humans on Earth, to both share and enjoy this planet's natural bounty, to live in ecologically sustainable fashion, and to maintain the biodiversity and resilience of life? This question will be addressed in the final chapter. It is at the heart of the nascent debate about the Sustainability Transition.

In the natural world, the tendency of populations to exponential growth is generally constrained by predation, by limits to food supplies, by infectious disease, and, in many animals, by density related changes in reproductive behaviour. As numbers approach the environmental limits and negative feedback increases, one of the following patterns (see Figure 7.3) occurs:

• Logistic (S-shaped) growth, in which immediate response to negative feedback results in an orderly asymptotic plateauing of numbers.
• Domed or capped growth, in which the response to negative feedback is delayed, thereby necessitating a compensatory die-off.

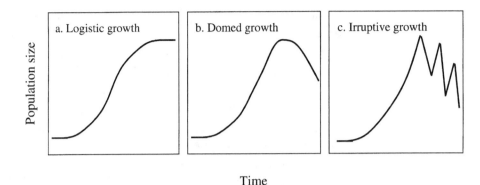

Figure 7.3 Three basic patterns of population growth: logistic, domed (capped) and irruptive (or 'Malthusian'). The equation for the logistic pattern of population growth is: $dN/dt = f(r.[K-N]/K)$. At any instant, the rate of population increase (dN/dt) is a function both of that species' intrinsic reproductive rate (r) and of the unused fraction of environmental carrying capacity available for that population ($[K-N]/K$). The equation thus highlights the contrasting notions of 'r' and 'K' species (see main text, pp. 206–8).

- Irruptive growth, with a ('Malthusian') chaotic post-crash pattern, again reflecting a delayed response to negative feedback.

The idea that the logistic, asymptotic pattern of growth prevails in nature was formalised by Raymond Pearl, an American biometrician, in the 1920s. This formulation challenged the widely assumed Malthusian scenario. Indeed, given the varied growth patterns observed in wild, domesticated and labora-tory-based species, it is clear that no single equation describes all population growth. Further, it is clear that humans have malleable social goals which usually over-ride biological forces. This distinguishes us from other species.

The debate over whether environmental crises are more likely on a local or global scale is, in reality, moot. Probably, the most exposed and least well-protected populations would suffer first. Hence, any global environmental crises that arise in future will tend to appear first as local or regional setbacks. Indeed, although it is difficult to attribute, this may already be happening as a result of humankind's destabilisation of the world's climate system. The increasingly disastrous consequences of intensified rainfall on precarious urban slum housing and village communities was underscored over a six-month period in countries including China, Bangladesh, India, Venezuela and Mozambique as the world moved turbulently into the year 2000. This larger-scale category of environmental hazard to human population health is the subject of chapters 10 and 11.

The impact of HIV/AIDS on population growth

Of the 57 million deaths that currently occur annually, an estimated 2.5 million are now from AIDS. HIV/AIDS has become the leading cause of infectious disease mortality in the world, and the fourth leading cause of death overall, after coronary heart disease, stroke and acute respiratory infection. In sub-Saharan Africa, HIV/AIDS has had devastating health, demographic and economic effects. Two-thirds of the world's approximately 40 million cases of the disease are in Africa, although it is beginning to spread more rapidly in much of populous Asia. The disease has now reduced life expectancy at birth in the worst affected African countries by a shocking 15–20 years.

Is the advent of HIV over the past two decades some sort of *natural* check on human population excess? The question is sometimes posed in these Malthusian terms, implying that such epidemics are nature's correctives. The question, posed thus, is potentially misleading. Nature has no grand plan, no intent. However, it is certainly true that when populations become malnourished, overcrowded, disorganised or otherwise stressed, infectious disease is more likely to break out. We have yet to see the full social and political history of HIV/AIDS written. However, it is certain that social and economic changes in parts of Africa were fundamental to the origins of this pandemic infectious disease, with heightened possibilities of transmission via increased rural–urban movement, long-distance trucking, and the economic and cultural powerlessness of women sex-workers. The extent and persistence of the crisis in Africa has also reflected the prevailing culture of denial, extending from policymakers to local communities, and opposition to condom availability by Catholic church leaders. This denial has been complemented by: (i) a tradition of sexuality in a patriarchal society whereby young women are available to older men, while younger men must make do with commercial sex (in South Africa, in 2000, one in every five school-girls over age 15 years was infected with HIV); (ii) the fatalism inherent in traditional religion and much local culture; and (iii) the heightened vulnerability of being poor, powerless, and often having other preexisting sexually transmitted diseases.[51]

Demographers initially thought that HIV/AIDS would have little demographic impact. Most victims were dying in or after their fourth decade of life, after completing much of their child-bearing. Men were dying more than women. However, that picture has changed. The heterosexual transmission of HIV is rife in poor Third World populations, and about half of infected mothers transmit the virus to their fetus or, perhaps, their breast-fed baby.

Further, recent studies of infected but otherwise healthy women have shown that HIV infection depresses fertility. Clearly, then, HIV/AIDS *has* affected population growth. Countries such as Botswana, Zimbabwe and Zambia have been particularly hard hit. Whereas developed countries were able to hold HIV prevalence in adult populations to below 1%, by the turn of the century the figure had reached around 20–25% in many sub-Saharan African countries.

One tragic aspect of the HIV/AIDS catastrophe in Africa is that the newly promoted hormonal methods of birth control – such as the widely used oral contraceptive pill in Kenya or the long-term injectable hormones used in South Africa – provide no protection against HIV infection. Those contraceptives are therefore also helping to reduce Africa's population growth via this inadvertent means.

Health consequences of modern reproductive interventions

In our celebration of today's repertoire of assisted reproduction techniques we should not forget that nature has its own quality control procedures. Defective eggs and sperm are unlikely to achieve fertilisation; defective embryos are discarded in early pregnancy; and many defective fetuses are expelled via spontaneous abortion. Some of our assisted reproduction techniques preclude this quality control. Further, some of the *ex vivo* manipulation and handling of germ cells may increase the risks of molecular damage or of disordered sequences of gene activation. The advent of intra-cytoplasmic sperm injection, which enables fertilisation of an egg with sperm from an otherwise infertile man, is illustrative of the sorts of risk involved. This procedure entails some increase in risk of the several genetic disorders that are associated with either low sperm count (e.g., Y chromosome deletions) or absence of the duct (vas deferens) that delivers sperm from testicle to prostate gland (e.g., cystic fibrosis).

The sparse epidemiological evidence available to date has not identified any obvious adverse consequences of assisted reproduction techniques – such as increased rates of congenital anomalies or child cancer. However, since most of the individuals born via these techniques have yet to reach adulthood, further follow-up is essential – including investigating their ability to produce healthy offspring. Research vigilance is needed.

By contrast, we have had four decades of experience with oral contraception. The Pill, comprising progestin and oestrogen, essentially acts by mimicking the body's own production of sex hormones. The progestin component (the hormone that naturally prepares the lining of the uterus for implantation of a fertilised egg) signals to the ovary not to ovulate. Curiously, whereas the Pill suppresses ovulation it does not suppress menstruation – although that could easily have been achieved. Its original designers believed, apparently without appreciating the infrequency of menstruation in the long ancestral history of human females, that monthly menstruation was 'natural'.[52] That is not so. Modern Western women have approximately three times as many menstrual cycles as do their ancient forebears. If only three of the modern woman's 35 years of reproductive life-span are spent either pregnant or breast-feeding, then the other 32 years yield over 400 menstrual cycles. Anthropologists estimate that hunter-gatherers and traditional agrarian women, with approximately five to six pregnancies and prolonged breast-feeding of each baby, have around 100–150 menstrual cycles.

The repeated cyclical proliferation of cells in the ovary and the lining of the uterus (endometrium) increases the probability of genetic mutation and cancerous change. International epidemiological data show that ovarian, breast and endometrial (uterine) cancers are essentially diseases of modernity. Ovarian cancer is thought to be increased by the repeated monthly microtrauma of follicle (egg) release and ensuing cellular proliferation as the ovary undergoes repair. Pregnancy and lactation reduce the risk of ovarian cancer. So too does use of the Pill, by suppressing ovulation. Indeed, a woman who takes the Pill for ten years reduces her risk of ovarian cancer by over half. Likewise, the risk of endometrial cancer is halved, via the action of progestin in preempting much of the oestrogen-induced thickening of the endometrium. However, because the Pill has been formulated to allow menstruation, the gentle monthly tides of progestin and oestrogen that it imparts cause repeated cycles of cellular proliferation of breast tissue. That proliferation, occurring particularly in response to progestin, increases the probability that a dividing cell will incur a random mutation that leads to cancer. Hence the longstanding concern that the Pill may increase the risk of breast cancer. However, with the modern low-dose Pill, there appears to be no overall significant increase in risk of breast cancer – although many studies over the past quarter-century have indicated a slight increase in risk in young women during and soon after use.

The Pill also increases the risk of deep vein clots which, though rare, can be life-threatening. On the other hand, the Pill confers much greater health gains by averting unwanted pregnancy and reducing the risk of ovarian cancer and a very common disease, coronary heart disease. On balance, the Pill is clearly good for health – but it might be even better if it did not induce menstruation (although the woman would then not know if she were pregnant, which could result in detrimental exposure of the fetus to contraceptive hormones).

Finally, in evolutionary terms, the stretching of post-reproductive life to three to four decades in modern women may pose some unusual risks and benefits to health. Studies have consistently shown that blood cholesterol level and hence the risk of coronary heart disease increase more rapidly in Western women after the menopause relative to the rate of increase in men (who nevertheless still have higher absolute rates of heart disease, in part because of their historically higher smoking rates). This post-menopausal increase in blood cholesterol reflects the decline in production of oestrogens. The fall in oestrogen levels also accelerates the loss of calcium from bones, thus prediposing to osteoporosis. Post-menopausal hormone replacement therapy (HRT) – itself a radical change in the hormonal lifecourse of modern women – is therefore opening new vistas of possible reductions in several diseases of older age. Nevertheless, the early evidence from controlled trials of HRT has not shown a reduction in heart disease. As an 'evodeviation' of modern human ecology, HRT is both a deliberate and generally beneficial intervention in the long hormonal life-course of women in late-industrial society with long life expectancy. It will be important to monitor closely for any other health effects, including changes in risks of breast cancer and autoimmune disorders (since oestrogens influence immune functioning).

Conclusion

Over the past two centuries, beginning in Western countries, both the age at death and the causes of death have changed dramatically. Average life expectancy almost doubled during the twentieth century. Population pyramids are changing their shape, becoming less bottom-heavy, as populations age. Over the past half-century, low-income countries have been following, variably, the same general path: declining childhood deaths, receding infectious diseases, longer life expectancies, and, when fertility rates also decline, ageing populations. Fertility remains moderately high in many poorer countries, and there is still considerable momentum in world population growth. There are therefore serious questions about the Earth's carrying capacity at a global level.

Confronted with the historically unfamiliar prospect of near-certain child survival, and living an urbanised lifestyle increasingly unsuited to large family size, we have extended our repertoire of fertility control methods. Those hormonal and surgical contraceptive methods, in turn, impart other benefits and risks to health. Reproductive behaviours change as populations become educated, wealthier and oriented to living longer lives. On the biologists' r-K continuum of breeding strategies, modern urbanising humans are moving towards an ultra-K strategy – investing more resources in fewer offspring as economic and social conditions become more secure. As infant mortality rates fall to around 1%, the potent age-old selective force of differential childhood survival recedes, rendering natural selection nigh a spent force within the world's high-income populations. Meanwhile, the repertoire of fertility assistance expands; and cloning is now on the horizon. So too is somatic gene therapy and, perhaps, the possibility of genetically modified humans.

Ageing brings inevitable changes to population health profiles. The organ that best differentiates the human species from all other animal species, the brain, is becoming a focal point of vulnerability in our lengthening lives. We face the prospect of an increased prevalence of dementia in ageing societies. This represents a particularly critical juncture in the long story of divergence between human biology, as evolved, and human culture, as acquired. With that same brain we may yet be clever enough to find ways to counter this distressing affliction of older age.

8

Modern affluence: lands of milk and honey

The transformation of death rates, birth rates and disease profiles around the world, over part or all of the past 150 years, reflects various radical changes in human ecology. In Western societies, this epidemiological transition had its roots in the late eighteenth century and has led to the replacement of the fluctuating ravages of infectious disease epidemics, famine and malnutrition by a more constant attrition by the noncommunicable diseases of adulthood. These are the 'diseases of modern civilisation'. Similar changes in disease profile are now emerging in much of the rest of the world, even as the poorer segments of those populations continue to be burdened by infectious diseases and malnutrition.

Earlier chapters have shown how the gains in material conditions of living, the advent of sanitation, the introduction of vaccination, gains in education, the nascent democratic process and general social modernisation all contributed to these great changes in disease and survival. Over the past two centuries in Western populations, infant and child mortality declined by an order of magnitude, life expectancy at birth doubled and, among adults, the average age at death increased by approximately 15 years. The later stage of this transformation, entailing the rise of noncommunicable diseases of middle and later adulthood, reflects the advent of mass markets, altered consumption patterns, changes in patterns of diet and physical activity, and the various other shifts in way of life that characterised twentieth-century Western populations. Similar changes are increasingly influencing the patterns of disease in developing countries.

The enormity of these changes can easily escape the casual observer. Noncommunicable diseases tend to rise and fall over the course of many decades. Hence, their time-scale is that of several generations, not of an individual life-span. Thomas McKeown pointed to the momentous decline in tuberculosis and measles mortality in England during the 1840–1950 period. During the twentieth century in high-income countries there were similarly spectacular increases in diseases such as lung cancer, coronary heart disease and diabetes. In recent decades there has been an apparent tripling in child asthma prevalence, a strong rise in sexually transmitted diseases, and now an escalation in the proportion of obese persons in urban populations every-where. This gathering wave of obesity will translate into greatly increased rates of cardiovascular disease, diabetes and other diseases within several decades.

The important point to stress here is that these are *population*-level shifts in the rates of disease occurrence. They reflect changes in human ecology – a resetting of the boundaries within which individuals live and make choices. Contemporary epidemiological research is primarily directed at identifying which categories of individual within a particular population get the disease in question. Such studies entail collecting information at the level of the individual, about personal behaviours, exposures and disease occurrence. Yet the more important question often refers not to individuals but to 'sick populations'.[1] Why has the disease rate in the population changed? To answer that second question satisfactorily, we usually need to have first explored the individual-level relationship in order to identify which exposures and behaviours cause that particular disease. For example, we need to know that excessive alcohol consumption, a high intake of saturated fats and extremes of temperature can precipitate fatal heart attacks *before* we set out to explain the rapid rise of coronary heart disease deaths in post-communist Russia, or the rapid fall in such deaths in post-communist Poland or German-occupied Norway during World War II. In general, the greater challenge is to understand why the disease rate has changed within the population, and to account for the (usually) uneven distribution of disease between socioeconomic, ethnic and other sub-groups within the population. These population-level patterns thus provide a reality check against which epidemiologists should test the explanatory power of their individual-level research findings.

A change in the incidence rate of a disease signifies a change in the population's circumstances, a change in its way of life. The epidemic of obesity and its associated health disorders in modern urban societies is not simply an aggregate of thousands of individuals' problems (even though that is how the health-care system tends to construe it). Rather, it is a manifestation of a shared change in way of life, entailing a systemic imbalance between the average amounts of energy ingested and expended.[2] Modern urban populations do not simply 'over-eat' relative to previous generations. The greater problem is that they are underactive. They drive cars to work and to the local shops; they sit at desks; they go up one floor by elevator; and they watch television in lieu of more active pursuits. Labouring exertion has been greatly reduced in both workplace and home. That is a pattern of daily life that would have been unimaginable 100 years ago. The result, unsurprisingly, is a rise in the prevalence of obesity.

This category of health problem has been described by Stephen Boyden as 'evodeviationary'.[3] That is, he says, the problem results from a deviation in human culture and behaviour away from the environmental conditions that prevailed during human biological evolution. This is an important notion, although it needs to be treated with caution. It is also actually a well-rehearsed notion. Edward Jenner, who developed vaccination against smallpox two centuries ago, wrote: 'The deviation of Man from the state in which he was originally placed by Nature seems to have proved to him a prolific source of Disease.'[4]

Jenner, however, was referring mainly to various infectious disease epidemics. He knew little of non-infectious diseases and nothing of biological evolution. Our ideas today about incongruities between environmental habitat and human biology are, we assume, more sophisticated. We understand more clearly, for example, that wide-ranging changes in human ecology such as alterations in diet, physical activity or reproductive behaviour can, by introducing unfamiliar stresses upon human biology, affect rates of disease. However – and here is the caution – whilst many such impacts on health are detrimental, they are not all necessarily so. After all, the hunter-gatherer diet would have exerted nearly all of its evolutionary selection pressures before the fifth decade of life, after which age it was rare to reproduce and rear children and adult survival was uncommon. In other words, natural selection in humans did not have to test the suitability of pre-agrarian diets for later adulthood. (Perhaps, then, the beneficial effects of the polyunsaturated n-3 fatty acids in slowing heart disease or preventing recurrence of heart attacks, described in chapter 5, have no *direct* precedent in human biological evolutionary experience.)

Because our field of vision is usually confined within a lifetime's experience and within our own culture, we may not perceive the larger-scale shifts in human ecology. Mostly those shifts occur on a multi-decadal timescale, often spanning several lifetimes.

Consider the Western diet, for example. How well do we realise that, over the past two centuries, the average levels of individual consumption of fat and refined sugar in Western society have increased fivefold and fifteenfold, respectively? Or that the increase in fat includes the addition of a substantial amount of 'unnatural' commercially hydrogenated unsaturated fat – the polyunsaturates that are described as 'trans' fatty acids on today's labelled margarine containers, and which appear to increase significantly the risk of coronary heart disease.[5] Or that the advent of technological changes in the grinding, sifting and milling of grains has caused a more than tenfold decrease in per-person cereal fibre consumption? Steel roller mills, developed in the 1870s, enabled the fractions of milled wheat grains to be separated efficiently, on an industrial scale – and so produce highly prized uniform-quality white bread, devoid of bran and wheat-germ and depleted of essential oils, vitamins and minerals. These various changes, arising over the course of a century or two, have transformed the modern human diet and, therefore, the pattern of disease.

Indeed, each of the two major revolutions in post-palaeolithic ways of living – the agricultural revolution beginning 10,000 years ago and the industrial revolution beginning around 200 years ago – radically changed the types of foods and nutrients available to human populations. First, hunter-gatherer diets based on plant foods (predominantly fruits, berries and fibrous vegetables) along with lean game meat and fish, were replaced by the early agriculturalist's cereal-based diets. Those early agrarian diets have typically contained relatively less fresh vegetables and fruit than did those of our pre-agrarian ancestors. The decline in vegetable and fruit intake with agrarianism reflected two things: an increased dependence on cultivating a restricted range of high-yielding seasonal foods, and the dispersal of human populations into temperate and colder climates.

More recently, in industrial society, we have developed energy-intensive technologies for food production, processing, transport and storage. These provide us with a year-round supply of foods that have artificially high concentrations of energy, fat and sugar. As societies industrialise, the consumption of starchy staples decreases, from around 50% or more of total food energy to 25% or less. Meanwhile, fat consumption increases from 10–20% of total energy up to 40%. Meat becomes a mainstay. Modern developed societies have thus radically reshaped their diet in ways that have contributed to the occurrence of various noncommunicable disease processes during the prolonged adulthood that now characterises most contemporary societies.

The variety of regional cuisines is shown in Figure 8.1. In Africa and much of Asia (excluding Japan and the small 'tiger' economies) over half of all dietary energy comes from cereals or, less often, starchy roots or fruits. By contrast, in Europe and North America, less than one quarter of total energy comes from cereals. The level of consumption of added fats, meat, dairy products, sweeteners and alcohol is generally inversely related to the consumption

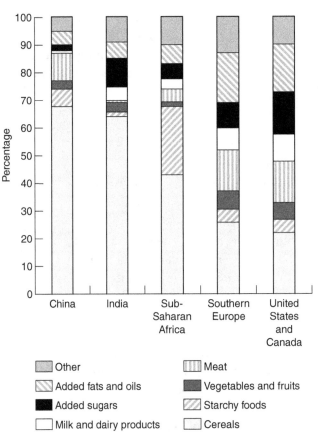

Figure 8.1 Contributions of major food groups to total energy intake in selected countries and regions.

of starchy staples. For example, less than 10% of total energy comes from meat in the low-income countries compared with 15–20% in countries such as Australia, New Zealand and North America. (Further contrast comes from various contemporary herders and hunter-gatherers, in whom meat protein intake is typically in the range of 20–35%.[6]) In public health terms (and indeed for gustatory pleasure) the Mediterranean diet is a shining beacon. From voluminous epidemiological research it is clear that the contemporary food culture of Italy, Greece and Crete provides substantial protection against cardiovascular disease and various diet-related cancers.[7] The diet contains abundant fresh fruit and vegetables, grain products (bread and pasta), olive oil (a monosaturated fat) and modest amounts of meat, fish and cheese. Alcohol, particularly wine (rich in antioxidant phenolic compounds), is drunk in low to moderate amounts, mostly with meals. While not low in total fat, the Mediterranean diet has relatively little saturated fat. It is part of a lifestyle that for many people still includes plenty of physical activity.

The kaleidoscope of disease in Western societies

In the previous chapter we noted that the high rates of cancers of the breast, ovary and uterus in Western women are largely due, variously, to recent reductions in fertility and the altered timetable of menarche and child-bearing, with consequent changes in hormonal experiences and in cycles of cellular proliferation. Many other recent shifts in human ecology have markedly affected patterns of health and disease. To take three obvious examples, our lungs are not equipped to handle cigarette smoke, our bodies are not designed to withstand the massive forces of car crashes, and our livers cannot process large amounts of alcohol. Many other aspects of our cultural evolution are to our advantage: we protect ourselves against injury and ill-health by wearing clothes, trading foodstuffs and by sleeping in secure housing. The improved nutritional circumstances of pregnancy and early childhood lay the foundations for good health in adulthood. It is this new, fluid, mix of changes in human culture, environment and behaviour that account for the kaleidoscopic changes of disease patterns in Western societies during the twentieth century.

The death rate from coronary heart disease began to rise early in the twentieth century. So too did the incidence of various gut disorders, including appendicitis and diverticulitis. In the second quarter of the century lung cancer mortality began to rise in men, to be followed after mid-century by a rise in women, mirroring the time-trends in their uptake of smoking. Stomach cancer deaths began a long decline in the second quarter of the century, as subsequently did peptic ulcer after peaking around mid-century. Cancers of the large bowel, of the prostate gland (in men) and of breast (in women) began to increase around mid-century, and those higher cancer rates have persisted. Meanwhile, the death rate from stroke declined from early in the twentieth century, especially after mid-century with improved treatment of high blood pressure and reduced dietary salt intake – and, as yet, despite the recent rise in the prevalence of obesity. During the last third of the century, coronary heart disease death rates began to decline in Western countries, albeit at different times in different countries.

Throughout most of the twentieth century there was a general rise in the rates of injury and death on the roads, as car usage proliferated. A total of 25 million road-accident deaths has occurred, mostly in industrialised countries. This is approximately the same number as died in the great disasters of the Spanish Flu of 1918–19 and the Chinese famine of 1959–60. From the 1970s, the advent of seat-belts, safer car design, drink-driving legislation, and urban traffic calming began to turn this tide. Meanwhile, less obvious and less talked about, mental health problems appear to have increased during the twentieth century. Such trends are not easily documented since changeable diagnostic criteria bedevil the statistics. Nevertheless, in 1990 major (unipolar) depression was estimated by the World Health Organization to be the world's fifth most burdensome disease category, and second only to coronary heart disease in the developed world. The prevalence of depression appears to be increasing in both developed and developing countries and it is projected to become the second most burdensome disease category in the world by 2020.[8]

Coronary heart disease: a case study

It is instructive to consider coronary heart disease, as exemplar, in more detail. There are striking differences between populations in patterns of cardiovascular disease – high blood pressure, coronary heart disease and stroke. These diseases are rare in elderly members of traditional hunter-gatherer groups. They are also infrequent in many contemporary Third World rural agrarian populations, such as in China. Historically, atherosclerosis may have been confined to societies' overfed and under-exercised élites: the disease is evident in mummies of Egypt's Pharaohs. Yet, despite recent declines, coronary heart disease and stroke are the leading cause of premature death in high-income countries, and are rising rapidly in urbanising populations everywhere. They currently account for almost a quarter of the world's annual total of deaths. The preeminent importance of social-environmental and dietary factors is reflected in the increases in heart disease in people migrating from low-risk to high-risk countries, as when the Japanese migrated to California early in the twentieth century, and when Italians and Greeks migrated to Australia after World War II. These migrant populations, nevertheless, have maintained a risk of cardiovascular disease that is substantially lower than that of their host population, and is commensurate with their retention of traditional dietary and other practices.[9]

The two most important causative factors in the rise of coronary heart disease in Western societies in the first half of the twentieth century were cigarette smoking and the 'early affluent' diet.[9] The epidemic of nicotine addiction began, approximately, during World War I in men and during World War II in women. The early changes in diet associated with modernisation and the emergence of mass consumption entailed a shift towards diets higher in animal foods (especially saturated fats) and refined carbohydrates and lower in vegetables and fruits. Blood cholesterol levels began to rise, creating the precondition for an epidemic of coronary heart disease. Indeed, the rise in mortality from this disease was sufficiently great in Finland and Australia to cause a transient decline in male life expectancy in the 1960s.

In the latter decades of the twentieth century, as mentioned above, coronary heart disease declined in high-income countries. It is still the single largest cause of premature death in those populations, but death rates have approximately halved in various countries such as the United States, Australia, New Zealand and Canada since the late 1960s. The decline began a decade ago later in the British population (who, for reasons not easily imagined, remained relatively more attached to their traditional cuisine). Declines in other countries of northwest Europe and Scandinavia also began in the late 1970s and early 1980s. Yet, frustratingly for epidemiologists, the reasons for the decline remain uncertain: was it dietary change (especially amount and type of fat), more prevalent consumption of alcohol (especially wine), reduced (and filter-tipped) smoking, improved fetal/neonatal nutrition, more effective medical and surgical intervention, or all of the above? While gains in maternal and child nutrition in the early decades of the twentieth century may have contributed to future reductions in cardiovascular disease for those generations,[10] the eventual downturn in coronary heart disease death rates largely occurred across all adult age-groups simultaneously, rather than being staggered across successive oncoming generations. This indicates that some change in adult circumstances was of particular importance.

In Europe there have been two interesting contrasts in the pattern of coronary heart disease. First, the Mediterranean European countries have long had much lower rates of heart disease than the northern countries of Western Europe. The apparent importance of diet has been underscored by the persistence of low rates in first-generation migrants from Italy and Greece after settling in higher-risk countries such as Australia and the United States (in some contrast to later generations within those migrant populations who adopted more of the host country diet). The French, too, though only 'Mediterranean' in the south, and famously partial to meat, rich sauces, cheese and cigarettes, have had lower rates of coronary heart disease than Britain, Germany and other northwestern European countries (although the gap may now be closing[11]). This, too, has been attributed, albeit inconclusively, to diet-related factors: the protective effects of red wine, a high intake of antioxidant micronutrients in fresh vegetables, and dining in a sociable and unhurried fashion that confers low-stress metabolic benefit.

Second, even as death rates from coronary heart disease began declining in Western Europe in the last quarter of the twentieth century; they continued to rise in the communist countries of Central and Eastern Europe during the 1970s and 1980s. In part this east–west divergence in coronary heart disease mortality reflected the fact that the epidemic of cigarette smoking largely began after World War II in the then-communist countries, when smoking rates (in men) were already plateauing in Western countries. In part the divergence may have reflected the increased dietary intake of saturated fats resulting from communist state-subsidised meat, milk and eggs, coinciding with the period of 'late dietary affluence'[12] in the West when consumption of these foods was declining and consumption of vegetable oils and fresh fruit and vegetables was rising again. Meanwhile, less certainly, there may also have been adverse cardiovascular consequences from a rise in stress-related hormones (especially cortisol) as social morale and community networks declined in those communist countries.

The plot thickened following the collapse of European communism in 1989. A diversity of heart disease mortality trends emerged – rates increased further in Russia and Hungary during the early 1990s, whereas they decreased promptly in Poland and, soon after, in the Czech Republic. The surprisingly rapid fall in heart disease mortality in Poland during those years, of the order of 20–25% in persons aged 45–64, accompanied a rapid change in the national diet.[12] State subsidies had been removed and markets were newly open to imported foods. The ratio of polyunsaturated fats to saturated fats in the Polish diet doubled between 1989 and 1990, as did the consumption of imported fresh fruit. The rapid fall in heart disease mortality could not readily be explained by trends in smoking, alcohol consumption, social stress, blood cholesterol levels or medical interventions. Most probably the change in diet averted fatal heart attacks in persons with underlying coronary heart disease, perhaps by reducing the tendency of blood to clot.[12] Note that the question at issue here is a population-level question: What happened within Polish society and its economy that altered the average risk of heart disease death? Of course, one could seek evidence, at the individual level, of the relationship between personal dietary habits and the occurrence of heart attack in modern Poland – and that, indeed, is what modern epidemiologists are very good at doing. But that would miss the point at issue here.

As we learn more about how individuals' genetic makeup affects their response to environmental exposures, we can understand better why it has often been difficult to demonstrate diet–disease relationships at the individual level. For example, is is well known that the change in blood cholesterol concentration in response to a given increase in dietary fat intake differs between individuals. The minority of individuals with the so-called Apo E4/4 genotype experience a much greater increase in blood cholesterol than do those with other Apo E allelic combinations.[13] In populations eating diets high in fat, particularly saturated fat, individuals with the apo E4/4 genotype evince a much greater-than-average increased risk of coronary artery disease. Hence, there is no simple one-on-one relationship between an individual's dietary fat intake and blood cholesterol level; the randomly distributed Apo E4 genotypes within the population blur the diet–cholesterol relationship. Interestingly, the E4/4 genotype occurs approximately twice as often in African and Asian populations (around 30%) as in Europeans (around 15%). Within Europe, it is twice as prevalent in Scandinavians as in Italians (approximately 20% versus 10%). Maybe part of the effect of the celebrated Mediterranean diet is actually due to Mediterranean genes that attenuate the impact of dietary fat upon blood cholesterol concentration?

WHAT ACCOUNTS, more generally, for this recent change in the pattern of diseases in developed countries? There have been two particularly influential attempts at an integrated explanation of these changes, both by British scientists.

In the 1970s, Dennis Burkitt and colleagues proposed that the high rates of various non-infectious diseases in Western societies reflected the advent of industrial processing, refinement and modernisation of the diet.[14] Burkitt, an English surgeon with long experience in eastern Africa, promoted particularly the 'dietary fibre hypothesis' to account for the serial emergence of diseases rarely seen in traditional rural African populations: appendicitis, dental decay, haemorrhoids, varicose veins, diverticulitis, and, later, diabetes, gallstone disease, heart disease and large bowel cancer. These diseases, he said, were attributable to two main types of change in the diet. First, the lack of fibre from cereal grains caused the various bowel disorders and varicose veins (the latter via the back-pressure due to chronic constipation on intra-abdominal veins and hence on the tributary leg veins). Second, the excess of refined simple sugars and saturated fats contributed (including via obesity) to diabetes and heart disease.

This was a stimulating hypothesis that launched a thousand studies, many of which reported supportive results. Yet this was never going to be an easy hypothesis to test in non-experimental studies of free-living humans. By comparison, questions about smoking and disease are relatively easy to answer – an individual either smokes or does not. With dietary fibre, however, the classification of 'exposure' is not 'yes' or 'no', but must be derived from complex dietary data. Further, dietary fibre intake does not vary in isolation: diets low in fibre tend to be low in some other things and high in others. These research difficulties aside, Burkitt's suggestion that agrarian African diets are optimal for human biology was actually based on a false premise. As we saw in chapter 2, human biology evolved predominantly for hunter-gatherer diets, not for the much more recent agrarian diets. Our ancestral foragers consumed the type of fibre present in leafy vegetables, fruits, and tubers, not the generally less fermentable type of fibre found in wheat, millet, sorghum and maize. For this reason it is not surprising that the many epidemiological studies of diet and disease in Western populations have not found the strong and generalised protective effect of cereal fibre that Burkitt hypothesised. For several diseases, including gallstone disease and chronic bowel disorders, dietary fibre does have a moderate protective effect.

In the 1990s, David Barker proposed that the particular temporal pattern of rise and fall in various 'Western diseases' was consistent with the changing patterns of diet over earlier decades, especially as it affected the nutritional status of young women before and during pregnancy.[10] Barker and colleagues have adduced a wide range of epidemiological and animal experimental evidence that, in general, supports the thesis. Their thesis is that the experiences of fetal life, especially as determined by suboptimal maternal nutrition, 'programme' fetal growth and metabolism in ways that enhance immediate survival, but which often compromise good health in adult life.[15] (This thesis, recall, was discussed in chapter 3 specifically in relation to the evolution of insulin sensitivity levels in hunter-gatherers adapting to the Pleistocene diet.) The adult risks of several major diseases, including heart disease, stroke, diabetes, respiratory diseases and, perhaps, allergic disorders, appear to be increased in low birthweight babies or, in some studies, in babies with thin bodies. These two types of growth deficit reflect undernutrition at different stages of fetal life, and affect, respectively, blood pressure and insulin action. The increased susceptibility to adult cardiovascular disease and diabetes, Barker argues, is the price paid for the marginally nourished fetus making necessary biological adaptations to sustain the developmental trajectory of the large nutrient-hungry brain. The wisdom of nature necessarily values brain-dependent survival in early life over bodily durability in expendable post-reproductive life.

Each of these theories invokes a primarily dietary explanation. The dietary fibre deficiency theory suggests the idea of a mismatch between human biological needs, as shaped by evolution, and the type of diet on offer in modern industrialised society. The 'fetal origins' theory embraces a different sort of 'mismatch', one that occurs when a growth-retarded fetus and low birthweight baby, adaptively attuned to surviving on a 'lean fuel', becomes an overweight individual in well-fed adult life. That latter theory has, most recently, undergone some broadening in light of epidemiological evidence of the importance of life-long influences that incrementally modulate biological function and the individual's risk of disease. The 'critical window' notion of the fetal origins theory is thus evolving towards a more integrated 'pathway', or lifecourse, model.[16]

Underlying Burkitt's dietary fibre hypothesis is the idea of a mismatch between ancient and modern human ecologies. Nevertheless, although modern 'Westernisation' has created disparities between ancient and present ways of living that augment various serious diseases, yet it has also doubled our life expectancy. This, of course, is primarily because of three major benefits to population health: infectious diseases have been substantially reduced; women are much less likely to die in childbirth; and various life-lengthening clinical treatments have emerged over the past half-century. As discussed in the previous chapter, we could extend adult life expectancy further if we were now to eliminate the health hazards of the late-industrial way of life in general. Further, to maintain those extended life expectancies will also require learning to live in ecologically sustainable fashion.

Consumption behaviours and disease risks

The advent of mass consumer behaviour in increasingly affluent developed countries during the twentieth century increased the comforts and pleasures of daily life. Its association with more generalised access to health care and modern medical treatment has contributed to gains in health. Meanwhile, however, there have been three main detrimental effects of this rise in consumerism. First, as note above, it has brought changes in lifestyle many of which have entailed risks to health. Second, in most countries it has increased the evident differences between rich and poor, especially with the rise of a highly visible middle class. This has contributed to tensions, political grievances and, in many countries, an exacerbation of health inequalities. Third, it has intensified the pressures on the wider environment, a topic explored in later chapters.

The first of these three detrimental effects is the focus of this chapter. There is an interesting underlying question here. What is it about human nature that predisposes to acquisition and consumption? Our instinct for self-gratification is clearly strong. It is an inevitable product of natural selection. Individual survival is underwritten by the drive to acquire desired, life-supporting, commodities. Dietary fats and sugars were important 'survival' foods during the long Pleistocene. Human taste-buds, building on longer mammalian evolutionary experience, have therefore evolved to have a keen sensitivity to such foods. Further, because these foods were scarce commodities in evolutionary terms, the brain seems oblivious to their high energy value; there are no instinctual constraints on consuming fats and sugars. So, it is no surprise that people are attracted to chocolate bars, or that the British gentility have made an icon of scones with jam (sugar) and cream (fat). A notorious treat for tourists visiting Glasgow, Scotland, is a deep-fried Mars Bar – a parody of consumer taste, of course, but not without evolutionary significance.

This pervasive drive to satisfy our brains' dopamine-driven pleasure centres casts an unsettling light on the more general problem of substance abuse. The use of drugs and alcohol as psychoactive substances is an age-old characteristic of human societies. Endogenous chemicals are necessarily involved in neurotransmission. Now, because certain exogenous chemicals can act similarly on the brain (nicotine mimics the neurotransmitter acetylcholine, triggering the release of pleasure-enhancing dopamine), and since humans are smart enough to find and process such exogenous chemicals, so we have generated a growing array of mind-altering drugs. Hunter-gatherers and simple agrarians have usually been limited in their access to steady supplies of pure psychoactive substances. However, with modern technologies, an internationally integrated drug trade, and an expanding urban market of thrill-seeking, bored, desperate or addicted persons, drug abuse has become a major global health problem. It has also created huge new opportunities for erstwhile marginal viruses, such as the hepatitis B and HIV viruses.

Conventionally, these changes in consumer behaviour, in exposure to the 'risk factors' of daily life, are referred to as 'lifestyle' changes. We must be wary

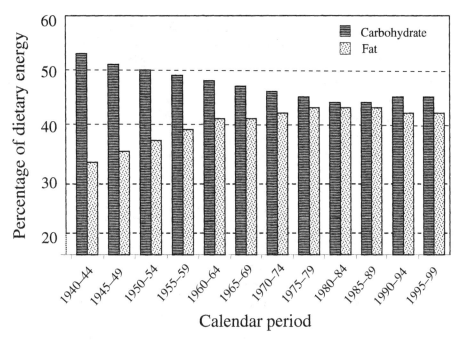

Figure 8.2 Changes in the percentage contribution of dietary carbohydrates and fats to the British diet, 1940s to 1990s. Until the 1990s, the percentage contribution of dietary fats to daily energy intake was increasing.

though. Individual behavioural choices are made within a social, economic and political context. They are often not 'free' choices, but are the product of situational constraints and influences. They reflect, say the sociologists, the political economy of the individual's and community's circumstances. We will look further at the question of socioeconomic inequalities in the next chapter.

Meanwhile, epidemiologists continue to glean important information about the immediate causes of disease by studying how these individual-level behaviours and exposures influence the occurrence of specific diseases. Modern epidemiological research has thereby yielded voluminous information about the role of individual behavioural risk factors in disease. The more important factors include cigarette smoking, alcohol consumption, obesity, high fat diets, high intake of salt, dangerous driving and unsafe sex. The major health outcomes attributable to these factors are shown in Table 8.1. Many protective behavioural factors have also been identified, including: fresh fruit and vegetables (protective against many cancers and cardiovascular disease), consumption

Table 8.1. Well-recognised individual risk behaviours and health outcomes

Risk factor	Main associated health outcomes
Cigarette smoking	Lung cancer, other respiratory diseases, various other cancers, heart and blood vessel disease
Alcohol consumption	Road trauma, injury and violence, cancers of mouth, oesophagus and larynx (especially in conjunction with cigarette smoking), breast cancer in women (still some uncertainty), liver cirrhosis, organic brain damage, hypertension at high intake
	Protective effect against coronary heart disease at moderate level of intake (but increased risk at high intake); enhanced socialising, stress alleviation
Physical activity	Prevention of weight gain, improvement in various metabolic characteristics (insulin sensitivity, blood lipid profile), release of mood-enhancing endorphins
Obesity	Hypertension, coronary heart disease, adult-onset diabetes (NIDDM), gallstone disease, breast, and endometrial and colon cancers, arthritis
High dietary fat	Obesity, atherosclerosis (esp. coronary arteries and cerebral arteries), some cancers (prostate, perhaps breast and uterine)
High dietary salt	Hypertension
Unsafe sex	Unwanted pregnancy (and abortion), sexually transmitted infectious diseases (including HIV and virally induced cancer of cervix)
Oral contraception	Reduced risk of unwanted pregnancy (and abortion), gallstone disease, reduced risk of ovarian cancer and endometrial (uterine) cancer, marginal (if any) increase in breast cancer, exposure to sexually transmitted diseases

of polyunsaturated oils from vegetable and marine sources (cardiovascular disease, arthritis), oral contraceptives (ovarian cancer) and hormone replacement therapy (osteoporosis, and perhaps cardiovascular disease).

This constellation of risk factors characterises the 'affluent' Western lifestyle. Currently, the prevalence of many of these risk factors is highest in the less-well-off segment of the population. In recent decades these same factors have become increasingly prominent as causes of non-infectious diseases in urbanising populations in developing countries and in the countries of Central and Eastern Europe.[17] Cigarette smoking causes an estimated 90% of lung cancers in developed countries, and around one-third of all cancers. Smoking has a greater absolute impact on cardiovascular disease, accounting for an estimated one-quarter of deaths from this common disease. Approximately half of all cigarette smokers in Western populations die before age 70 as a result of their smoking. As the transnational tobacco industry powers its way into developing countries, assisted by the prevailing 'free trade' ethos and its own devious ability to obfuscate scientific evidence and sidestep import duties, approximately 150 million extra deaths will occur worldwide over the coming quarter-century because of the smoking epidemic.[17]

Despite the many new insights from epidemiological research into the health risks posed by these factors, it has generally proved difficult to modify individual behaviours. In the 1980s, health agencies in Western societies directed much effort into public education campaigns that exhorted individuals to adopt healthy behaviours. Success was limited, and even that was largely confined to higher socioeconomic groups.[18] Meanwhile, on a broader front, shifts in behavioural norms (for example, in relation to both active and passive smoking) and in consumer preferences (for example, in relation to low-fat products) have resulted in various health-promoting changes in community behaviour. This experience underscores the fact that effective solutions are most likely to come from healthy public policies that attune society's commercial, educational, marketing and city-planning practices to the health needs of the population. For as long as we mistakenly view 'health' as the province solely of the health sector, we forfeit major opportunities to achieve a health-supporting environment. The current WHO Director-General, Gro Harlem Brundtland, states the argument well: 'Every minister is a health minister.'

Dietary energy, physical activity and obesity

As 'Westernisation' encroaches upon non-Western cultures, so the various adverse health consequences of these historically unfamiliar lifestyles are becoming more prevalent. Many poor urban populations in Third World cities, as noted previously, now face the dual risks of 'traditional' infectious diseases and those of the noncommunicable diseases associated with smoking, unbalanced diets and sedentary living.

The substantial increase in the prevalence of overweight and obese persons in urban populations everywhere over the past several decades is one obvious manifestation of this mismatch between past and present lifestyle. The underlying cause of this trend is the radical change in the balance of energy intake and energy expenditure in contemporary populations relative to earlier generations. Average levels of dietary energy intake in Western societies actually fell during the twentieth century, but not as fast as the decline in physical activity levels. That decline is embedded in the way of life of late industrialisation. The net result is that people are still eating more than they require for their limited energy expenditure.

Elsewhere in the world the problem is often compounded by a rapid transition from traditional diets to the quasi-Western diet of 'early affluence'. In Brazil, the energy-density of diets increased during the 1970s and 1980s, as the fat content rose from around 20% to 30% in the richer areas and from around 15% to 25% in poorer regions. During that same time obesity increased markedly in prevalence in urban populations, and has more recently begun to emerge as a problem in the urban poor. Since dietary fat has a high energy content, the increased fat content of the Brazilian diet may well have caused much of the increase in average personal energy intake.

China too has undergone a very rapid nutrition transition over the past quarter-century. National household surveys prior to the 1990s indicated that the great majority of Chinese ate diets in which less than 10% of energy came from fat. The traditional, predominantly rural, diet was high in complex carbohydrates and dietary fibre, low in fat, and high in vegetables and fruit. Animal foods (often fish) were a garnishing; feasts were an occasional luxury. Today, however, most urban Chinese and many rural residents derive over one-quarter of dietary energy from fat, while for the wealthiest the figure exceeds 40%. There has been a consequent divergence in health profiles between China's richer and poorer people, with obesity and chronic diseases increasing in the rich (although the rates are still low by international standards) while malnutrition persists in the poor. Chinese health authorities have responded by attempting to encourage the urbanising middle class to revert back to soybeans and away from animal foods. Yet, at the same time, China's urban transport policies are moving away from reliance on walking and bicycling towards expanded use of cars and buses. As ever, it is easier for governments to encourage personal diet-modification policies than to reengineer urban landscapes and transport systems or to reorient school-children away from television and video games to outside physical activity. China still has the possibility of moving from a traditional high mortality regime (dominated by high rates of infectious disease) to a low mortality regime (such as in Hong Kong and Japan) without traversing the terrain of high rates of avoidable noncommunicable diseases in adulthood. But this will require enlightened social policies and cultural steadfastness.

THE WORLD HEALTH ORGANIZATION forecasts an emerging worldwide epidemic of obesity in the early decades of the twenty-first century.[19] In a world in which one in every seven persons is seriously malnourished, this also underscores the disparity in food availability between the rich and poor countries. Within developed countries, the increase in obesity has been greatest in the less affluent. Surveys indicate that people in lower socioeconomic strata tend to eat more energy-dense convenience-food diets, have less access to recreational facilities, and have a poorer understanding of the causes of obesity. In contrast, in developing countries the rise in obesity is currently most evident in the urban middle classes.[2]

Obesity is not a benign condition. It induces metabolic and physiological disturbances that cause various serious noncommunicable diseases – particularly high blood pressure, cardiovascular disease, diabetes, certain types of cancer and arthritis. Scientists usually define obesity in terms of the body mass index (BMI): the ratio of body weight to height-squared. In healthy lean persons in Western society the average BMI is 23. Those with a BMI of 30 or over are deemed to be obese. The proportion of obese persons has approximately doubled in Western countries since the early 1980s.[2] In the late 1990s, nearly 50% of Australian men were overweight (i.e., BMI over 25) and 15% were obese. In Britain in the 1990s the prevalence of obesity also reached 15%, twice what it was in the early 1980s, while in the United States the figure reached 40% in some segments of the population.[2,20] In Western populations the risk of those several noncommunicable diseases diseases, and indeed the overall death rate, increases markedly as the BMI rises above 25.[21] In urbanising populations in low-income countries the rise of obesity (Figure 8.3) is contributing to the broad increase in these same diseases.

This increased prevalence of obesity is occurring because an increasing proportion of people are taking in more energy than they are expending. Over hundreds of millennia, humans had to expend considerable energy to find or catch food, then to grow food, and, later, in urban settings to do mostly physical work to earn money to buy food. All that changed extremely quickly in Western societies during the latter half of the twentieth century with the advent of automated manufacture, labour-saving devices and sedentary recreation, especially television. In London, as second-car ownership increased, the average weekly distance walked by school-children declined by one-fifth between the 1980s and 1990s

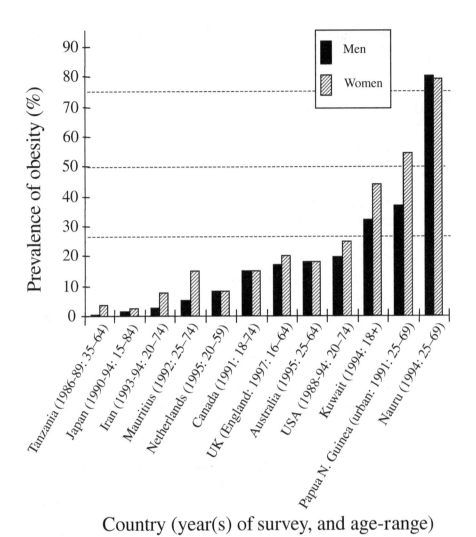

Country (year(s) of survey, and age-range)

Figure 8.3 Prevalence of obesity in samples of adult populations around the world during the 1990s. The relatively low figure for the Netherlands suggests something protective about the Dutch way of life, whereas the extreme experience of Nauru reflects the adverse consequences of a rapid disruption in diet and physical activity patterns following the rapid accrual of wealth. In some contrast to the rest of Europe, a high proportion of daily journeys in the Netherlands are taken on foot, bicycle or public transport. The Nauruans, in the second half of the twentieth century, experienced rapid gains in wealth from the mining of their unusually rich phosphate deposits (from bird guano). In addition to these many adult population surveys, there is accruing evidence of rapid increases in child obesity in urban environments. As yet we know little about the long-term health consequences of this type of life-long excess in body weight.

and the prevalence of childhood obesity rose. Londoners also cycle much less and travel by car much more than they did several decades ago. The inevitable consequence has been an imbalance between energy in and energy out. In Europe, the daily adult consumption of calories actually decreased by around one-third during the middle and later decades of the twentieth century. However, this reduction in energy intake was less than the reduction in energy expenditure. Meanwhile, over the latter stages of the twentieth century, food energy intake has tended to increase again. For example, average daily caloric intake has edged up in US adults since 1980, while physical activity has not increased. Like feed-lot cattle, modern urban humans are well fed but little exercised. Like feed-lot cattle they develop more quickly and grow larger.

IN NATURE, the body weight of humans and other vertebrate animals often fluctuates on a seasonal basis. In West Africa, studies of rural women show an annual variation in seasonal weight of around 5% between the harvest and non-harvest months. Fat (adipose) tissue is where nature stores surplus energy for mobilisation in needy times. Polar bears, for example, have evolved to depend on massive seasonal obesity to tide them over the long periods of time when the Arctic ice is either too thick or too sparse for them to be able to stock up on seal meat.

Hunter-gatherers normally vary between leanness and moderate weight. Obesity, even if achievable, is not compatible with a physically active and mobile life.[22] Indeed, the primary year-round task for most hunter-gatherer bands is to avoid hunger and starvation. In those often marginal circumstances, over hundreds of thousands of years, human biology, behaviour and culture naturally evolved ways of boosting the intake and storage of food energy. Hence we have evolved a biologically based strong craving for survival foods – that is, energy-dense foods such as high-fat organ meats or depot fat from animals and sugar-laden foods such as honey. The nomadic Israelites of the Old Testament looked forward to 'the land of milk and honey' and to living off 'the fat of the land'. Throughout the more recent history of agriculture-based societies, it has been the cherished prerogative of the privileged class to be plump. Some cultures deliberately fatten their rulers; others fatten their marriageable young women. Cultural priorities have varied, of course. Classical Greek and Roman sculpture, such as the Venus de Milo and Aphrodite of Melos, present non-corpulent beauty. On the other hand, classical and romantic European painters from Rubens to Renoir have often portrayed naked female corpulence as a symbol of sexual attractiveness and fertility.

The corpulence on those European canvases is typically most evident in buttocks and thighs. This is a form of obesity we would now recognise as being free of serious health risk. Studies have shown a clear difference in noncommunicable disease risk between those with apple-shaped 'central', or abdominal, obesity and those with pear-shaped 'peripheral', buttocks-hips-and-thighs, obesity. The former pattern of body fat deposition is associated with metabolic disturbances of insulin and corticosteroid action that increase the risk of diabetes, hypertension and heart disease.[23] Certain populations, particularly South Asians, may be constitutionally, perhaps genetically, predisposed to central obesity.[24] The evolutionary explanation for any such genetic predisposition remains obscure.

Meanwhile, fashions of female body shape in Western society change cyclically. In the 1990s, emaciated pubescent super-models may have helped nurture extreme dieting patterns in suggestible teenagers.[25] There was an apparent associated increase in the frequency of abnormal food-denial behaviours, often culminating in anorexia nervosa and bulimia. The risk to health from this extreme thinness is well known; young people occasionally die from the self-imposed starvation of anorexia. Minor levels of thinness, on the other hand, carry few risks to health – so long as future food supplies are guaranteed.

Meat-eating, vegetarianism and disease risks

During most of humankind's agriculture-based existence, meat has been a luxury food. As discussed in chapter 2, this was a major departure from the many millennia of substantial meat dependence in hunter-gatherer populations. The sparseness of animal protein in the Western diet began to change later in the nineteenth century with the opening up of the American west and the growth of the meat industry, facilitated by automated disassembly lines in abattoirs, the advent of refrigeration and the advance of the railways. Refrigerated shipping gave European consumers access to new expanses of pastoral land in Australia, New Zealand and Latin America. In those newly stocked countries, eating two to three meat meals per day became a cultural norm.

The German biochemist Von Leibig made the important discovery in the mid-nineteenth century that animal protein promotes growth. Subsequently, the United States established a system of state-funded agricultural universities to foster meat and dairy science as the cornerstone of a new era of human nutrition. Since the 1930s, generations of schoolchildren in Britain, Australia and New Zealand have been brought up on meat and milk as the key to growth, health and soldierly fitness. However, debate persists about the balance-sheet of health risks and benefits of meat-eating. Early epidemiological studies of vegetarians suggested that meatless diets reduced the risks of death from various major diseases – including coronary heart disease, stroke, and cancers of the bowel, breast and prostate. A recent synthesis of the results of five large studies following up vegetarians and non-vegetarians showed that the vegetarians were 24% less likely to have died of coronary heart disease. Interpretation of these findings is bedevilled by the fact that vegetarians tend also to display other health-enhancing behaviours, such as being non-smokers, teetotallers and physically active. Studies of vegetarians in England indicate that the health benefit associated with meat avoidance is primarily due to such diets being low in saturated fats.[26]

The important role of a high dietary intake of saturated fats as a cause of heart disease has been confirmed in numerous epidemiological studies. Further, various experimental studies in which people have been randomly allocated to eating diets either high or low in saturated fats have found that the low-fat diet lowers the particular fraction of blood cholesterol (LDL-cholesterol) most strongly implicated in coronary heart disease. Meanwhile, we understand better that the meat versus fat debate is confounded by the differences in the types of fat in wild and domesticated meat, and by the particular properties of the n-3 (or omega-3) fatty acids in fish oils. We will therefore look at the biochemistry of dietary fats in a little more detail.

The fat that we eat is absorbed from the intestine as fatty acids. The basic structure of these molecules, with their energy-containing chemical bonds, was discussed in chapter 5. Plants, terrestrial animals and fish each display distinctive profiles of fatty acids. Now, let us briefly summarise the story of the hominid diet from earlier chapters. The diet that our australopithecine ancestors ate during 3 million pre-Pleistocene years was mostly plant foods. Subsequently, from around 2 million years ago, early humans ate increasing amounts of lean game meat, fish and shellfish. This wild meat contained relatively little fat, and most of it was unsaturated structural fat – unlike the yellowish saturated fat in the marbled strips of fat in corn-fed American beef. The fat from domesticated animals, dairy foods and eggs is much more saturated. A further complication, mentioned earlier in the chapter, is that the commercial partial hydrogenation of vegetable oils produces *trans* fatty acids (the natural form being the stereo-isomeric *cis* form) that appear to increase coronary heart disease.[5] Hence the preference by today's educated consumers in

Western society for margarine and other oil-based products with low *trans* fatty acid content.

Some of these saturated fatty acids are known to increase the concentration of cholesterol in the blood. Saturated fats account for around two-thirds of the elevation in blood cholesterol in Western populations compared to non-Western populations on traditional diets. In contrast, the naturally occurring plant and seafood *cis* unsaturated fats generally lower blood cholesterol levels. Olive oil, which comprises predominantly the monounsaturated oleic acid, appears to lower blood concentrations of the atherogenic ('bad') LDL cholesterol while raising that of the protective ('good') HDL cholesterol. Safflower, sunflower and soybean oils all contain polyunsaturated fatty acids (of the n-6 alpha-linoleic group) that lower total blood cholesterol, but they do so by lowering both the LDL and HDL fractions. Meanwhile, like olive oil, the particular attribute of the n-3 fatty acids, derivatives of alpha-*linolenic* acid and popularised in fish oil, is that they lower the LDL cholesterol *and* raise the HDL cholesterol.

Diet and cancer

Cancers occur in all higher vertebrate animals. They arise when, improbably, one lineage of cells within a tissue or organ acquires rogue characteristics that turn it 'malignant'. This clone of cells ignores the normal constraints on cell proliferation, and begins to invade adjoining tissues and, later, more distant tissues. The abnormality is the result of genetic damage to the original cell line. The immediate cause of the damage is either exposure to a genotoxic agent that produces a critical mutation, coupled with a failure of the usually prompt genetic repair mechanisms, or, rarely, via heritable mutations.

Increasingly, though, science is looking beyond this mechanistic explanation to explore the biology of cancer in terms of stimuli that increase cellular proliferation.[27] After all, mammalian DNA repair mechanisms have been well-honed by evolutionary pressures. Of the approximately 10,000 oxidative 'hits' that occur each day to the DNA in *each* of our cells, nearly all are repaired. Mutations thus accumulate only slowly with ageing. There is therefore only a small probability of damaging DNA in exactly the way that leads to a viable cancer-related mutation, and which is accompanied fortuitously by other critical mutations that are prerequisite to malignancy. A more plausible role for most 'carcinogens' is to increase cell proliferation. This can occur via chronic inflammation, as with persistent asbestos fibres in the lungs, *Schistosomiasis haematobium* in the urinary bladder, hepatitis, *Helicobacter pylori* in the lower stomach and duodenum, and perhaps long-term inhalation of cigarette smoke. It can occur with sex hormones, either endogenous or exogenous, that impinge excessively on hormone-dependent tissues, particularly breast, endometrium and prostate. It can also occur if viruses such as the near-ubiquitous Epstein-Barr virus (EBV) are released from normal host immunological controls (as happens in HIV/AIDS) allowing them to induce a proliferation of lymphoid B-cells and hence the occurrence of lymphoma.

Worldwide, the dominant causes of human cancer are dietary deficiencies or excesses, cigarette smoking and several types of virus (which cause, in particular, cancers of the cervix, liver and lymphoid tissues).[28] Other environmental and occupational chemical exposures, ionising radiation, ultraviolet radiation, alcohol, tobacco chewing and various drugs account for most of the remainder. As a population's average life expectancy increases, the proportion of all deaths due to cancer increases. In developed countries the proportion is around one-fifth. As with heart disease, there are huge variations in the incidence of specific cancers between populations. Cancer of the oesophagus, for example, varies several hundredfold between high rates in the Iranian Caspian hinterland and parts of China, on the one hand, and low rates in certain Western countries. Cancers of the stomach, liver and uterine cervix are common in many poor countries. Cancers of the breast, prostate and colon predominate in rich countries. Lung cancer has been rising in most of the world, and will continue to do so in women everywhere and in men in developing countries. In developed countries, approximately one-third of all the cancers are due to dietary factors and one-third are due to smoking.[28]

IN EARLIER DECADES and centuries, various clinicians had observed that the risk of cancerous disease reflected patterns of eating. Excess consumption and undernutrition were both invoked. Moral overtones could sometimes be heard: gluttony, meat-eating and sloth were incriminated. In the 1950s and 1960s, the idea that dietary factors might be a major cause of cancer was rather a novel idea. It was clear enough that alcohol consumption increased the occurrence of cancers of the mouth, throat and oesophagus. But few epidemiologists in the Western world were inclined to consider whether dietary imbalances might influence risks of prominent cancers, such as those of bowel, breast, lung and prostate. That was a time when the laboratory-based model of chemical carcinogenesis prevailed: cancer was regarded as the result of specific chemical or physical (e.g., radiation) factors that damaged the genetic material of cells, occasionally causing some of them to become uncontrollably malignant.

The diet-cancer connection was put on a firmer footing in the 1970s following several broad-brush epidemiological analyses of diet-related trends and fault-lines in international cancer patterns.[29] Dennis Burkitt, mentioned earlier in this chapter, concluded from his observations in Africa that the Western high-fat low-fibre diet caused various 'diseases of Western civilisation', including large bowel cancer. An immediate consequence of this was that the causation of large bowel cancer was viewed afresh, as likely to reflect the physical, biochemical and bacteriological consequences of insufficient dietary fibre – the complex carbohydrate material that partially undergoes bacterial fermentation within the colon. Cancer-inducing chemicals, if present in the fibre-deficient digested material, would be less diluted, would move more slowly within the bowel, and would thus come into greater contact with epithelial cells of the bowel lining. Further, the species profile of the billions of bacteria in the colon would be disturbed by the change in their own carbohydrate dietary fare. This change in bacterial demography would alter the chemical characteristics of the faecal material and the fermentative production of volatile fatty acids (some of which appear to stabilise colon epithelial cells against excessive proliferation). Some of the 'functional foods' in modern supermarkets, such as 'live' yoghurt with lactobacillus, purport to maintain a healthy profile of gut bacterial species.

At about the same time it was becoming clear that another major cancer of economically developed countries, breast cancer, was predominantly due to hormonal influences. There was diverse evidence at both international and local levels. Low and high risk populations of women have different sex hormonal profiles. As Japanese migrant women in America underwent increased risks of breast cancer so their hormone profile changed. Individual women in developed countries with breast cancer, compared to cancer-free women, tended to have begun having children at an older age and to have had fewer children, an earlier onset of menstruation, higher endogenous oestrogen levels, and greater body weight. Further, experiments in healthy adult women showed that a change in dietary fat intake, or in alcohol consumption, affected the sex hormone profile; while, similarly, vegetarian and meat-eating women had different levels of active oestrogenic hormones. Overall, there is broad evidence that breast cancer and cancers of the endometrium and prostate are influenced by sex hormones, insulin and other hormones – and those, in turn, by diet, physical activity level and obesity. In large part, then, changes in the incidence of these cancers reflect changes in human ecology.

So, over the final quarter of the twentieth century, a more integrative, biologically based view of the causation of cancer emerged. Clearly, chemical carcinogens are important causal factors in many cancers – chemicals encountered in cigarette smoke, in the workplace, and perhaps in contaminated drinking water, urban air and overcooked meat. But, increasingly, cancer is viewed as a disease caused by shifts in the normal checks and balances on the cell's genetic integrity, proliferation and programmed cell death ('apoptosis'). That is, the proliferation of mutant cells can be facilitated by subtle shifts in the biochemical and hormonal milieu. This perception of cancer and its causation has led us to consider cancer prevention within a wider ecological context. Hence, our ideas about dietary strategies to reduce cancer incidence now focus more on seeking a better balance of foods and nutrients. This is the dominant theme in the conclusions of the comprehensive international report on diet and cancer published in 1997 by the World Cancer Research Fund. That report, compiled over four years by a panel of fifteen cancer scientists from nine diverse countries, concluded that the overall cancer rates could be reduced by the reorienting of national cuisines towards a diet based on foods of plant origin.[30]

THE DIET-AND-CANCER story remains incomplete and complex. We have identified various dietary risk factors, biological mechanisms, and the importance of age of dietary exposure. But as well as seeking specific carcinogenic culprits in the diet there is a need to identify the *type* of diet which, on balance, alters the overall risk of cancer. For example, is the traditional Mediterranean diet a low-risk diet relative to others in the Western world? Likewise, the vegetarian diet? Perhaps dietary diversity *per se* may hold the key. Agrarian diets in poor rural populations around the world are typically monotonous and limited, and are therefore a likely source of increased cancer risk because of micronutrient deficiencies which impair cellular stability, antioxidant defences and repair mechanisms.[31]

There is, too, a larger evolutionary framework within which to consider diet and cancer. Oxygen, released by plant photosynthesis, has accumulated in the atmosphere during the second half of Earth's existence. This oxygen has proven a double-edged sword. On the one hand, having decimated earlier anaerobic life-forms, it then allowed the evolution of more efficient, aerobic, metabolism. On the other hand, oxygen's high reactivity can damage macromolecules. Terrestrial plants have therefore evolved antioxidant defences against this oxidative assault. This metabolic armour depends on certain elements (such as selenium and zinc) and on the synthesis of complex molecules (vitamins A, C and E). Not surprisingly, many of these micronutrient elements and vitamins have also become, through coevolution, the 'passive' antioxidant defences of the animals that eat those plants. Leaves and ripening fruits, being the metabolically active parts of the plant, contain high levels of antioxidant vitamins. In contrast, seeds comprise dormant genetic material and energy stores, with typically lower antioxidant concentrations. Because the primate-hominoid diet that shaped human biology was mostly one of (antioxidant-rich) leafy vegetables and fruit, it is a reasonable prediction that human health will be served optimally by a diet high in antioxidants. Yet most modern human populations have a relatively low intake of fresh fruits and vegetables. Hence, the daily oxidative assault from our oxygenated environment may be less well countered, thereby increasing the risk of carcinogenesis. This may help explain the now compelling evidence that a high intake of fruit and vegetables reduces the risk of many types of cancers.[32]

Globalisation, commodities and health: the larger view

It is clear that altered patterns of living and consumption reflect social and economic change in society at large. That change is now occurring on a larger scale as various globalising processes influence populations everywhere. 'Globalisation' refers to the various contemporary processes of increasing global interconnectedness. Economic globalisation and the rise of liberalised markets in international trade and investment is a central feature. Two other important domains are technological globalisation, especially of information and communication technologies, and cultural globalisation, entailing the dissemination of dominant ideas, images and values. Globally coordinated advertising, transnational media ownership, technological innovation and new international marketing opportunities, in conjunction with urbanisation, are increasingly driving modern consumer behaviours.

The balance-sheet of gains and losses to population health from globalisation is complex, and includes both the benefits of wealth creation and the nexus between these processes and the large-scale environmental changes that humans are now imparting to the ecosphere.[33] Many traditional, locally attuned, health-supporting 'wisdoms' with respect to diets, physical activity patterns, local crafts and so on have been jeopardised by aspects of globalisation. The phenomenon is well exemplified by the intensified, and often devious, global promotion of tobacco products.

Cigarettes into the Third World and Central and Eastern Europe

It would be remiss to finish this chapter without a brief look at the origins and now the globalisation of one of the great modern changes in human behaviour and one that is a scourge of population health everywhere. Historians will look back with some fascinated incredulity at the spread of cigarette smoking in the twentieth century. They will see several threads to this calamitous story: the power of biological addiction, the limp and ineffective attempts by revenue-dependent governments to curb smoking, and the immoral and dishonest role played by the powerful and wealthy tobacco industry.[34] They may be surprised at how many of us, at least via our pension funds, were shareholders in this death-dealing industry.

Tobacco, for use as snuff and in pipe smoking, was introduced into England in the early seventeenth century, following the early American colonial investments in tobacco growing in Virginia. However, it was to take a further two centuries before the idea of cigarettes emerged in Europe and North America, and three centuries before cigarettes became available as a mass-produced item. During the French Revolution the masses defied the aristocratic affectation of using nasal snuff by smoking little hand-rolled cigars – or 'cigarettes'. By the 1850s, Turkish-rolled cigarettes were being sold by the fledgling Philip Morris company in England, and cigarettes became available to British troops in the Crimean War. Before long, several entrepreneurial Americans recruited skilled cigarette rollers from Europe. Soon the automated Bonsack cigarette-making machine had been invented, and this, in the astute business hands of James Buchanan Duke, led quickly to a massive increase in cigarette production and huge commercial profits. Intense politicking followed in the first decade of the twentieth century. The US Congress, petitioned by objectors, declared itself unable to constrain this new alleged health hazard. The Anti-Smoking League grew in strength; yet nicotine was removed from the control of the Food and Drug Administration. Fifteen US states banned the sale of cigarettes for health reasons.[35]

The modern mass-produced cigarette, however, was already on the move. By 1918 there was an entire generation of addicted young men in Britain and the United States who had received cigarettes while fighting World War I. General Pershing had petitioned the US authorities for extra cigarettes and bullets for the US army. By the 1920s cigarette smoking was established as normal adult behaviour in Western society – and a status symbol for the fast set. Within several decades manufactured cigarettes far out-numbered handrolled cigarettes. The foundations for one of the twentieth century's greatest public health scourges had thus been laid. One out of every two cigarette smokers dies prematurely from a tobacco-related disease.

By the end of the twentieth century smoking was causing an estimated 4 million deaths per year, rising to a projected 10 million deaths per year by 2020.[17] Of today's 1.2 billion smokers, more than four of every five live in low- and middle-income countries. Meanwhile, the tobacco transnationals are pushing deeper into the new and lucrative markets of the Third World and Central and Eastern Europe, aided by the modern world's socially and environmentally blinkered 'free trade' rules.[36] The tobacco industry has other powerful allies. Thailand's attempts in the late 1990s to resist the entry of the international tobacco industry provoked strong-arm threats of trade sanctions by the US Government, acting on behalf of powerful US tobacco interests (who have 'invested' heavily in the US Congress).

The acceptance by Britain's prestigious Cambridge University, in 1996, of a Chair of International Relations endowed by the British American Tobacco company is a measure of the extent to which such corporate interests and their values – even an industry as notoriously dishonest and manipulative as the tobacco industry – are becoming integrated into the social and political fabric of modern, market-driven society. There is now extensive evidence indicating that British American Tobacco, in 2000, was involved during the 1990s in the international smuggling of cigarettes, thereby avoiding import taxes.[37] One wonders what Cambridge University's professor of international relations would make of this.

Conclusion

The accrual of wealth, increasing access to energy sources, new modes of transport and communication, greater literacy, increased life expectancy and the rise of urban consumerism have transformed our ways of living in modern societies. Changes in reproductive behaviour, diets, levels of physical activity, and the mass use of addictive substances have been at the heart of the 'lifestyle revolution' in Western populations. In the light of a half-century of increasingly sophisticated and wide-ranging epidemiological research we have a much better understanding of the ways in which these consumption patterns, behaviours and urban environmental circumstances affect the risks of non-communicable diseases.

This knowledge, applied at the population level, can help us understand the panoramic changes in patterns of health and disease around the world in recent times. Meanwhile, there are other, deeper currents that influence the tides of health and disease. One such underlying influence is that of urbanisation – the progressive shift of human populations away from countryside and village and into towns and cities. This has become a defining characteristic of modern human ecology. It, too, has great consequences for patterns of health and disease, and is the subject of the next chapter.

9

Cities, social environments and synapses

> If we still believe that cities are the most complicated artifact we have created, if we believe further that they are cumulative, generational artifacts that harbor our values as a community and provide us with the setting where we can learn to live together, then it is our collective responsibility to guide their design.   Kostoff S, 1991[1]

Towns and cities are at the heart of human history. Even so, they are a relatively recent product of cultural evolution, and a radical transformation of the human habitat. As urbanisation gathers momentum around the world, the urban environment increasingly dominates the landscape of human social interactions and physical exposures. Life in cities presents a complex profile of gains and losses for human health.

Settled living first occurred in the Fertile Crescent of the Middle East as early agrarianism emerged. The consequences for infectious diseases and nutritional disorders have been explored in chapters 4 and 5. Equally importantly, the advent of settled agrarian living transformed humankind's social and economic relations, resulting particularly in the concept of 'property' – occupied farm-land, permanent dwellings, and a local market for exchanging surplus products. As rural settlements grew into larger villages, the increasing productivity of the land allowed the development of social stratification. As Charles Darwin remarked in his journal, commenting on the equality that he observed in the primitive inhabitants of Tierra del Fuego during his voyage on the Beagle: 'It is difficult to understand how a chief can arise till there is property of some sort by which he might manifest his superiority and increase his power.'[2]

Towns first formed around 7,000 years ago in the Fertile Crescent, soon to be followed by the emergence of large cities and city-states. In the land of Sumer (the Kuwait and southern Iraq of today) the organisation of urban society was accompanied by the beginnings of monumental architecture, sculpture, cylindrical seals for authenticating accounts on clay tablets, and, around 5,000 years ago, the world's first writing. These early Mesopotamian cities, such as Ur, Uruk and Babylon, were the seat of centralised hierarchical societies in which rulers, priests, scholars, soldiers, bureaucrats, technicians and artisans lived in a symbiosis with a large, subordinate and impoverished peasantry. Early Mesopotamian artwork portrays the 'priest-king' in diverse poses: in prayer, as victorious warrior, or as ensuring the abundance of the harvest and the fecundity of livestock.

By around 3,000 years ago there were only four cities in the world with an estimated 50,000 or more inhabitants, including Thebes and Memphis in Egypt. By 2,000 years ago, when world population approximated 200 million people, there were still only about 40 such cities. Most of humankind continued to live in rural villages until the new European forces of mercantilism, industrialisation and intercontinental imperialism thrust city living to the fore. Even so, less than 5% of world population lived in urban environments in 1800. Today, however, this figure has reached 50% and by 2030 the proportion will be 65%.

This ongoing move from countryside to city is as momentous a change in human ecology as was the ancient move from hunter-gatherer itinerancy to agrarian settlement. The current worldwide migration into cities reflects various factors: the lure of jobs, the contraction of rural employment in the face of increasingly mechanised food production, the flight from food insecurity and other forms of insecurity, and the search for variety and stimulation. Cities, despite their crowds, aggravations, squalor and hazards, remain centres of glamour, wealth, dreams and hope. Urbanisation may also reflect a basic social instinct. Humans, with their emotions, speech and cognition, are evolutionarily oriented to social existence and the sharing of experiences. Anthropologists tell us, however, that the functional interactive group size for hunter-gatherer humans is no more than 100–200.[3] Aristotle, too, doubted 'if a very populous city can ever be properly governed'. Nevertheless, via our various legal, moral and technical reinforcements, we mostly manage to live satisfactorily in these large and complex communities.

Cities are a cultural artefact, occurring late in humankind's story. We thus differ from other social creatures such as ants, bees and termites. The winnowing processes of natural selection have imbued those organisms with a hardwired instinct for building their 'cities'. For example, each of the giant termite mounds that stand 3–4 metres tall in northern Australia is the product of programmed construction by tens of thousands of toiling termites. Elliptical in cross-section, the mounds are oriented side-on to minimise exposure to the midday sun. The vertical ribbing maximises the cooling effect of passing breezes. The termites are not experimenting, nor are they casually improvising; they are doing the bidding of their genes. We humans, however, carry no genes for city building. Through inspiration, trial-and-error and the evolution of technology, we have found how to live in settled communities, build houses and large public buildings, transport ourselves around our cities, import and distribute food and material needs, and dispose of wastes.

THE URBAN ENVIRONMENT is a spontaneous, changeable and historically unfamiliar habitat. We continue to reinvent ways of city living. It is therefore no surprise that cities pose an array of risks and benefits to health and wellbeing. In the twentieth century we looked back at nineteenth century European cities, with their inner-city cesspools and their dark satanic mills, with fascinated horror. Later in the twenty-first century our successors may well look back with similar bemusement on the huge, largely treeless, major cities of the late twentieth century, congested with private motor cars and veiled in air pollutants. They may also be struck by the massive 'ecological footprints' of today's cities, with their high levels of consumption and waste generation.

Cities provide physical security, cultural and social diversity, excitement and fulfilment. They are the dominant source of employment in modern economies. They can improve access to health-care and schooling. Urban living typically reshapes family and social relations, and offers extensive contact networks. However, in sprawling Third World shanty towns life is often crowded, unhygienic and physically precarious. Cities also create the possibility of mass consumer markets. Urban populations represent vast captive markets, easily reached by advertising, recruited into patterned behaviours, subject to peer-consumer pressures and enticed to visit seductive shopping malls. This urban consumerism has many health consequences, as dietary patterns change, levels of physical activity decline, smoking rates increase and, for poorer people, as the sense of relative material deprivation is heightened.

The modern era of urbanisation began in Europe and North America. However, most of the change is now going on in non-Western countries. The majority of the world's very large cities with populations over 15 million are in poorer countries such as India, Pakistan, China and Brazil. Mexico City now has over 20 million inhabitants, 4 million cars and perhaps the world's worst air pollution. When the pollutant levels become too high in Mexico City industrial production is halted and people are urged to stay indoors. This, however, is just one of many health hazards of the contemporary urban environment. Many large Third World cities have vast, struggling urban-fringe populations that typically face a double health jeopardy – first, the diseases of poverty, especially infections, injury, the hazards of unsafe drinking water, solid waste accumulation and toxic wastes;[4] and second, the chronic adult health disorders and diseases that result from the late-industrial urban lifestyle, such as obesity, diabetes, heart disease and lung cancer. In 1996 the UN Centre for Human Settlements said of sub-Saharan Africa in its *Global Report on Human Settlements*:

the deterioration in the built environment is sharply in evidence throughout most of urban Africa. As more of the urban population was forced into unplanned settlements on the outskirts of large cities, or into more crowded living space in an already deteriorating housing stock in the more established 'high density' areas; as a lower proportion of the populations had direct access to clean, piped water, regular garbage disposal and good health services, the quality of life for the vast majority of the population deteriorated during the 1980s and 1990s.[5]

Over the next three decades 2 billion more people will be added to the world's urban population. The volume of resources consumed and of pollution created will grow exponentially. Yet it is likely that half of this expanding urban population will be living in shanty towns, without running water, electricity or sanitation. The environmental, social and public health problems graphically described above for African cities exist also in many large cities of Latin America and Asia. On current trends, therefore, the proliferation of urban populations portends additional environmental pollution, massive pressures on adjoining and distant ecosystems, a continuation of the diseases of poverty, and a world polarised into very rich and very poor. On an optimistic view, emerging trends in economic liberalisation and political transparency may lead to material advances and to reductions in poverty. In reality it appears that economic globalisation, in its current form, is widening the rich–poor gap, increasing employment insecurity, and extending urban slums and shantytowns.

Beyond these material problems there is the interesting question as to the suitability of cities as the social, emotional and spiritual habitat for a species whose Pleistocene genes have attuned it to open spaces, trees, grasslands, personalised contact networks and the presence of other animal species.[6] Do suburban gardens (or window boxes) and the family dog provide sufficient compensation? In the 1890s the pioneering sociologist Emile Durkheim wrote of the anomie and alienation that is the experience of many urban dwellers.[7] Today's social scientists continue to debate the optimal size and form of cities, having generally agreed that the scale of modern cities is not appropriate to human social and biological needs. Among urban planners and urban dwellers there is now increasing discussion of the ideas of liveability and sustainability. The broader issues of how social environments influence patterns of health and disease will be discussed, albeit briefly, later in this chapter.

Industrialisation, cities and health: recent history

The history of urbanisation and human health is well illustrated by Great Britain, the first country to begin industrialising. As England's larger cities underwent a rapid population growth in the late eighteenth and early nineteenth centuries, a new underclass of powerless factory workers and their families was created, drawing particularly on dispossessed rural workers. As noted in earlier chapters, conditions in the cities were squalid, malnutrition was widespread, infectious diseases rife and death rates typically exceeded birth rates. Nevertheless, urban populations were able to expand because of immigration from the countryside – where the impacts of closure of the commons, the aggregation of landholdings and the mechanisation of agriculture had produced an earlier impoverished underclass. This continued stream of rural immigrants, coming from environments in which they had been much less exposed to the 'crowd' infectious diseases of childhood, replenished the urban pool of young adults at risk of early death.

The first urban public health crisis, in 1840s England, prompted the creation of the Health of Towns Commission. This, as we saw in chapter 6, was linked to Edwin Chadwick's drive for urban sanitation along with other public health legislation in mid-nineteenth-century England. Meanwhile there were advances in nutrition, housing, general social modernisation and other important public health interventions such as smallpox vaccination. These advances, as we saw in chapter 7, dramatically reduced deaths from infectious diseases. These health-enhancing urban planning ideas were carried forward by Benjamin Ward Richardson, an English physician-sanitarian. In 1875, he proposed 'Hygeia', the ideal city with a population of no more than 100,000 persons, medium-density settlement, well-ventilated smoke-free housing, networked sewers, tree-lined streets, parks, public transport and community-based facilities for the sick and disabled.[8] Richardson's ideas were influential in both Britain and North America. Accordingly, the Canadian government's Commission on Conservation aspired to cities that were both pleasant and health-promoting. Toronto in the 1920s, for example, undertook systematic city-wide pasteurisation of milk supplies, chlorination of drinking water supplies and educational programmes in 'municipal housekeeping' (family hygiene, sanitation, nutrition and child-rearing).

With industrialisation, cities throughout the Western world began to expand. In earlier centuries, cities had been more compact. They were often circumscribed by fortified walls, and had much smaller populations. Mediaeval London accounted for a mere 700 acres. The visitor to Italian cities such as Florence or Siena readily senses the original human scale of those old walled cities. The public buildings, churches, main piazzas, galleries and museums are all within a 15-minute walk of one another. These, like Athens and Rome, were 'walking cities'. As industrialisation advanced in nineteenth-century Europe the influx of rural poor impelled many middle- and upper-class people to move out to newer, more salubrious suburbs, serviced by radial roads, horse-drawn street-cars and railways. In this process, particularly evident in England, lay the origin of suburban sprawl.

Late in the nineteenth century, electrification appeared. In the United States in 1890, around 80% of urban railways were horse-drawn. By 1900 the proportion had shrunk precipitously to around 1% as electrified tram and light-rail systems took over. Whereas London had begun building its steam-engine undergound railway in the 1860s, from around 1900 other Western cities built electrified underground railways which enabled rapid movement of even larger numbers of people. City life was becoming more energy intensive; urbanism was gaining momentum. The urban mortality penalty was receding. Gains in life expectancy, reflecting the greater numbers surviving childhood, now allowed urban populations to grow of their own accord, no longer dependent on rural replenishment.

THE EARLY TWENTIETH century saw suburban sprawl continued, assisted by the extension of suburban railway systems. As factories relocated towards the periphery of cities, the non-residential city centre became transformed into a hub of financial and commercial activity. The residential flight to the suburbs continued, soon to be abetted by the advent of the private motor car. In the United States in the 1930s, urban mass transit systems were purchased and then dismantled by a conspiratorial cartel of car manufacturers. The future of American cities was thereby secured for the private motor car. 'Automobile cities' had arrived. Indeed, the foundations for a century of automobile-dependent city growth had already been laid.[9] The long and harrowing history of urban epidemics and their associated miasmas had imbued town planners with a fear of crowded living. Likewise, the squalid environmental hazards of early industry and food processing had led to a preference for keeping housing, factories and markets apart. Where possible, then, low-density urban development was favoured, with differentiation of zones. Here was the inspiration for the auto-dependent cities of North America and Australia.

The striving for healthy cities in Western countries dissipated during the 1930s recession and World War II, and was then overshadowed by the prosperous post-war era of automated production, industrial expansion and mass consumerism. Consequently, the quality of the urban environment in developed countries declined. Investment in public transport contracted; indeed, over half of downtown Los Angeles is now occupied by streets, freeways, parking facilities and garages. During the 1980s and 1990s the decline of inner-city areas and public housing estates created major social problems. Rising unemployment, persistent pockets of poverty, a contraction in social services and urban infrastructural decay all contributed to an environment where alienation and violence naturally arise. In contemporary New York and London around 1% of the population 'sleep rough' on the streets or in emergency shelters. The combination of a vulnerable underclass, structural unemployment, well-organised criminal networks and increasing supplies of high-grade heroin and cocaine from rural Third World sources has triggered a rising epidemic of drug addiction, accompanied by increases in property crime and infectious disease transmission.

The resultant residential decline of the inner city is now being widely countered, in developed countries, by inner-urban renewal programmes. However, unless done in a varied and socially equitable fashion, urban renewal may simply reverse the residential relationship of rich and poor, consigning the disadvantaged to the remote outer suburbs, underserviced by public transport.

Overall, then, we are at a crossroads in our planning and management of cities. Urbanisation has occurred over the past several centuries in response to mercantilism, industrialisation and the labour-saving mechanisation of agriculture. The move to live and work within large urban-suburban environments has been made possible by fossil fuels, electrification and motorised transport. Modern communications and the international deregulation of trade and financial transactions have further boosted the role of cities as the hub of globalised private enterprise. Meanwhile, for many people in the developed world city life has become more difficult, more stressful and less conducive to good health.

The health impacts of urbanisation

The range of urban environmental influences on health is great. The benefits of ready access to health care and educational facilities have been noted earlier in this chapter. The historical deficit in life expectancy in industrialising cities relative to surrounding rural populations has been eliminated in high-income countries. Nevertheless, there are many characteristics of contemporary city life that increase the risks of various diseases and health disorders.

The urban environment potentiates the spread of infectious diseases via crowding, patterns of human mobility and contact (sexual and other), and the persistence and spread of unhygienic conditions in slums and shanty-towns. Research in Kwa-Zulu Natal, South Africa, has shown that the vector-borne infection schistosomiasis, which spreads via infected water-snails, is infiltrating into urban areas via the migration of the rural population to shanty towns around the cities. Similarly, rural-to-city migration and insanitary living conditions have caused filariasis (elephantiasis), a disease transmitted by mosquitoes that breed in contaminated pools of water, to spread in Recife in northeast Brazil. Cities also affect patterns of infectious diseases in the developed world, especially sexually transmitted infections and the poverty-associated diseases such as tuberculosis and cholera. The incidence of childhood tuberculosis in the residentially crowded sections of the Bronx in New York City is six times higher than the city's average, while in London tuberculosis rates are markedly higher in the unemployed and in those living in cheap rented accommodation.

Urban living also influences a number of non-infectious diseases. The worldwide increase in obesity discussed in chapter 8 is essentially a manifestation of urban living, combining reduced physical activity with more abundant energy-dense diets. Such diets, along with increased mechanisation in the workplace affect body weight, blood pressure and other precursors of cardiovascular disease. Research in Kenya, for example, has shown that, when people move from rural western Kenya to Nairobi, their blood pressure increases as do their weight and dietary salt intake.[10] Cities can amplify social isolation, contributing to the depression that often accompanies old age. Cities also contain nodes of violence, criminality and drug dependence among the poorer, jobless and socially marginalised sub-populations. For such reasons, adult life expectancy among black men in Harlem, New York, is less than in men in Bangladesh.

Many of these influences on health can be viewed within the larger framework of urban human ecology. Of particular interest are the more systemic aspects of the urban environment that, by acting at the population level, affect the *rates* of disease or death in the urban population overall. An example, pre-viously mentioned in chapter 1, is that of the relationship between heatwaves, the form of cities and the resultant excess mortality. The conventional (and perfectly respectable) question that an epidemiologist might ask is: 'What type of individual is most likely to die during a heatwave?' Meanwhile, at the collec-tive population level, an equally interesting question is: 'What characteristics of the urban environment influence the extent of excess mortality during a heat-wave?' The two questions are complementary; they address different phenom-ena, at different levels. The latter question is overtly an 'ecological' enquiry about the characteristics of the human urban habitat that increase the popu-lation's vulnerability to thermal stress. It holds the promise of genuine and long-term primary prevention of excess mortality, via improvements in the design of cities.

A few more details about the relationship between heatwaves and mortality will illustrate how various aspects of urban ecology influence patterns of health.

Heatwaves and mortality: systemic versus individual factors

The Pleistocene hunter-gatherers in equatorial Africa lived in a reasonably equable climate. The subsequent human colonisation of other continents exposed populations to a great variety of climatic regimes, often with strong seasonal contrasts. Houses, settled living and the growth of cities have enabled some modulation of exposures to those weather extremes. However, many of today's large cities tend to amplify extremes of temperature. In particular a 'heat island' effect occurs in summer, because of the expanse of brick-and-asphalt heat-retaining structures, the treeless expanses of inner cities and the physical obstruction of cooling breezes. Temperatures therefore tend to be several degrees centigrade higher in inner-city areas than in the leafier suburbs and the surrounding countryside, and night-time cooling is thereby dimin-ished. In winter the downtown area in some cities, with its street-canyons of tall buildings, funnels chilly winds which cause a further drop in temperature. This is sometimes called a 'cold island' effect.

Severe heatwaves typically cause a transient rise in the death rate, particu-larly in the elderly, the sick and the frail. Some of the deaths are due to heat stroke, when the body is unable to counter adequately the extreme heat load. Most of the deaths occur in persons with advanced heart or blood vessel disease or chronic lung disease. The mortality impact of heatwaves is typically greatest in the centre of large cities, where not only is the temperature highest but often the residents are poor and without air-conditioning.

In July of 1995, in the United States, more than 460 extra deaths over the course of a week were certified as due to the effects of the extreme heatwave in Chicago when temperatures reached 40°C. The rate of heat-related death was much greater in blacks than in whites, and in persons who were bed-ridden or otherwise confined in poorly ventilated inner-city apartment-block housing. One week later that same severe heatwave arrived in England and Wales where it caused a 10% excess of deaths during a 5-day period, particularly adult deaths from heart attack, stroke and respiratory disease. In Greater London, where daytime temperatures were higher and night-time relief was less than in the countryside, the mortality increased by around 15%. Concurrent rises in air pollution during the heatwave could account for no more than half of the excess deaths.[11]

Studies in both the United States and Europe have indicated that urban populations living at lower, warmer latitudes are less affected by summer heat extremes than are urban populations living further north. However, those northern populations are less affected by winter cold extremes. Each population is most vulnerable – because of housing design, clothing, behaviour and physiological adaptation – to seasonal weather extremes of the kind that is least familiar in that location. A further issue, from studies in the United States and Germany, is that over the past few decades urban populations in temperate zones have been experiencing progressively fewer excess deaths during summer heat extremes. This may reflect the increasing availability of air-conditioning. It may also reflect the decline, since around 1970, in the prevalence of cardiovascular disease, a major source of individual susceptibility to heatwaves. (If so, then populations in low-income countries, where coronary heart disease is now on the increase, may become *more* vulnerable to dying from heatwaves in future.)

Urban transport systems, cars and health

The character of modern cities has, as already noted, been substantially shaped by automobile dependence. Private car ownership and travel has increased spectacularly over the past half-century. This has undoubtedly created new freedoms and opportunities. By the year 2000 there was a total of 600 million cars in the world, plus 15 million commercial vehicles, increasing by around 10 million per year. China, with over 2 million cars, will have around 4 million by

2010. In the absence of affordable underground trains or light rail systems in cities in low-income countries, the demand for private cars is rapidly increasing. In São Paulo, where the population of 17 million now owns around 5 million cars, the proportion of motorised trips taken by car has doubled over the past quarter-century, from around 25% to 50%.

Our relationship to urban traffic is complex. Each driver reasons that if only other people would drive less, then he/she could drive more easily and enjoyably. Our cities have evolved through phases of dismantling tram systems, discontinuing light-rail services, blighting footpaths with parking meters, and building massive freeway systems. Now we attempt to counter the problem by creating inner-city pedestrian malls, restricting city parking, disfiguring the roads with traffic-calming bumps, and introducing road-pricing schemes that use toll-gates or high-tech electronic tolls. In cities in the Netherlands and Denmark the provision of extensive tracks and parking facilities for bicycles during the 1980s has greatly boosted cycling, and the proportion of daily journeys taken on foot or by bicycle is well above the European average.[9] The city of Portland, Oregon, voted in the early 1990s against putting a modern freeway through the city. Instead, they opted for a light-rail system and restrictions on downtown car-use. Today, as un-American as it might seem, the citizens of Portland are proud of their new public transport, clean air and lower-stress lifestyle.[9] Meanwhile, elsewhere, both manufacturer and consumer continue to conspire against the disincentives to private transport. In the United States 'dashboard dining' is becoming popular, as car design incorporates pull-out devices for holding coffee cups and macro-muffins to enable commuters to eat breakfast in the morning traffic jam. In car-paralysed central Bangkok wealthy commuters have television sets, telephones and toilets in their enlarged cars. In wealthy countries, many suburbanites aspire to an out-of-town image by driving absurdly large four-wheel drive vehicles, many of which go 'off-road' only when parked on the footpath besides an up-market clothing shop.

Urban transport systems have wide-ranging consequences for health.[12] Cars clearly confer certain health benefits. These include the greater safety of late-night transport (especially for women) and reduced social isolation for the elderly and other people who find public transport difficult to use. On balance, however, the impact of cars upon urban population health is negative. Urban traffic poses two major, well-recognised, public health hazards: physical trauma and air pollution. Globally, there is a rising toll of fatal and non-fatal injuries, affecting pedestrians, cyclists and car-users. There are approximately 1 million deaths from car crashes each year, most of them in developing countries. In developed countries, injuries and deaths on the roads are now declining, as the design of cars and roads improves, as seat-belts become mandatory and as drink-driving laws become tougher.

Exhaust-gas emissions contribute greatly to urban air pollution, particularly the formation of photochemical smog during summer. In Mexico City, for example, three-quarters of the air pollution is caused by motor vehicle exhaust. The wide range of documented health consequences reflects the diversity of pollutants: nitrogen oxides, fine particulates, carbon monoxide, various volatile organic chemicals and lead. Epidemiological studies indicate that these exhaust emissions increase the incidence of assorted respiratory diseases, including asthma attacks, and of coronary heart disease. The latter may be induced by the inhalation of very fine particulates which apparently cause inflammation of the respiratory epithelium, the resultant release of acute-phase proteins into the bloodstream and, hence, an increased tendency of blood to clot. In low-income countries, lead emissions from leaded gasoline remain a cause of impaired child intellectual development. The study of these various health impacts is difficult since air pollution is a complex exposure, the measurement of cumulative personal exposure is difficult, and coexistent risk factors such as smoking and occupational exposures abound. Further, levels of urban air pollution change over time: in many high-income countries, exhaust emissions are falling (as shown in the downward slope of graph B in Figure 6.1), whereas they are rising in most lower-income countries as urban traffic proliferates in the presence of less stringent environmental standards.

There are several less-well-recognised health impacts of cars. They cause fragmentation of neighbourhoods and intrusive noise. Sleep disturbance near roads and highways is a common complaint and source of mental stress. As discussed in chapter 8, increasing reliance on cars has reduced the level of physical activity, causing a rise in obesity in urban populations. It is not surprising that the Dutch, who have restricted their car use in favour of trams and bicycles, have both a manifest sense of urban community and Europe's flattest trendline in the rising prevalence of obesity over the past two decades.

In our redesign of cities in the twenty-first century, prime consideration must be given to the role and form of urban transport.[9] It is not just that motor vehicles have caused various types of adverse health impacts, along with physical and social environmental blight. They also contribute greatly to the mounting global pressures on the world's atmosphere and future climate. We have begun to solve the traffic-associated public health problems of road trauma and noxious exhaust gas emissions. We have yet to solve the problems of physical inactivity and greenhouse gas emissions. Solutions will depend on lessening the need for private motoring, switching to non-carbon fuels, and creating convenient public transport systems.

The urban environment and mental health

The nineteenth-century American philosopher Henry David Thoreau said that cities are places where millions of people are lonely together. While this is rather an over-statement, much anecdotal and survey evidence indicates that many city-dwellers do not feel engaged in a community; they feel disconnected from other people. Migration from countryside to city usually entails moving from a rural community-type society to an urban association-type society. The former is conservative, hierarchical and stable; it entails extended kinship and long-term friends. Association-type life in the cities brings social fluidity and more liberty; friendships are often ephemeral, and the sense of community is typically reduced.

An important and general influence on population health is the form and extent of social cohesion. At the individual level, it has long been evident that access to social networks and social support influences a person's prospects for good health and survival. Now we are beginning to understand how, at the group level, both social cohesion and the levels of material assets and equity can influence the population's overall health. That topic is considered further in the next section. First, though, how does the urban environment affect the pattern of mental health disorders?

Among city-dwellers, it is the poor, the socially marginalised and the isolated who are particularly vulnerable to mental disorders.[13] Many studies in North American cities have shown that the contour of mental disorders closely follows the contour of poverty in inner city areas. On the one hand, crowding and lack of privacy and control over one's living space may cause aggressive behaviour, child and spouse abuse, or drug and alcohol abuse. On the other hand, isolation and loneliness, without family or social support, may cause depression, suicide or drug and alcohol abuse. However, caution is needed here. First, causality might be 'in reverse'. Individuals with mental disorders may become detached from friends and community. Longitudinal studies are therefore required to clarify the sequence of events. Second, the diagnostic classification of mental health disorders is often difficult, and culture-dependent. Many researchers have assumed that the incidence of major psychiatric illnesses varies little between populations and cultures, even though the profile of symptoms may differ.

Recent studies, however, indicate that the occurrence of mental health disorders depends greatly on the cultural, social and economic context.

In developed countries, higher rates of psychiatric disorders have generally been reported in urban versus rural populations. In contrast, some studies in developing countries have found higher rates of psychiatric morbidity in rural than in urban populations – as, for example, have been reported for China and Taiwan.[13] If these urban-versus-rural differences are real, might they reflect differential probabilities of migration between city and country according to the individual's mental health status? In fact there is some evidence of a tendency for restless, agitated and psychotic people to move from rural districts to city centres, where anonymity may fulfil a desire for social isolation.[14]

Several studies have found a higher prevalence of schizophrenia in urban populations than in rural populations. This, some argue, is because of the 'geographical drift' of pre-schizophrenics into the cities. However, a large study of 50,000 Swedish army recruits showed that the incidence of schizophrenia is two-thirds higher among young men brought up in cities compared to those with a rural upbringing – indeed, the risk of schizophrenia was proportional to the size of town of upbringing.[15] What sort of environmental factor causes schizophrenia? This remains contentious, although apparently some aspect of the early-life social environment imprints upon the immature brain.[16] Whatever the actual causal factor, the origins of schizophrenia almost certainly entail an interaction between genes and environment. The notion of a 'nature versus nurture' dichotomy is misleading (as Shakespeare recognised in *The Tempest* in describing the anti-social and menacing Caliban as one 'upon whose nature nurture will not stick').

Neurological studies reveal that, in schizophrenics, part of the prefrontal cortex (the most recently evolved grey matter, acquired by the *Homo* lineage in the past half-million years) is imperfectly linked with other cortical and limbic system centres. This deficient neural linkage impairs cognitive coherence. Various other anti-social behaviours reflect disordered functioning of the brain's limbic system, the neural circuitry that controls how we emote, experience sensations and remember. Perhaps it is not surprising that the enormous complexity of our recently evolved cerebral cortex, especially the prefrontal cortex and its myriad connections, results in occasional malfunctions. Many of evolution's improvisations are imperfect. While disorders of the psyche are disabling for the individual – and discomforting for family and friends – yet, considered at the population level, this might be viewed as a small price for the human species to pay for the wonders and benefits of the unique *virtual reality* that constitutes human consciousness. In other words, we incur the hazards of neurological complexity in return for the facilities of abstract thought, artistic creativity, interpreting the ideas and intentions of others, imagining other scenarios and planning the future.[17] Clearly, natural selection has allowed the human species to pay that price.

Ecological footprints of urban populations

Cities also impinge on human health via a larger-scale and less immediate pathway. Since urbanism entails intensified and concentrated economic activity, cities have a great impact on the wider environment. There are, of course, major ecological benefits of city living: cities confer economies of scale, of proximity and of the shared use of resources. However, life in today's cities entails great 'externalities'. Urban populations depend on food grown elsewhere, on raw materials extracted from elsewhere, and on having their wastes disposed of elsewhere. Cities, as ecosystems, thus have inputs of energy and materials and outputs of waste; they have a large 'ecological footprint'.[18] Oil and gas supplies usually come from distant sources. Londoners drink wine from southern Australia, South Africa and Latin America. In Tokyo the disposable chopsticks come from the Malaysian jungles. So, too, the year-round fresh fruits and vegetables that modern affluent Western consumers now take for granted: the out-of-season green beans from Kenya and citrus fruit from Brazil. The population of 4 million in Sydney, Australia, consumes approximately 1 million tonnes of food annually, almost 1 billion tonnes of water, and generates 500 million tonnes of sewage and 35 million tonnes of carbon dioxide.[9]

A study of the environmental resources – wood, paper, fibre, food (including seafood) and waste-absorbing 'sinks' – consumed by 29 cities of the Baltic Sea region is illustrative.[19] For supplies, those cities depend upon a total area of forest, arable land and marine ecosystems several hundred times greater than the total area of the cities. A similarly large area is required to absorb the wastes. In Vancouver, Canada, the almost half-million residents, occupying just 11,400 hectares, actually require the ecological services of 2.3 million hectares (Table 9.1).[18] The ratio of 207:1 for the 'overshoot' of the urban population is substantially greater than the ratio of 12:1 for the population of the parent region, the Lower Fraser Basin as a whole. Neither ratio would be sustainable if applied to the world population.[20]

The externalities of urban living include increasing contributions to the world's problems of greenhouse gas accumulation, stratospheric ozone deple-

Table 9.1. Ecological footprints of Vancouver and the Lower Fraser Basin, Canada

Geographic unit	Population	Land area (hectares) (a)	Ecologial Footprint (hectares) (b)	Overshoot Factor (b/a)
Vancouver City	472,000	11,400	2,360,600	207
Lower Fraser Basin	2,000,000	830,000	10,000,000	12

Source: Rees W, 1996[18]

tion, land alienation and degradation, and coastal zone destruction. The urbanised developed world, with one-fifth of world population, accounts for three-quarters of all greenhouse gas emissions. Contemporary urbanism is thus contributing mightily to the process of global environmental changes – and, as we shall see in chapter 10, this jeopardises the health of current and future generations.

The social environment, inequalities and health

The social and economic conditions of life have a fundamental influence on health. This may sound rather obvious. After all, we know that impoverished and poorly educated African populations have particularly high rates of HIV/AIDS, that suicide rates go up when unemployment levels go up, and that in each society poor people die younger than the rich. Nevertheless, much of the research that epidemiologists do, and much of the popular discussion about health and disease, is about the risks incurred by individuals because of their specific personal behaviours or exposures, such as cigarette smoking, occupational asbestos exposure, mobile phone use and eating high-fat diets. We rarely stand back from the detail and assess the larger contextual influences on the health of communities or whole populations.

This focus on individual risks to health reflects the priorities of contemporary epidemiology (as discussed in chapter 8). Most of that discipline's modern methods have developed in the United States, where the prevailing view of 'society' is somewhat reminiscent of Margaret Thatcher's remark in the 1980s that there is no such thing as society *per se*; there are only individuals and families. The emphasis is on the individual. Hence, in much recent epidemiological research the focus of attention has been on individual free-range consumers who are assumed to exercise personal choices in the market-place, on the roads and in bed. There has been less interest in studying the more elusive, but more fundamental, social influences on the health of populations.[21]

During the 1990s a lively debate arose among epidemiologists over the appropriate focus of research into the causes of disease. Should the epidemiologists' task include asking distal ('upstream') questions about the social, cultural and economic determinants of health? After all, the proximal ('downstream') risk factors such as cigarette smoking and unsafe sex are not randomly distributed within the population. Different groups within society therefore incur different risks because of their particular circumstances: their material conditions, level of disposable income, personal autonomy, value systems, peer and commercial pressures, knowledge and attitudes.[22] This is not a new idea, but it is one that has been somewhat eclipsed in recent years. The sociologist Emile Durkheim proposed in the late nineteenth century that it was a society's characteristics at large that determined the suicide rate.[23] The rate, he said, was not simply the aggregate of individual suicidal tendencies. Rather, it reflected characteristics of the population: the underlying social values, the types of social relations, and the moral significance accorded to the act of suicide. Individual-based explanations, said Durkheim, were inadequate.

There are two dimensions of complexity here that must be addressed by researchers. The first task refers to deciding on the appropriate level and type of analysis of disease causation. The second task refers to how we envisage the evolution of health risks over time; over the course of a life.

THE FIRST TASK, basically, is to get an appropriate balance between an emphasis on social (upstream) or behavioural and biological (downstream) processes. Here there is unresolved debate. In some respects these two levels of analysis are complementary, as we saw above in relation to studying heatwaves and mortality (and as we saw in chapter 8, in discussing the iterative relationship between epidemiological studies at population and individual levels). Likewise, at the population level, a generalised decline in the occurrence of early childhood infections may have predisposed recent generations of children to asthma, while, at the individual level, the determinants of asthma attack may be parental smoking or exposure to high local levels of ambient air pollution. However, one of the legacies of the biomedical model – which, as offspring of the 1880s germ theory, has dominated twentieth-century ideas about the causes and processes of disease – is the assumption that causation is specific and observable within the individual. Hence, there is an expectation that important causes of disease will both act at and have direct biomedical manifestations at the individual level.

The recently rejuvenated debate over the causes of socioeconomic inequalities in health, in developed countries, has thrown into sharp relief three different ways of thinking about disease causation: the psychosocial, the materialist and the 'political economy of health'. These three conceptual models, discussed below, both compete with and complement one another. The debate is an important one because the long-observed inequalities in health between rich and poor in Western countries have been increasing over recent decades. In Britain, for example, the social class differential in lung cancer death rates widened markedly during the third quarter of the twentieth century and has subsequently persisted. The inverse social class gradient in coronary heart disease death rates in Britain approximately doubled over the later decades of the twentieth century (Figure 9.1). In the early 1970s the rate of premature death from coronary heart disease was 1.2 times greater in men in the lowest social class than in the highest social class; by the early 1990s the ratio had increased to around 2.2.[24] Now, this could be the result of a class-related divergence in adult life experiences over approximately that same period from the 1970s to 1990s, or it could be the result of early-life or cumulative lifelong differences between social classes. In each case, the mortality difference could have arisen either because of divergent psychosocial experiences and levels of life-stress, with resultant pathophysiological disturbances. Or it could have arisen because of differences in the material conditions of life, such as access to health care, types of diet eaten, occupational exposures or peer-influenced smoking habits.

Underlying these 'psychosocial' and 'materialist' explanations is a more fundamental analysis of the influence of culture, politics and social structure. Applying a political-economy perspective, this analysis examines patterns of health and disease in terms of power relations, opportunities and the dissemination of knowledge.[25] It takes account of the political and cultural history of the population. This type of analysis is analogous to economist Amartya Sen's elucidation of the root causes of hunger in the world – that is, the notion of whether or not individuals have 'entitlement' to food, by dint of land ownership, money to spend or particular social status (e.g., Buddhist monks who receive food from the community).[26]

The psychosocial model is well illustrated by the follow-up studies of Whitehall civil servants by Michael Marmot and colleagues, documenting health differences between hierarchical occupational grades.[27] Across the four main

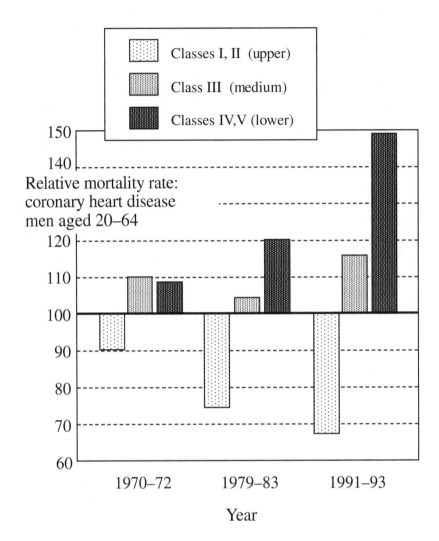

Figure 9.1 Increase in the social-class-related gradient in death rate from coronary heart disease in men aged 20–64 years in England and Wales during the period 1970–93. Social class is based on usual occupation; rates are adjusted for age differences. For each of the three time periods, the whole-population rate is set at 100 for ease of comparison. During this past quarter-century, death rates from coronary heart disease declined in Britain as they did in other Western countries. The decline began earlier and occurred faster in the upper social classes than in the lower classes. Hence the widening of the class gradient.

occupational grades there is a threefold inverse gradient in coronary heart disease mortality – that is, the lowest grade has a death rate three times higher than the upper grade. This gradient appears to be only partly explained by differences in individuals' conventional biomedical risk factors. What else in their social-environmental experience could be contributing? The essence of the psychosocial approach lies in studying how individuals' psychosocial experiences (as a function of their status, control, job satisfaction and so on) translate into neurological, hormonal and immunological responses that then influence the disease process. As we will see below, there is evidence from primate studies that status and chronic situational stress affect blood cortisol levels and, in turn, the pathogenesis of cardiovascular disease. The psychosocial model thus offers an explanation of how seemingly elusive social experiences, unequally shared in society, can translate into biomedically based health inequalities. The focus of this model is the individual experience, and biological consequences, of the workplace environment, of hierarchical status, or of a personal sense of relative income deprivation. It may invoke 'social capital' as a determinant of health outcomes, but it does so in a way that emphasises informal (horizontal) networks of support for individuals within the community.

Critics of the psychosocial model point out that this approach does not explore how these socioeconomic class-related differences arose. Nor does it seek an understanding of who benefits, and at whose cost. In contrast, the broader political-economy perspective, invoking the notion of the 'social production of disease', seeks explanations at the community or population level in terms of social conditions, economic relations and the particular history of that population.[25] Specific disease outcomes are paid less attention, in large part because the weight of evidence indicates that, even if some particular diseases are greatly reduced, the overall death rate changes little so long as social conditions persist. Therefore, although this perspective affirms the power of history and social context, and the generic health gains that would flow from improvements in equity, autonomy and material circumstances, it is unable to provide an itemised agenda specifically for public health intervention.[25]

The materialist model brings these ideas about the importance of the underlying structural conditions of life into somewhat sharper focus. It also draws upon the important idea that health deficits accumulate across the individual's life-course. Thus, the physical conditions of daily life, the quality of housing and diet, access to knowledge about risks to personal health, occupational exposures, and access to formal health care all influence, cumulatively over time, the individual's health outcomes. These material conditions also contribute to collective levels of health-related knowledge, motivation and opportunity within local communities.

These, then, are the contending points of view in seeking to understand how unequal social experiences translate into health inequalities. Their respective proponents often overstate the differences between these models. After all, in many respects the models are complementary. Yet the differences in emphasis *are* important, since they carry differing implications for social policy. Does one, on the psychosocial thesis, advocate the strengthening of community networks, the amelioration of community relations and the alleviation of work-stress and hierarchical tensions in the workplace? Or does one advocate, from a materialist perspective, a redistribution of wealth and opportunity, a more equitable access to basic facilities (including health care), and an improvement in the physical conditions of living and working? Or both? Further, should remedial efforts be directed primarily at the social experiences of adults, or should longer-term investment be made in optimising the material conditions of childhood, adolescence and adult life?

THE SECOND TASK – that is, how we envisage the evolution of risks to the individual's health over time – was introduced in chapter 8 in discussing how the experiences of fetal and infant life influence various adult risks of disease. The evidence suggests that suboptimal nutrition and growth in those early stages are important. Suffice it to say here that as the long-running follow-up studies of cohorts of children from mid-twentieth century yield results, and as studies of primates provide further corroborative findings, so we will understand more clearly how the risks of adult disease are pre-conditioned early in life.

The pattern of neuroendocrine responses to social stimuli and stressors, in particular, is affected by early-life family and social experiences. Undoubtedly, the choice of a high-fat diet in adulthood will influence the occurrence or progression of coronary heart disease. However, its actual biological impact on the coronary arteries will be modulated by the form and function of those vessels as a consequence of their growth pattern during fetal life and by the individual's socially-patterned, learned response to social stressors and the resultant levels of the stress hormone cortisol in the blood.

There is more to this complex topic of social inequalities in health than the above two tasks. The issue is central to human social ecology, reflecting how deficiencies in our social structures and relationships influence patterns of population health. The next several sections therefore consider further aspects of the topic.

Inequalities, hierarchies and health: causal pathways

Socioeconomic gradients in various aspects of health have long characterised settled human societies. We noted in chapter 5 the evidence of disparities in nutritional status and life expectancy between rich and poor in early agrarian communities. On the other hand, as recounted in chapter 4, infectious disease epidemics in Europe's urban populations were great levellers for many centuries. Then, in the wake of the industrial revolution, large class-related differences in life expectancy emerged in nineteenth-century industrial England. In the United States, death rates in men are inversely related to socioeconomic status across fourteen classes, for whites and blacks separately.[28] In Australia, life expectancy in Aborigines (approximately 55 years) is a stark two decades less than for non-indigenous Australians.

This inverse socioeconomic gradient applies similarly to many types of disease. However, for some diseases the gradient is in the opposite direction. Thus, among cancers, those of the stomach, cervix and lung generally occur at higher rates among poor individuals, while cancers of the breast and prostate typically occur at higher rates in society's better-off members. This pattern is also evident at the level of national populations within greater Europe: the poorer nations (Russia, Central and Eastern Europe and Portugal) have higher rates of the cancers of 'poverty' than do the richer nations.[29]

Explaining these socioeconomic differences in health status is a complex task. A primary question is: Does being poor cause poor health, or vice versa? Commonly, causality flows in both directions. In relation to the former direction of flow, from wealth status to health status, three additional questions arise:

(1) Is the effect of socioeconomic disadvantage due to psychosocial stress and its biological consequences or to material deprivation (poor diet, lack of access to health knowledge and health care, occupational hazards, etc.)? This issue has been discussed in the preceding section.

(2) Is part of the 'socioeconomic effect' due to high levels of avoidable personal risk behaviours, such as smoking, excessive alcohol consumption and being overweight?

(3) To what extent does a relative lack of social capital, as a collective deprivation, exacerbate the health risk of socioeconomic disadvantage? (And is this separate from the contextual experience of social class, race, and gender?)

Untidily, the answer appears to be that all of the above are relevant. This should not surprise us since we are talking about an intrinsically complex system: human society, its internal social linkages, the shared and longitudinal experiences of its members, and a diverse set of disease outcomes.

It is an easier task to identify socioeconomic differences in specific exposures that account for observed health differences. For example, differences in smoking habits underlie the very strong class gradients for lung cancer deaths in Britain (and may help to explain the recent widening of the class gradient in coronary heart disease in Figure 9.1). Before the 1950s, lung cancer did not show a social class gradient in either men or women, reflecting the fact that class differences in smoking emerged only decades after the habit became common, initially in men, in the inter-war period. However, since mid-century the lung cancer death rates were clearly higher in the lower social classes, and the downturn in rates began a decade or so later in those classes. Whereas that gradient for lung cancer is readily attributed to differences in adult smoking, the inverse socioeconomic gradients for stomach cancer and stroke appear to depend more on early-life experiences.[30] The inverse social class gradient for stomach cancer may well reflect a greater prevalence of early-life colonisation of the stomach and duodenum by the bacterium *Helicobacter pylori* in poorer people – an infection that apparently induces chronic inflammation and reduced gastric acidity, thereby enhancing the formation of carcinogenic chemicals within the stomach.

It remains difficult to give a full account of the socioeconomic gradient in coronary heart disease. Various studies have shown that the inverse gradient applies across the full spectrum of society; it is not merely the poor and the uninformed who are at increased risk. So it is apparently not just a matter of more cigarette smoking and fattier diets in the lower socioeconomic stratum. Indeed, in the above-mentioned Whitehall follow-up study of British civil servants, only about half of the threefold inverse gradient in heart disease mortality could be explained by the measured differences in the main known risk factors: blood pressure, blood cholesterol, relative weight and smoking.[27] This observation and similar research elsewhere suggests that social hierarchies have important health consequences – even when everyone has secure employment. Hence, research within this domain has begun to focus on the neurohormonal consequences of social status, control and associated life stress.

In seeking neurohormonal explanations for empirically observed differences in health outcomes to the workplace environment, this line of research is reestablishing connections with the mid-twentieth century ideas of Hans

Selye, René Dubos and others. Selye, exploring the direct response of the human organism to stressors in the immediate environment, pointed out that the modern human social environment contains additional stressors to those faced by traditional hunter-gatherer living.[31] Some of these stressors, being chronic and embedded in social relations, are not resolvable via our innate 'fight-or-flight' responses. If a person's biological responses are excessive or insufficient, entailing changes in stress-related hormones (particularly cortisol, secreted by the adrenal gland), then disordered biology or disease follows. For example, a range of studies has shown that individuals who have a low sense of control at work, a low effort-to-reward ratio (i.e., unsatisfying work) and a chronic sense of subordination have a higher risk of disease, especially cardio-vascular disease.

These characteristics of the workplace capture, in microcosm, some of the experiential aspects of living within a social hierarchy. Hierarchical structures characterise most human societies at large. However, they are not exclusively a product of human culture; they are inherent in wider nature. Diverse animal species exhibit various types of stratification, focused on priorities in feeding and breeding. The stratification may entail either a rigid caste system of the kind seen in ant and termite colonies, or a more fluid, contestable and socially reinforced hierarchy as seen in birds and mammals. Jane Goodall's pioneering work with chimpanzees in Africa in the 1970s made clear that the within-family hierarchical behaviours that we sometimes glimpse in zoos is funda-mental to life in the wild.

Studies in primates, as in humans, indicate that social hierarchies affect pat-terns of health. Experiments in free-living baboons and in monkey colonies appear to implicate status-related levels of unresolved stress as a conditioning factor for organic disease.[32] For example, the loss of social status in monkeys rehoused with dominant animals was associated with a fivefold increase in coronary artery atherosclerosis.[33] However, the situation is not straightfor-ward. In stable hierarchies of animals the low-status individuals are under chronic stress, whereas in unstable hierarchies it is the (temporarily) high-status individuals that are stressed.

In Kenya, studies of free-range olive baboons by Robert Sapolsky, an American primatologist, show that the dominant males have a different pattern of endocrine response to stress compared to the subordinate males. The surge of adrenalin and cortisol into the bloodstream is shorter lived in the dominant males. However, in the subordinate males, who do not expect to dispel the threat nor regain control quickly, the cortisol levels stay raised as their low-level anxiety persists. While this pattern of differential response is evident within a hierarchically stable group of baboons, when the hierarchy is destabilised it is the erstwhile dominant males who now register some prolongation of the stress reaction. This pair of findings is revealing because it makes clear that the cortisol profile of the dominant individuals is crucially dependent on social context. Meanwhile, studies in macaque monkeys show that, for a given high intake of dietary fat, there is a severalfold greater extent of coronary atherogenesis in the low-status monkeys compared to the high-status monkeys. Evidently something about the hormonal status of the low-status individual potentiates the vessel-damaging effect of high blood cholesterol levels. These primate studies thus suggest that low social status and chronic stress are conducive to cardiovascular disease, via higher blood pressure and readier atheroma formation. As always, however, extrapolation of the results of animal studies to the human situation must be done with caution. Not only are there inter-species differences, but the configuration of the social context is of critical importance.[34]

No amount of political correctness can dispel the fact that social hierarchies, in nature, are intrinsic to the evolutionary process. Greater reproductive success goes to the more 'fit'. However, since humans have a unique culturally based capacity for modifying, indeed over-riding, biology, so the *possibility* exists of achieving an egalitarian society. We have not yet managed to translate that possibility into an enduring reality. The case for doing so is strengthened by the accruing evidence that social inequalities are bad for health – both that of the disadvantaged individual and that of society at large.

Two lines of recent research have shed further light on how social hierarchies and relationships might affect patterns of health and disease. One has examined macroscopic patterns in national and sub-national populations, characterised by differing levels of income inequality and social capital. The other refers to studies of recent mortality trends in the countries of Central and Eastern Europe.

Health inequalities: evidence at the population level

Within populations, wealthier individuals live longer. Scaling up this observation, one might therefore expect wealthier populations to have higher average life expectancies. Although that is broadly true, it is not a linear relationship. As national per-person income rises so does average life expectancy, but the curve begins to flatten out above an income level of approximately US$5,000 (Figure 9.2). The fact, however, that it does not actually flatten out among the

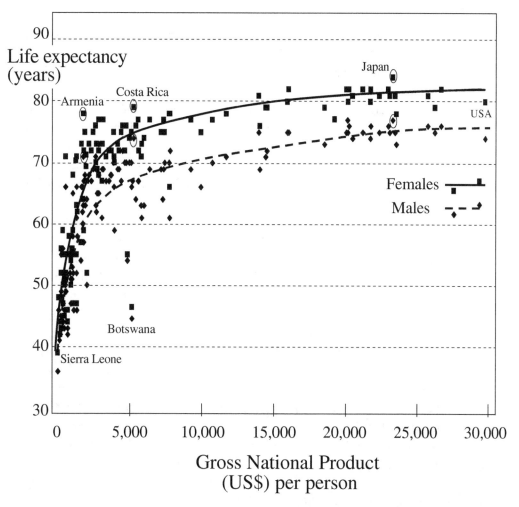

Figure 9.2 Relationship between gross national product (GNP) per person and life expectancy in 133 countries, for males and females separately. GNP is in $US, adjusted for purchasing power parity. At higher income levels, the gain in life expectancy becomes less sensitive to an increase in wealth. Further analyses have shown that those countries above the fitted line tend to have more equal internal income distributions than do those below the line.

There is a similar (but inverted) relationship between per-person GNP and child (under-5) death rates. In countries with per-person GNP over about $10,000, there is little further reduction in child mortality below 5–10 deaths per 1,000 live births. Below that GNP figure, the rate increases, reaching around 250 per 1,000 live births in the poorest countries. (In some poor countries, young girls have higher death rates than boys because of culturally based discriminatory behaviours, especially with food and access to health care.)

high-income countries indicates that material conditions can exert a significant residual influence on a wealthy nation's health outcomes and hence life expectancy.[35]

Among these high-income countries, nevertheless, life expectancy is more closely related to the *distribution* of income within each population than to its average level.[36] The more egalitarian countries such as the Scandinavian countries, Japan, the Netherlands and Switzerland have higher life expectancies than do countries with large income differentials such as the United States, Britain and West Germany. Richard Wilkinson has demonstrated that the relationship is fairly robust: it is evident no matter what cut-point is used to differentiate high and low income earners within each population – that is, it is independent of whether the cutpoint refers to the share of total national GDP that goes to the bottom 20%, 30%, 40% (etc.) of income-earners. The relationship has also been observed at the state level in the United States.[37] (However, this inter-provincial relationship is not evident within several other developed countries with, on average, less skewed income distributions than the United States.)

How might income inequality *per se* affect a population's average level of health? Is it that the greater the sense of an individual's relative deprivation within society, the more likely is that individual to smoke, eat poorly, and take or encounter physical risks? Or, alternatively, might there be some property of the population, associated with income distribution, that is not reducible to the individual level – something that influences the general 'tone' of health within that population? Returning to the discussion of the 'McKeown thesis' in chapter 7, might it be that those societies that share their wealth more equitably also tend to invest more in social infrastructure and facilities, increasing the stocks of social and human capital?

At that population level, indices of socioeconomic inequality appear to reflect something about the society's internal dynamics: the patterns of social interaction, the quality of social capital, and the profile of access to information and health-sustaining medical care. Survey research in the United States indicates that people living in states with greater inter-individual differences in income report that they experience their social environment as more hostile and mistrust other people.[37] This suggests that income inequality somehow erodes social coherence in a way that impairs population health. Supportive evidence has been adduced from a study of the community of Roseto in Pennsylvania, United States.[38] Earlier in the twentieth century this egalitarian and richly socially networked Italian migrant town had unusually good health indices relative to the general American population. Then, as social structures eroded, as young people moved to bigger cities, and as competitive individualism increased, so the relative health advantage of Roseto declined. Since dietary habits and other material circumstances also changed, assigning causation is not straightforward. Nevertheless, various commentators have concluded that, early on, there was a beneficial community-level influence on the health status of Roseto.[36]

Meanwhile, at the individual level, income distribution affects a person's actual material assets as well as the sense of relative deprivation. Both may affect social cohesion. The debate about level and type of mechanism continues.

Social cohesion and health: Central and Eastern Europe

The bleak mortality experience of Central and Eastern Europe (CEE) in recent decades raises similar population-level questions. Since the 1960s there had been a widening gap in mortality between the East and West, with life expectancy in the West improving steadily, while life expectancy in the East had plateaued or, in men, even declined (see Figure 9.3).[39]

During the 1970s and 1980s the CEE countries experienced increasing death rates, especially in young and middle-aged men, from many causes, including heart disease, stroke, respiratory infections, and accidents and violence.[39] It has not been possible to explain the striking east–west divergence in death rates during those decades simply in terms of individual-level risk behaviours (such as smoking and drinking) or exposure to environmental pollutants. It is fairly clear that deterioration in dietary patterns within the Soviet bloc, such as excessive intake of animal fats and deficient intake of antioxidants in fresh fruit and vegetables, contributed to the divergence. However, the health deficit was so marked relative to the adjoining Western Europe that something more fundamental was probably also occurring. Perhaps the centralised state control of daily life, the poverty of community networks and suppression of individual initiative induced a collective learned helplessness and community disengagement.[40] Hungary fared particularly badly. Not only were premature death rates from coronary heart disease and various cancers very high during the 1980s and 1990s, but suicide rates escalated over several decades as did deaths from alcohol-induced liver cirrhosis. The alcohol consumption levels in Hungary were about one-third higher than in other CEE countries. Further, Hungary experienced an extreme loss of social morale in association with substantial inequalities in material and health-care circumstances.

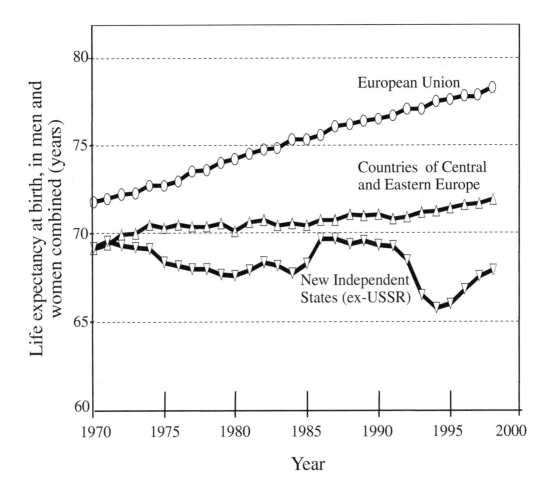

Figure 9.3 Time trends in life expectancy, for men and women combined, in Western Europe, Central and Eastern Europe and the new independent states (ex-USSR). For each grouping, figures have been averaged across member countries. The lower graph reflects the experience that was shown in more detail for Russian women in Figure 1.4. State campaigns against excess alcohol consumption in Russia and its satellite countries during the later 1980s and the greater optimism associated with glasnost policies under Gorbachev may both have contributed to the temporary rise in life expectancy. This, however, was followed by a transient plunge in life expectancy, especially in Russian men, following the collapse of communism and the onset of economic and social disorder. Meanwhile, the countries of Central and Eastern Europe fared better in the early 1990s than did the new independent states. Poland and the Czech Republic made rapid gains in life expectancy, although others, such as Hungary, experienced setbacks.

After the collapse of communism in this region in 1989, there were striking falls in life expectancy. In 1994, life expectancy at birth in the former communist countries of Central and Eastern Europe was 71.3 years compared to 77.3 in the countries of Western Europe. Between 1990 and 1994 life expectancy in Russia among men fell from 64 to 58 years, while among women it fell from 74 to 71 years. In Russia, after the dissolution of communism in 1989, social disintegration and individual frustration underlay the dramatic surge in premature male mortality, some of which is attributable to the excessive alcohol consumption that occurred during 1990–95.[41] However, analysis of regional mortality in Russia shows that the decline in life expectancy was also clearly correlated with local labour turnover, crime rates and unequally distributed income.[42]

There is much other historical evidence that social, cultural and political characteristics of a society influence the population's susceptibility to disease. For example, following European settlement the pattern of emergence of coronary heart disease and the change in life expectancy in indigenous Amerindian, Maori and Australian Aboriginal populations reflected not only the characteristics and changes in the social structures of those populations but also the characteristics of the settler populations with which the indigenous populations interacted.[43]

Cities, societies and synapses

Building cities is a triumph of our cerebrally based culture. It is therefore an irony that some aspects of family and social relations within the modern urban environment may adversely affect childhood brain development and, in turn, adult biological functioning and health. In particular, socially learned patterns of response to life stress are laid down in early life. The resultant cohesiveness of neuronal networking within the young individual's brain affects subsequent adult coping and competence. Further, early educational experiences affect the 'plasticity' of the brain, and perhaps its resilience against later-life dementias.[44]

There is mounting evidence that deficits in parenting and other aspects of family life, in social networks, and in the richness of early environmental stimuli can cause critical deprivations in the early-life maturation of the brain. The neonatal brain comprises billions of nerve cells, mostly still 'unwired'. There is an intense process of 'sculpting' the neuronal content of the young brain: connections are made between cells; unconnected cells are abandoned;

neuronal pathways are established and are then consolidated by repeated experience and stimulation. The baby begins to see, to recognise, to smile, to change body position, and then – most human of all – to respond to words. Primitive grasping reflexes that echo our primate past, where a lax grip might result in a fall from the tree, are quickly replaced by newly acquired motor skills. The infant brain has flexibility; the capacity for learning is vast; and the balance and richness of social and environmental stimuli are of crucial importance. More generally, there is a growing recognition that the environments and experiences of early life, including the fetal period, are reflected in biological changes that increase the risks of dysfunction throughout the life cycle – a process that has been termed 'biological embedding'.[44]

The importance of these early-life processes is corroborated by recent research that reveals an intimate linkage between the nervous and endocrine systems. Cells of the two systems have some identical receptors on their membranes, and various messenger neuropeptide (hormone) molecules are thus able to coordinate the responses of the two systems via the bloodstream. For example, the lymphocytes of the immune system have cortisol receptors which, when activated by increased cortisol in the bloodstream, damp down immune activity. Further, nerve fibres of the autonomic nervous system (which mediates the body's 'fight–flight' physiological response) intimately entwine the lymphoid tissues of the immune system. It thus appears that our immune system contributes to the body's integrated reaction to perceived stress. Overall, then, we are beginning to appreciate the myriad ways in which the early-life social environment, especially within the modern urban setting, can influence cognitive development, stress reactivity and immune system functioning – and hence wellbeing and health.

A FINAL ISSUE to consider is the optimal size of cities and urban populations. Animal behaviourists write about optimal population size in the wild, and how various physiological and behavioural mechanisms stabilise population size. In the early 1970s, ideas emerged about the decentralisation of urban populations into small village-like settlements of about 500 people, aggregated into larger communities of around 50,000. In this way, 'human-scale' communities would replace the social and ecological problem of the modern, ever-expanding, megalopolis. They would have their own internal sense of identity, shared responsibility and cooperation. However, critics argued that such small and self-contained settlements would breed social pressures and moral coercion, would recreate the pettiness, rigidity and tedium of life in small villages.

Others foresaw intellectual and cultural constraints, antithetical to the magnificent urban expression of human creativity and striving.

The creation of small cohesive communities, nurturing a sense of belonging, must also be balanced against considerations of efficiencies of scale. That is, considerations of social sustainability must mesh with those of ecological sustainability. In general, ecological considerations require greater population density, well-planned green areas, and better transit, biking and walking areas.[9] Moving sewage and solid waste away from its origin to adjoining environmental sinks may have sufficed for small European cities, but Victorian-style sanitary engineering solutions to the problems of contemporary cities are no longer adequate. In the globalised world of the twenty-first century, we will need to modulate our design of cities. This will entail bringing back nature, via urban greenery, gardens and horticulture. It will require intra-urban community facilities on a human scale, for high-density 'urban village' nodes, separated by parklands, recreation facilities and garden plots, and connected by light-rail transport. Energy generation and transport will depend increasingly on environmentally benign technologies.

Urban population density can be increased by redesigning cities as aggregates of semi-detached 'urban villages', facilitating local self-sufficiency. The urban village concept, which originated in Europe, is now attracting more attention in North America and Australia. This type of urban environment is more integrated, less car-dependent and more oriented to the notion of 'urban commons' than is low-density privatised suburbia.

Conclusion

City living has become the dominant feature of modern human ecology. Cities are *sources* of ideas, energy, creativity and technology, and can, with luck, become the proving ground for enlightened, congenial multicultural living. However, they have also continued to be *sinks* for human poverty, inequality and environmental health hazards. Homelessness, social exclusion and severe privation are evident in cities in North and South. Meanwhile, as fossil fuel combustion increases, as consumer expectations rise and as human numbers increase hugely, so cities are acquiring increasingly large ecological footprints. In these several respects, urbanisation has recently become both socially and ecologically somewhat dysfunctional. This situation poses risks to the sustainability of good health.

We are social animals, craving comfort, security, variety and opportunity. Worldwide, cities have proliferated rapidly over the past two centuries; we are becoming a predominantly urban species. We cannot reverse this mighty trend in urbanisation, the culmination of 10,000 years of history. However, we *can* modify our urbanism – the way we live in cities – to fit better the needs of human biology and the needs of the ecosphere. Indeed, our predecessors in nineteenth-century cities achieved great modifications in pursuit of safer and healthier environments. We must now extend, quantum-like, that achievement to embrace the needs of sustainability.

Tackling these large-scale social environmental problems of cities will only become possible if done in conjunction with reducing socioeconomic inequalities and the local environmental hazards afflicting the poorer sections of most cities. 'Healthy Cities', as recently promoted by the World Health Organization, are an excellent idea. Ecologically sustainable cities, based on low-impact technologies, social enlightenment and the sharing of 'urban commons', are an even better idea.

10

Global environmental change: overstepping limits

Human alteration of Earth is substantial and growing. Between one-third and one-half of the land surface has been transformed by human action; the carbon dioxide concentration in the atmosphere has increased by nearly 30 percent since the beginning of the Industrial Revolution; more atmospheric nitrogen is fixed by humanity than by all natural terrestrial sources combined; more than half of all accessible surface fresh water is put to use by humanity; and about one-quarter of the bird species on Earth have been driven to extinction. By these and other standards, it is clear that we live on a human-dominated planet.   Peter Vitousek and colleagues, 1997[1]

The spectrum of environmental health hazards has changed over recent centuries, most markedly in the Western world. In the eighteenth century the dominant, familiar hazards were malnutrition, occasional famine and infectious diseases. Later that century, food shortages receded as agriculture began to modernise. The urban crowding and squalor due to early industrialisation in the nineteenth century ensured the continued dominance of infectious diseases. Subsequently, however, in the twentieth century, the spectrum of environmental hazards changed; the expansion of industry, the synthesis of organic chemicals, the intensification of agriculture and the advent of motorised transport increased the levels of local pollution in air, water, soil and food. Meanwhile in low- and middle-income countries recent economic development has supplemented the persistent environmental problems of diarrhoeal disease, malnutrition, and vector-borne infections with the newer health hazards of industrialisation. The Bhopal disaster, in India in 1984, underscored this plurality of environmental hazards faced by the urban poor.

Historically, then, most environmental health problems have entailed specific risks within a local context. Today, however, there is an additional and larger-scale environmental health problem.[1] We are depleting or disrupting many of the ecological and geophysical systems that provide life-support: nature's 'goods and services'.[2] The world's climate system, for example, has begun to change because of humanity's burgeoning emissions of greenhouse gases. From detailed national environmental inventories and economic indices, the World-Wide Fund for Nature has estimated that the aggregate consumption pressure by humans is now growing at around 5% per year, and that this has caused a one-third decline in Earth's natural ecological resource base since 1970.[3] This process, if unabated, will inevitably affect human population well-being and health.

Intriguingly, the great German writer and some-time environmentalist, Goethe, foresaw the present environmental crisis in his play, *Faust*, published in 1832.[4] He foresaw that the industrial revolution and the resultant economic growth would lead to increasing exploitation and subjugation of the natural world. Faust, whom Goethe presents as the representative modern man, embarks on an ambitious project of economic progress, symbolised by the building of a great dyke to reclaim land. The play warns that this human intervention may have unforeseen and tragic consequences. Nature, Goethe tells us, reacts according to laws of its own, laws which humans can never fully predict. Faust, however, with a blindness born of hubris, wagers with the Devil that he can succeed – that he can push back nature for humanity's benefit. The Devil knows better.

Larger footprints – and larger risks to health

For 2 million years, humans have mostly lived and consumed within the limits set by local environments. When natural limits were reached, hunter-gatherer bands occupied adjacent frontier land. As numbers grew and environments changed, human ingenuity was used: agriculture, irrigation, trading, island-hopping, and developing new cross-bred strains of animal and plant species. To survive long term a society had to live predominantly off nature's 'interest', leaving natural 'capital' mostly intact. Durable societies thus had a productive, not an extractive base, to their economy. As we saw in chapter 1, where extraction, depletion and destruction predominated, disasters often occurred – as with the eventual drastic shrinkage in the Polynesian population on Easter Island.

Today's global population is no longer living predominantly on nature's interest. Many non-renewable resources are being depleted: fossil fuels, species, and all of the land that is paved over by urbanisation and transport systems. Likewise many very slowly renewable resources are being depleted: soil, groundwater, various fisheries and stratospheric ozone. These global environmental changes (summarised in Figure 10.1) that we have set in train

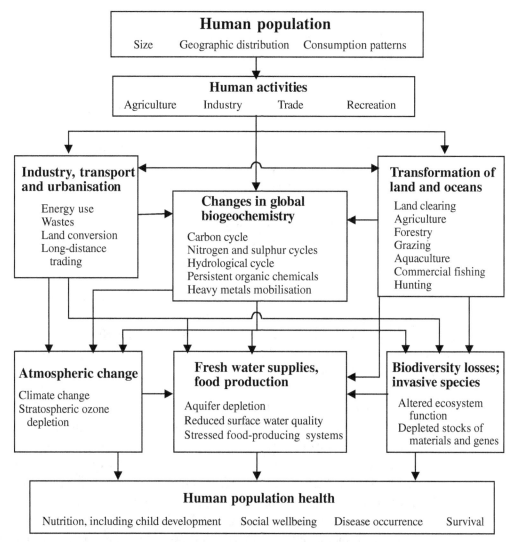

Figure 10.1 Pathways by which human actions directly and indirectly affect Earth's physical and ecological systems, thereby posing risks to human health. The diagram has five sequential layers: (i) characteristics of human societies; (ii) types of economic activities; (iii) arenas of direct impact on the environment; (iv) resultant global environmental changes (including global biogeochemistry box); and (v) health impacts.

Global climate change – which currently attracts much attention – is one of a number of large-scale human-induced environmental changes. These various changes in Earth's biophysical systems: (i) influence one another (e.g., warming of the lower atmosphere exacerbates ozone depletion in the stratosphere), and (ii) affect human health cumulatively and often interactively.

signify that we are living beyond Earth's limits. This has great implications for the sustainability of economies and urban societies, for creating political tensions and for human population health.

The increasing shortages of fresh water well illustrate the problem. Currently, more than half the world's population – some 3 billion people – lack access to proper sanitation, and 1 billion lack safe drinking water. Low-cost, community-based initiatives, such as have been implemented in parts of India, Bolivia, Ethiopia and Tanzania, could greatly improve water availability, but progress has been slow. Meanwhile, population growth, agricultural irrigation and industrial expansion are escalating the demand for water. Approximately 40% of the world's population, living in 80 countries, now face some level of water shortage. The vast underground aquifers in many countries are being used faster than they are naturally replenished, causing water tables to drop on every continent. For example, under the north China plain, which produces nearly 40% of the nation's grain harvest, the aquifer has been falling by 1.5 metres a year. Half of China's 600 cities now face water shortages, as demand grows by around 10% annually. The waterways under most pressure include China's Yellow River basin (that great river now fails to reach the China Sea for 3–4 months each year), the Zambezi River in Africa and the rivers that lead into the Aral Sea in Central Asia.

Humans currently use half of the world's accessible run-off water and, via agriculture and forestry, a quarter of the total water that passes through rain-fed plants species. The latter can be increased only a little. New dam construction could increase the former by around 10% by 2025.[5] Expensive options such as desalination, high-precision drip agriculture and even towing icebergs will be needed to meet the widening supply-and-demand gap. Otherwise, within the next two decades the increase in global demand for water will outstrip available supplies, and, by 2025, the number of people living in frankly water-stressed countries would increase tenfold to 3 billion.[6] Already the shortage of water, along with land degradation, is contributing to regional food production difficulties and the increase in environmental refugees. The total number of refugees in the world, now approaching 30 million, approximately tripled during the 1990s.

THE BASIC EQUATION describing human impact on the environment contains three main factors: the size of the population, the level of material wealth and consumption, and the types of technology that are used.[7]

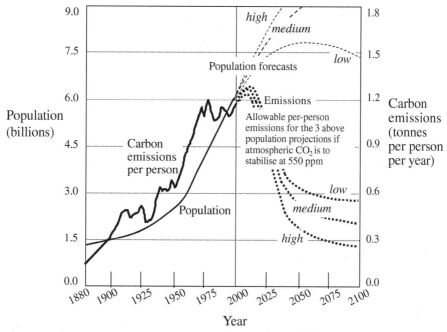

Figure 10.2 Time trends and projections in population size and world average per-person carbon emissions. Note the substantial reduction in carbon emissions that will be required if, in coming decades, a larger world population is to restrict atmospheric carbon dioxide levels to a 'safe', ecologically tolerable concentration (550 ppm = twice preindustrial level).

('Consumption', it is important to note, differs from 'use'. In general, consuming is done on a once-off basis, with the generation of wastes. We consume coal, but we use energy – since energy cannot be created or destroyed, although it can change its form.)

The global climate change problem, reflecting population size, level of energy use and power-generating technology, illustrates well the three-factor equation. Historically, during the twentieth century, as world population increased by just under fourfold and as the average per-person consumption of fossil fuel, via power plants, factories and internal combustion engines, increased by over threefold, so the annual human-made emissions of carbon dioxide increased twelvefold (see Figure 10.2).[8] Atmospheric carbon dioxide concentrations have duly increased by about one-third, to 370 parts per million (ppm). If the world were to limit atmospheric carbon dioxide to a doubling of its pre-industrial concentration (that is, from 275 ppm to 550 ppm) – which would induce a level of climate change that scientists think might be tolerable to most ecosystems – then with a projected population of 10 billion by 2100 the per-person carbon dioxide emissions would need to approximate those of the 1920s. That would entail a massive 70% reduction below today's level of emissions. (For comparison, note that the 1997 Kyoto Protocol, under the UN Framework Convention on Climate Change, was for an average 5% cut, and was confined to developed countries.)

Overall, much of the threat to ecological sustainability and, hence, to future human health comes not from continued population growth but from an increase in consumption levels. Environmental pressures would thus rise if the production and consumption practices of today's wealthy countries were generalised to low-income countries. When the world population reaches 10 billion later this century there will on average be about one productive hectare of 'ecological footprint' per average person – and yet that future world population will presumably wish to live like Californians, not Calcuttans. Californians currently require an average of 8–9 hectares of Earth's surface to provide the materials for their lifestyle and to absorb their wastes.[9]

The arithmetic of our 'patch disturbance', described in chapter 1, is rapidly becoming global. The capacity of the ecosphere to absorb extra anthropogenic carbon dioxide has clearly already been well exceeded. Regional water shortages are emerging. The widespread deforestation of hillsides has eliminated the water-holding capacity of forests and their fibrous litter-rich floors such that heavy rains now convert to massive floods – as happened in Central America under the deluge of Hurricane Mitch in 1998. The replacement of traditional mixed crop, multistrain, agriculture with landscape-wide monocultures has forfeited genetic resilience, thereby increasing vulnerability to plant disease epidemics. The loss of natural biodiversity, as ecosystems are over-harvested, cleared or paved over, is being supplemented by an accelerated introduction of 'invasive' species.

The general conclusion thus becomes obvious. Radical alternative technologies and a much greater commitment to international equity will be required if we are to achieve a smooth transition to an ecologically sustainable world. Rich countries, as the main source of new knowledge, technologies and wealth, must lead this effort. Minimising the probabilities of long-term harm to human health will be a key consideration – and is the main focus of this chapter. However, we will look first at the historical origins of these changes in type and scale of human impact on the environment, particularly within European society.

Europe: a long history of environmental exploitation

Wonders are many on earth, and the greatest of these
Is man, who rides the ocean . . .
He is master of the ageless earth, to his own will bending
The immortal mother of gods . . .
He is lord of all living things,
There is nothing beyond his power.

Sophocles, *Antigone*

As schoolchildren in South Australia, 'the driest state in the driest continent', we earned money during weekends picking olives from orchards on the bare hilly outskirts of Adelaide. Earlier generations of Greek and Italian migrants had encouraged the spread of olive trees in a terrain and climate that closely resembled the Mediterranean coast. However, that 'Mediterranean' landscape of Greece and coastal Turkey, extolled in countless tourist brochures, is actually the end-product of massive environmental degradation over several thousand years, caused by the pressures of expanding populations, urban settlement, pastoralism and timber-harvesting.[10]

From the second millennium BC, the ancient mixed forest of evergreen and deciduous trees around the Mediterranean was cut down for land clearance, firewood, housing construction and shipbuilding. Subsequent overgrazing by sheep, cattle and, finally, goats, ensured that vegetation was reduced to a low scrub of tough, inedible, plants. An estimated 90% of the forests that once stretched from Morocco to Afghanistan 4,000 years ago have thus succumbed to human pressures. In Greece, large-scale land degradation appeared around 650 BC, early in the age of the city-states, as settlements expanded. The hills of Attica were denuded of trees within a half-century. Several farsighted Athenian civic leaders sought to counteract deforestation and overgrazing.[11] Nevertheless, the military demands of the Peloponnesian War later in the fifth century BC transformed much of the countryside into treeless plains, causing soil erosion and flooding. Early in the following century Plato, in the *Critias*, wrote graphically:

What now remains . . . is like the skeleton of a sick man, all the fat and soft earth having wasted away . . . There are some mountains which have nothing but food for bees, but they had trees not very long ago . . . and boundless pasturage for flocks. Moreover, it was enriched by the yearly rains from Zeus, which were not lost to it, as [they are] now, by flowing from the bare land into the sea. But the earth it had was deep, and therein it received the water, storing it up in the retentive loamy soil, and . . . provided all the various districts with abundant supplies of springwaters and streams.

Similar problems arose in Italy several centuries later. In about 300 BC, Italy and Sicily were still well forested, but land and timber were coming under population pressure. Soil erosion consequently increased greatly, and several river-mouth ports silted up and had to be abandoned. By the reign of the Roman emperor Claudius, in the first century AD, Rome's main seaport, Ostia, had silted up irretrievably. In the second century AD, the Roman emperor Hadrian restricted access to Syrian forests to protect the remaining trees. But over the ensuing centuries environmental deterioriation occurred throughout Italy, northern Africa and Asia Minor as soils eroded and rivers silted up. This may have been exacerbated by an increase in heavy rains and flooding as the world's climate cooled during the third to fifth centuries AD. Antioch today lies under around 9 metres of water-borne silt from the surrounding deforested hillsides of those centuries.

The demands of the vast Roman Empire turned much of the Mediterranean littoral into granaries for feeding urban and military populations. Coastal Libya, for example, was initially a flourishing agricultural province. But several centuries of intensive agriculture, extending into the vulnerable hillside soils, led to land degradation and the gradual northwards encroachment of the southern desert. After Rome fell, nomadic tribesmen and their flocks moved into these erstwhile cultivated areas of northern Africa and the land degradation continued.

EUROPE STRUGGLED THROUGH the Dark Ages for the next half millennium. Islam and the Moorish empire maintained and extended learning in the south. The Norsemen began to stir in the ninth century, creating a network of colonies and trading centres around northern Europe and the Arctic Circle. The climate grew warmer (see, again, Figure 5.1). The Christian Church, provisioned by the Holy Roman Empire, spread northwards and became an organising framework for Europe's feudal societies. Populations began to expand. The clearing of temperate forests accelerated in the late Middle Ages and the burning of coal increased. Additional carbon began to circulate in the biosphere. By 1500, Renaissance Europe had burst onto the world stage with new political, artistic and commercial energy, seafaring preeminence, and many new and imported technologies. Within a century or so its leading natural philosophers would be arguing that, through science and technology, the natural world could be brought under control, improved and rendered more productive. This age of heroic intent was the seedbed for the flowering of classical science that occurred in the late seventeenth century, leading in turn to the Enlightenment and the ensuing industrial age.

The impact of humans upon the natural world was about to undergo both a change of scale and locus. The human ecological footprint was extending to other components of the ecosphere. By the twentieth century we had begun to disrupt the layers of the atmosphere, deplete the deep-ocean fisheries, and disrupt the ocean floor. We were beginning to deplete vast aquifers, accelerate the loss of biological diversity, release non-indigenous species into every corner of the earth, and disrupt the global biogeochemical cycles of nitrogen and sulphur. We continued to synthesise an array of organic chemicals some of which endangered other species. As we reached the last four decades of the twentieth century various Western scientists began to sound an alarm.[12] It was becoming clear that we were begining to live beyond the planet's limits. By the year 2000 that had become an indisputable fact. This is a remarkable turn of events: the activities of just one species are actually now altering the basic conditions of life on Earth.[1] Hence, the health impact of human interventions in the environment no longer occurs only via the direct and usually immediate consequences of local exposures. We now face complex and large-scale environmental hazards to health, within longer time-frames, as a result of our increasing impairment of Earth's life-supporting capacity.

Global environmental change: how big a health hazard?

The fact that the future will resemble the past makes science possible. The fact that the future will differ from the past makes science necessary. (Richard Levins, 1995)[13]

Addressing the above question poses an unusual challenge to science. The hazard at issue entails global environmental changes, evolving over future time, and often extending beyond the range of human experience. Simple extrapolation from our past experience may therefore be misleading. We simply do not know exactly how agricultural production will be affected by fresh water shortages and altered patterns of temperature, rainfall, pests and diseases that go beyond the historical range. Nor can we estimate accurately the extent of diarrhoeal and other infectious disease outbreaks that would occur in poorer populations under conditions of increased warmth and greater rainfall intensity. Besides, the health impacts of these global environmental changes will be modulated by demographic, economic, social and technological changes as societies evolve. The whole exercise is therefore intrinsically uncertain. Yet the question cannot be ducked: public and policy-maker want to know the likely consequences for human society of present activities and trends.

Scientists are most comfortable when making empirical observations about the present and past real world. Patterns and regularities can be discerned, and relationships can be inferred. That, classically, is the essence of scientific research. Most epidemiological research, too, is of that kind. Nevertheless, epidemiologists often enquire about the likely *future* health impacts of current trends in exposure. For example, what will be the harvest of premature deaths from the ongoing global increase in cigarette smoking? The task, however, becomes much more difficult when the 'exposure' entails a complex process of environmental change, displaced into the future. Scientists must rely upon the body of knowledge and theory from past research and experience to estimate, cautiously, the range of plausible consequences. This in turn requires the development of mathematical models to enable computer simulations of how future scenarios of environmental and social change will affect various outcomes: infectious diseases, food production, freshwater availability, coastal inundation, exposure to extreme weather events, ultraviolet radiation-induced health effects and so on.

The UN's Intergovernmental Panel on Climate Change (IPCC) has taken an interesting pluralistic approach to this task of scenario development. The IPCC has developed a set of plausible alternate future worlds, defined by several key characteristics such as the extent of globalised integration versus regionalised autonomy, and the extent of market-dominated consumption and growth versus an orientation to conservation and sustainability.[14] As illustrated in Figure 10.3, each of these future worlds, for the 2050s, has an associated level of greenhouse gas emissions, and hence of global climatic conditions, reflecting estimated population size, level of economic activity, and political commitment to restraining greenhouse gas emissions.

THERE ARE TWO main categories of large-scale environmental changes. There are those that are truly global, because their manifestations are integrated over most or all of the world even though their origins are multiple and local. The accumulation of greenhouse gases in the lower atmosphere is an obvious example. The other main members of this category are:

- Stratospheric ozone depletion.
- Disruption of global elemental cycles (especially nitrogen and sulphur cycles).
- The worldwide dissemination of persistent organic pollutants.

The second category comprises those changes that arise on a local scale but which have now become so widespread within the world that, like a gigantic patchwork quilt, they are now worldwide problems. That category includes:

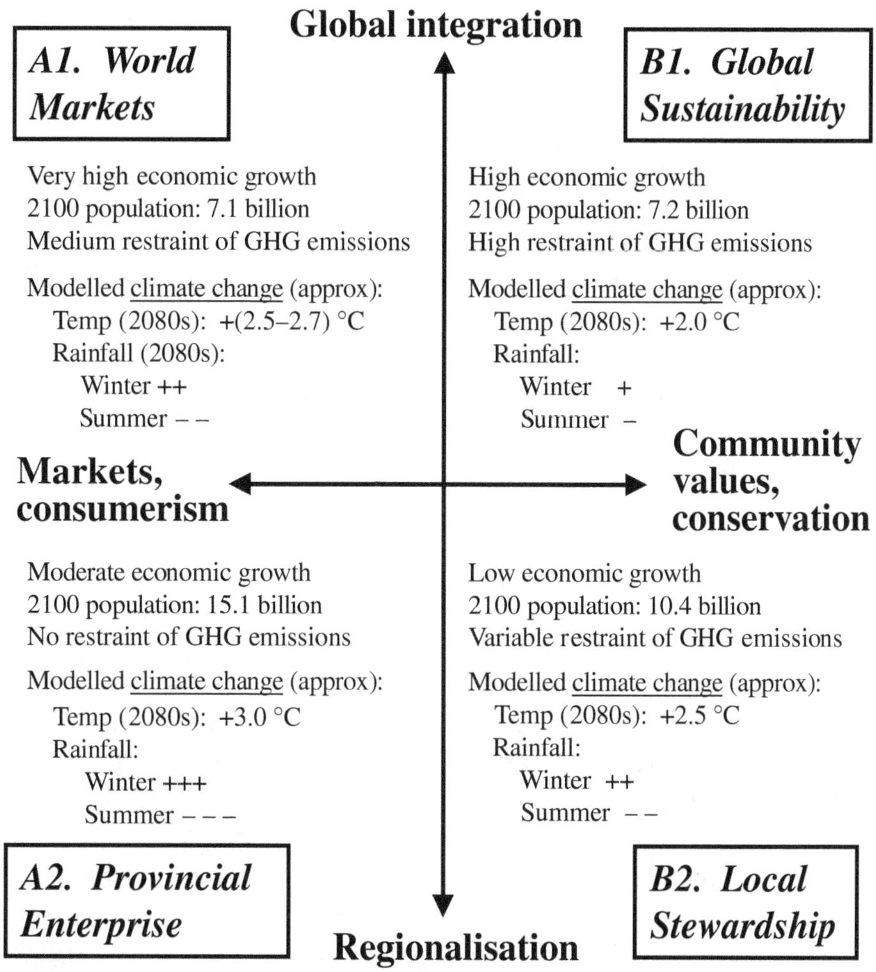

Figure 10.3 Four plausible 'future worlds', taking into account possible combinations of economic, political and demographic change over the coming half-century. These worlds, in turn, yield different levels of greenhouse gas (GHG) emissions and, hence, different estimated global temperature increases. These 'future world' scenarios were developed by a multidisciplinary group of scientists within the UN's Intergovernmental Panel on Climate Change. Computer modelling of climate change caused by these 'future worlds' indicates that the A2 (Provincial Enterprise) world with an emphasis on market-based economics and consumption and little international coordination would experience the greatest warming and change in patterns of rainfall. The B1 (Global Sustainability) world would experience the least climate change.

- Loss of biodiversity (populations, genetic strains, and species).
- Increasing exchange of potentially 'invasive' species.
- Land degradation.
- Depletion and disruption of fisheries.
- Depletion and contamination of freshwater (especially underground aquifers).

To illustrate the systemic nature of the environmental changes we are now causing, consider our impact on the world's carbon cycle. Carbon, the basis of life on earth, circulates continuously between air, vegetation, soil and oceans. Animal life accounts for a minuscule proportion. Meanwhile, vast and essentially immobile stores of carbon sit underground in fossilised deposits of coal, oil and methane gas, and under the oceans as limestone sediment. Alongside the several hundred billion tonnes of carbon that circulate naturally through the biosphere each year, humans annually now release an extra 7–8 billion tonnes, primarily via fossil fuel combustion and forest clearance. (That, on average, is almost 1 tonne of excess carbon per person per year. In fact, the distribution is very uneven: Americans, Australians and Canadians contribute around 7 tonnes per year, while the those living in Africa and South Asia contribute, on average, a fraction of 1 tonne.) Some of that extra carbon is absorbed by the planet's 'sinks' – the forests and oceans. The rest, approximately 3 billion tonnes, accumulates in the lower atmosphere as extra carbon dioxide, the main anthropogenic greenhouse gas.

The buffering capacity of nature's sinks is limited. Indeed, in a warmer world, scientists predict that the initial increase in carbon uptake via photosynthesis will plateau, while the rate of carbon release via plant and soil respiration will rise. Some computer models suggest that climate change will cause much of the mighty Amazonian forest (if still standing) to dry out and die, and thereby release its sequestered carbon, later in the twenty-first century. Perhaps this is the sort of triggering process that led to some of the run-away changes in the world's climate in past aeons. We are very uncertain of these things; they are outside the tidy frame of compliant empirical science.

The following sections explore how each of these types of large-scale environmental change could affect the health and survival of human populations. It is important to stress that these environmental changes do not act in isolation of one another. An editorial in the British newspaper *The Guardian* in April 2000, in relation to the then ongoing famine in Ethiopia, made the point well. It stated:

Five of the last six Belg rains have failed, indicating disruption of Ethiopia's chronically unpredictable rain patterns due to climate change. The population has doubled since 1985: plots are being subdivided and a pattern of leasing land has resulted in soil degradation – yields are falling, soil is being washed away. Since the late 1980s, even in a good year 5–6 million people have depended on food handouts for survival. This is exacerbated by the third largest number of HIV-AIDS victims (3 million) in the world.[15]

Global climate change and its health impacts

Whoever wishes to investigate medicine properly, should proceed thus: in the first place to consider the seasons of the year, and what effects each of them produces, for they are not all alike, but differ much from themselves in regard to their changes. (Hippocrates, in *Airs, Waters, and Places*)[16]

Climatic cycles have left great imprints and scars on the history of humankind. Civilisations such as those of ancient Egypt, Mesopotamia, the Mayans, the Vikings in Greenland and European populations during four centuries of Little Ice Age have all both benefited and suffered from great climatic cycles. Historical analyses also reveal widespread disasters, social disruption and disease outbreaks in response to the more acute quasi-periodic ENSO (El Niño Southern Oscillation) cycle.[17]

This great El Niño cycle, much studied by scientists in recent decades and now a household word around the world, entails natural reversals in equatorial currents of warm surface water and moist air across the Pacific Ocean. The flows are normally from east to west, but during an El Niño event the warm moist air flows eastwards, bringing torrential rains to coastal Peru and neighbours, and the warm Pacific Ocean waters move east, inducing rises of 3–4 °C and suppressing the upwelling nutrient flows for coastal fisheries. Meanwhile, a wide swathe of the low-latitude world to the west of the Pacific, from eastern Australia to northeast Brazil, experiences drought. These El Niño events occur approximately every five years, and their occurrence is correlated with extreme weather disasters, variations in agricultural yields and fluctuations in various infectious diseases. Other, lesser climatic cycles such as the North Atlantic Oscillation also have recurring impacts on natural systems and human societies.

Much of what we know about the acute impacts of climatic variation on human health comes from studies of El Niño events. Further, climate scientists suspect that global climate change will alter the patterns of climate variability and may induce an increase in frequency or intensity of the El Niño cycle.[18]

The documented increase in frequency, duration and intensity of El Niño over the past quarter century, in association with a global temperature rise of around 0.4 °C, is suggestive but not yet conclusive. During the 1990s the tempo of extreme weather events and disasters around the world increased, and by 2000 many climatologists were convinced that a new regime of less stable weather was emerging, under the influence of the climate change process.

To appreciate the potency of these extreme events consider the great El Niño of 1877–78, one of the strongest such episodes on record.[17] An estimated 10 million people perished in northern China and 8 million in India due to famines. Up to 1 million people also died in northeast Brazil, and droughts caused food shortages in famine throughout Africa. Meanwhile, Tahiti was struck by a 'terrible hurricane'. In the United States, large and persistent temperature and precipitation anomalies were recorded from mid-1877 to mid-1878. In the unusually mild and humid summer of 1878, one of the most severe outbreaks of mosquito-borne yellow fever affected the southern United States. The economic and human toll was enormous: in the city of Memphis, Tennessee, up to 20,000 people died out of about 100,000 cases of the disease. Similarly widespread impacts have accompanied recent El Niño events. In 1982–83, the floods on the western coast of South America caused a tripling in the incidence of acute diarrhoeal diseases and acute respiratory diseases in Bolivia and in Peru, and great increases in infant mortality due to malnutrition. Flooding in the Horn of Africa associated with the El Niño of 1997–98 was linked with an upsurge of cholera deaths due to disrupted sanitation and contaminated water supplies. Meanwhile, the burning of millions of hectares of forest in Indonesia was amplified by drought due to that El Niño episode. The resultant smoke haze spread across the Southeast Asian region, causing sharp rises in respiratory illness in the worst affected areas.

The diseases caused by Hantaan viruses provide another example. These viral diseases have been known in rural Asia for centuries, but they have now spread elsewhere because of economic and ecological changes that have increased contact between rodents and humans. The prolonged El Niño event of the early 1990s initially caused drought conditions in the southwest United States. This led to a decline in vegetation and in animal populations, including the natural predators (owls, snakes and coyotes) of the deer-mouse. When heavy rains occurred in 1993, inducing proliferation of grasshoppers and pinon nuts, there was an unchecked tenfold expansion in the deer-mouse population. These rodents harbour a virus that can be transmitted to humans via dried excreta and which causes hantavirus pulmonary disease – first described at that time.[19] This disease has subsequently spread to many contiguous US states, western Canada, and much of Latin America (especially Argentina).

Globally, there were more extreme weather events during the 1990s than in the rest of the twentieth century. In November 1998 Hurricane Mitch devastated Honduras and adjoining countries, killing 14,000 people. A year later, in eastern India, tens of thousands died in the powerful cyclone that hit Orissa. The following month, 20,000 people were killed in the massive La Niña floods in Venezuela, and many more in the giant cyclones that struck Mozambique and Madagascar in early 2000. At the same time, following a record-breaking drought, widespread and extreme forest fires afflicted Portugal. Scientists are increasingly certain that the ongoing human-induced change in world climate will bring greater climatic variability.[18] While it is not possible to attribute particular individual weather disasters to human influence on the climate system, it will be reasonable from here on to regard each extreme weather event as containing at least some human-induced component.

THE MOST WIDELY DISCUSSED aspect of global environmental change is human impact on the world's climate. Scientists predict that our increasing generation of greenhouse gases, principally carbon dioxide emissions plus various other heat-trapping gases such as methane (from irrigated agriculture and oil extraction) and various man-made halocarbons, will change the world's climate.[18] This will warm the world's surface. Indeed, most climate scientists suspect that this process has contributed to the strong recent uptrend in world average temperature. During the twentieth century, world temperature increased by approximately 0.6°C as the concentration of carbon dioxide in the lower atmosphere rose (Figure 10.4). There were, of course, other natural influences on world climate during the twentieth century – including an increase in volcanic activity during the third quarter of the century, the massive Mount Pinatubo eruption in 1992 and a slight overall natural increase in solar activity (which may have accounted for around one-sixth of the century's observed temperature increase, predominantly in the earlier decades). Without radical changes in technology and in international political and consumer will, the concentration of greenhouse gases will approximately double during the twenty-first century.

This unprecedented prospect has led to a large international scientific effort, to assess the evidence. This work is being carried out by the Intergovernmental Panel on Climate Change (IPCC). The IPCC, established within the UN framework in 1988, comprises many hundreds of scientists from diverse disciplines, charged with advising national governments on the causes and processes of

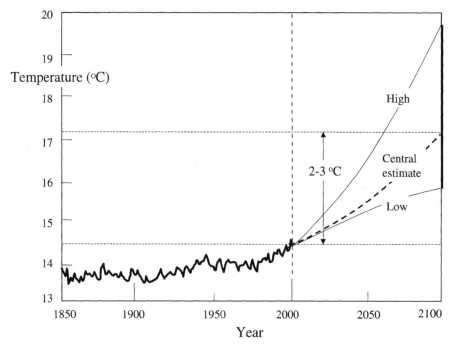

Figure 10.4 Global temperature record, since instrumental recording began in 1860, and projection for the coming century, according to Intergovernmental Panel on Climate Change. The wide range around the projection reflects uncertainties about aspects of the climate system and uncertainties about future human economic activity and technology choices. World temperature has increased by around 0.4 °C since the mid-1970s, and now clearly exceeds the upper limit of natural (historical) variability.

climate change, its likely impacts and their associated costs, and ways of lessening the impacts. The IPCC's Third Assessment Report (2001) forecasts an increase in average world temperature of approximately 2–3 °C over the course of the twenty-first century (see also Figure 10.4).[18] This increase, the report points out, would be much more rapid than any naturally occurring temperature increase that has been experienced by humans since the advent of agriculture around 10,000 years ago. It is also becoming clear that there is enormous inertia in the climate system. Recent modelling of climate change shows that even if we manage to arrest the build-up in atmospheric greenhouse gases by around 2070, the seas would continue to rise slowly for another 1,000 years as the extra heat permeated and expanded the oceans. By that time the rise would have approximated 1.5 metres.

The anticipated surface temperature increases would be greater at higher latitudes, greater on land than at sea, and would affect the daily minimum, night-time, temperatures more than daily maximum temperatures. Alaska, northern Canada and northern Siberia, for example, could warm by approximately 5–6 °C during the twenty-first century.[18] Indeed, the temperature increases that have already occurred above the Arctic Circle have disrupted polar bear feeding and breeding, the annual migrations of caribou and the network of telephone poles in Alaska (which had previously been anchored in the ice-like permafrost). Global climate change would also cause rainfall patterns to change, with increases over the oceans but a reduction over much of the land surface – especially in various low-to-medium latitude mid-continental regions (central Spain, the US midwest, the Sahel, Amazonia) and in already arid areas in northwest India, the Middle East, northern Africa and parts of Central America. Rainfall events would tend to intensify, increasing the likelihood of flooding. Regional weather systems, including the great southwest Asian monsoon, could shift.

There is, glaciologists tell us, a slight possibility of large sections of the Antarctic ice-sheet melting or sliding into the oceans, thus raising sea-level by several metres.[18] However, it appears that disintegration did not occur during the warm peak of the last inter-glacial period, around 120,000 years ago, when temperatures were 1–2 °C higher than now. Nevertheless, substantial melting of Antarctic ice appears to have occurred in a previous interglacial. Another possibility is that the northern Atlantic Gulf Stream might weaken, or even shut down, if increased melt-water from Greenland disturbs the dynamics of that section of the great, slow and tortuous 'conveyor belt' circulation that distributes Pacific-equatorial warm water around the world's oceans. North-western Europe, relative to same-latitude Newfoundland, currently enjoys 5 °C of free heating from this heat-source.[20] If weakening of the Gulf Stream did occur over the coming century or two, Europe may actually get a little colder even as the rest of the world warms.

A CHANGE IN WORLD CLIMATE would influence – indeed, is already influencing – the functioning of many ecosystems and the seasonal cycles and geographic range of plants and creatures.[21] Likewise, there would be health impacts in human populations. Some of those impacts would be beneficial. For example, milder winters would reduce the seasonal winter-time peak in deaths that occurs in temperate countries, while in currently hot regions further warming might reduce the viability of disease-transmitting mosquito populations. Overall, however, scientists assess that most health impacts would be adverse.[21] That assessment will be strengthened by evidence of early health impacts – something that epidemiologists anticipate emerging over the coming decade.

The more direct type of health impact of climate change would include those due to changes in the seasonal weather extremes. Climatologists estimate that an increase of 2 °C would approximately double the frequency of heat-waves in temperate zones. An accompanying increase in weather variability would increase this frequency further. Since the peaks of excess mortality caused by extremes of heat and cold affect particularly the elderly and the sick, the average impact on life expectancy may not be great. Nevertheless, since populations everywhere are both ageing and urbanising, this impact would assume considerable aggregate importance. Other direct-acting effects would include the respiratory health consequences of altered concentrations of bio-organic pollens and fungal spores and of air pollutants such as photochemi-cally produced ozone which form more readily at warmer temperatures. The anticipated increase in storms, cyclones and floods in some regions would have various adverse health consequences. The massive physical, psychological and social devastation caused by Hurricane Mitch in Central America in 1998 illus-trated the potentially great toll of extreme weather events.

Less straightforward, but likely to be more serious, are the indirect health effects of climate change.[21] Most of these would result from the disruption of complex ecological systems. These include alterations in the geographic range, seasonality and intensity of vector-borne infectious diseases; altered transmis-sion of person-to-person infections, especially food-poisoning and water-borne pathogens; the nutritional consequences of regional changes in agricultural pro-ductivity; and various consequences of rising sea levels. The health of popula-tions would, of course, also be affected by refugee movements and by conflicts over climate-affected shortages of agricultural and water resources.

Infectious diseases

Many infectious diseases that evolved originally in sparse populations of herbi-vores, primates and early hominids required assisted passage for the infectious agent, via insect, rodent or other 'vector' organism. Those organisms, especially free-living mosquitoes and flies, are typically very sensitive to climatic condi-tions: temperature, humidity and rainfall (surface water). Interestingly, various palaeoecological studies have linked ancient changes in world temperature, during and between ice-ages, to changes in the geographic range of insects of

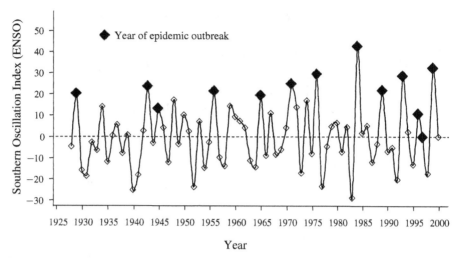

Figure 10.5 Relationship between El Niño events and Ross River virus epidemics in southeast Australia, 1928–99. This and many other vector-borne infectious diseases are very sensitive to variations in temperature, rainfall and humidity. For this reason scientists anticipate that the transmission of diseases such as malaria, dengue fever and various types of encephalitis will be affected by global climate change.

the kind that are vectors for today's diseases in humans. The development of the infectious agent within the vector is often extremely temperature-sensitive, accelerating at warmer temperatures. It is no surprise, then, that the fluctuations in temperature and rainfall that accompany El Niño events have caused recurrent outbreaks of malaria in India, Pakistan, Kenya, Venezuela, Colombia and elsewhere.[22] In the Asia-Pacific region, El Niño fluctuations appear to affect the occurrence of dengue fever (the world's most prevalent vector-borne viral disease, spread primarily by the *Aedes aegyptii* mosquito, and causing an estimated 100 million cases annually in tropical and sub-tropical countries) and, in Australia, Ross River virus disease (Figure 10.5).[21]

It is a reasonable expectation that climate change, via a shift in background climate conditions, will affect the spatial and seasonal patterns of the potential transmission of various vector-borne infectious diseases. These would include malaria, dengue fever, the various types of viral encephalitis (brain infection), schistosomiasis (or 'bilharzia', spread by water-snails), leishmaniasis (spread by sand-flies in South America and around the Mediterranean coast), onchocerciasis (West African 'river blindness', spread by black flies) and yellow fever (also spread by the *Aedes aegypti* mosquito). The key phrase in this discussion is *potential transmission*. It is important to estimate how the intrinsic disease-transmission properties of the world might alter in response to climate change. Indeed, such research is in the classic tradition of experimental science, which seeks to hold everything else constant while estimating the effect induced by varying just one key factor. Such estimations can be made in which climate change is that one key factor, as putative determinant of the future transmissibility of infectious disease. Nevertheless, we know that the *actual* transmission of diseases such as malaria is, and will be, much affected by economic and social conditions and by the robustness of public health defences. Hence, we also need to develop methods of modelling that incorporate other foreseeable contextual changes. This is a tall order, but we have no other way of exploring the likely future risks of climate change to human health.

The main anticipated impact of climate change on the potential transmission of vector-borne diseases would be in tropical regions. In general, populations on the margins of endemic areas in tropical and subtropical countries would be most likely to experience an increase in transmission. Indeed, malaria is currently resurgent in many countries where, several decades ago, it had been greatly reduced with vector control measures. Climate change may compound that process – as it may also do with dengue fever. That disease, like malaria, has also increased substantially in recent decades, and has done so particularly in Central and South America. This appears to reflect a combination of increasing population mobility, urbanisation, poverty and regional warming, along with a slackening of mosquito control programmes. Meanwhile, in temperate zones, climate change may also affect diseases such as tick-borne viral encephalitis (which occurs in parts of Western Europe, Russia and Scandinavia) and Lyme disease (discussed in some detail in chapter 4).

Estimation of climate-induced future changes in the potential transmission of malaria illustrates well the uses, and limitations, of computerised mathematical modelling. Considered overall, such models project that, for standard scenarios of climate change, the geographic range of potential malaria transmission would undergo a net, albeit small, expansion – for example, that an additional 3–4% of the world's people (i.e. several hundred million people) would live in regions of potential transmission of malaria in the second half of the twenty-first century, while seasonal transmission would increase in many currently malarious areas.[23] Modelled projections have also been made for dengue fever and schistosomiasis. Interestingly, in many regions global warming may actually diminish the geographic range of schistosomiasis transmissibility because warmer water would reduce the viability of certain major species of water snail.

These models have unavoidable limitations. They are limited by incomplete information about the biological and ecological processes that they attempt to model; by difficulties in finding relevant historical data against which to validate them; and by their inability to simulate fully the rich tapestry of social, economic, demographic, behavioural and technological changes in human societies that will inevitably accompany the future course of climate change. They therefore do better at modelling the risks of potential transmission than the rates of actual transmission. Nevertheless, they represent the best that science can do to foresee the direction and approximate magnitude of the climate-induced shifts in risk that future populations will face.

CLIMATE CHANGE WOULD also influence various directly transmitted infections, especially those due to contamination of drinking water and food.[21] The usual summer peaks of salmonella food poisoning are likely to become both higher and wider in a warming environment. The major existing problem of food safety in the modern world will thus face an extra stress from climate change.

Not only are many bacteria and protozoa sensitive to temperature, but patterns of rainfall can disrupt surface water patterns and the quality of drinking water. The occurrence of infectious diseases such as cryptosporidiosis and giardiasis, spread via contaminated drinking water, would therefore be influenced by a change in climatic conditions, particularly if extremes of rainfall and drought intensified. Fascinating recent evidence suggests that the spread of cholera is facilitated by warmer coastal and estuarine waters and their associated algal blooms. Detailed microscopic studies reveal that the tiny aquatic planktonic organisms – the base of the marine food web – act as a natural environmental reservoir and amplification system for the cholera bacterium.[24] So we must add an ecological dimension to our understanding of cholera: transmission is not simply person-to-person via direct faecal contamination of local drinking water. Thus, the warming of coastal water, such as occurs periodically off Peru and Bangladesh, may facilitate the entry of cholera into local communities via seafood.

Food production, hunger and malnutrition

Yields of food, especially cereal crops, are sensitive to temperature, rainfall and soil moisture. Climate change would result in a mixed global picture of regional gains and losses, reflecting the local balance of changes in temperature, soil moisture, carbon dioxide 'fertilisation', and alterations in crop pest and pathogen activity. The gains would tend to be in temperate zones, while the losses would be in tropical and subtropical zones where food-insecure populations already exist.

Scientists use dynamic crop growth models to simulate the effects of climate change on cereal crop yields. These models comprise equations that represent the important physiological processes responsible for plant growth, and how those processes are affected by temperature, rainfall, soil moisture, the fertilising effect of atmospheric carbon dioxide, other soil characteristics, management practices and genotypic features. However, they do not (cannot?) include the climatic modulation of plant pests and pathogens. One major study has estimated that standard scenarios of global climate change, linked with plausible future scenarios of demographic, economic and trade-liberalisation changes, would result in a mixed picture of changes in cereal grain production.[25] There would, at least initially, be gains in yield of 5–10% in several temperate regions (much of Western Europe, Argentina, Japan, China and Canada); there would be downturns of similar magnitude in various already food-insecure regions, including South Asia, parts of the Middle East, parts of Africa and Central America. Overall, climate change could result in tens of millions of additional hungry people by the 2080s, especially in sub-Saharan Africa. The resultant malnutrition would increase the risk of infant and child mortality and cause physical and intellectual stunting. In adults, energy levels, work capacity and health status would be compromised.

There are two further issues to consider here. First, climate change may also increase climatic variability, and hence the occurrence of extreme weather events in many regions of the world. The economic demographer Tim Dyson, mostly an optimist about the future prospects for feeding the world, speculates that the increasing volatility of harvests in North America during the 1990s may have been caused by incipient climate change.[26] Second, the impacts of climate change upon plant pests and diseases have received little attention so far. Yet, as with human infectious diseases, this could be an important problem area. Consider an event in 1976, when the extreme heat and drought of summer in Europe led to the import of potatoes from Mexico. Unfortunately they carried a new strain of the infamous *Phytophthera infestans*, the fungal blight and organism that caused the Irish potato famine. The hybridisation of that new strain with the extant older strain in Europe has recently created new fungal variants that threaten European potato crops, necessitating huge amounts of (soil-damaging) chemical fungicide.

Climate change would also influence marine and freshwater food yields. Approximately one-sixth of all protein consumed by the world population is of aquatic origin, and in many developing countries it accounts for the majority of animal protein. While short-term weather impacts and seasonal rhythms have long been recognised by the fishing industry, decadal-scale shifts in climate have only recently been acknowledged as a factor in fish and marine ecosystem dynamics. Various life-stages of fish populations are sensitive to temperature, including spawning, growth rates (in part because of temperature influences on food availability), migratory patterns and breeding routes. The influence of temperature is evident in the fluctuation of catches of Pacific salmon and sardines in synchrony with large-scale climate variations and ocean processes, and the fluctuations in catches of Atlantic cod, Peruvian anchovies and, in the mobile western warm pool of the Pacific, of skipjack tuna.[22]

Sea-level rise: impacts on coastal regions and populations

Oceans would expand and most glaciers would shrink in a warmer world. The sea-level is forecast by IPCC scientists to rise by approximately 40 centimetres by 2100.[18] This *rate* of rise would be several times faster than has occurred over the past century. It would be superimposed on rises and falls that coastal populations are already experiencing for other reasons. For example, Venice is slowly sinking; much of Bangladesh is sinking because of depletion of freshwater aquifers by tubewells; and Finland is still rebounding upwards because of its release from massively heavy ice-sheets that melted 12,000 years ago.

Since over half of the world's population now lives within 60 kilometres of the sea, a rise in sea-level could have widespread impacts on public health, especially in vulnerable populations. A half-metre rise (at today's population) would approximately double the number who experience flooding annually from around 50 million to 100 million. Some of the world's coastal arable land and fish-nurturing mangroves would be damaged by sea-level rise. Rising seas would salinate coastal freshwater aquifers, particularly under small islands. A heightening of storm surges would damage coastal roadways, sanitation systems and housing.

The countries most vulnerable to sea-level rise include Bangladesh and Egypt, with huge river delta farming populations, and Pakistan, Indonesia and Thailand, with large coastal populations. Various low-lying small-island populations in the Pacific and Indian Oceans, with few material resources, face the prospect of wholesale displacement. (In response to the threat of climate change, they have organised themselves into a political bloc, and have devised the collective acronym, AOSIS, the Association of Small Island States. They are thus nominally and literally the obverse of an oasis: tiny foci of land surrounded by water.) As mentioned above, even if atmospheric greenhouse gas levels are stabilised later this century the world's seas will keep rising for over 1,000 years. Our environmental incursions are taking us into unexpectedly deeper waters.

Stratospheric ozone depletion, ultraviolet radiation and health

To the ancients, the sky was the expansive realm of the gods, inaccessible to puny humans. A brief 100 years ago, the few scientists who studied environmental pollution and disruptions of ecosystems would have been incredulous at suggestions that, by the late twentieth century, humankind would change the composition and function of the stratosphere. Yet, after 8,000 generations of *Homo sapiens*, it is actually our generation that has witnessed the onset of this extraordinary process.

A billion years ago, living organisms could not inhabit the land. Life was confined to the world's oceans and waterways, relatively protected from the incoming solar ultraviolet radiation. Today terrestrial species are shielded by Earth's recently acquired mantle of ozone in the stratosphere 15–30 kilometres above us, absorbing much of the solar ultraviolet. That stratospheric ozone (O_3) is a byproduct of the slow build-up of oxygen (O_2) in the atmosphere once widespread photosynthesis got underway in the oceans and waterways. From around 400 million years ago, the last tenth of Earth's history, aqueous plants were able to migrate onto the now-protected land and evolve into terrestrial plants. Animal life followed, eating the plants. And so the succession has evolved through herbivorous and carnivorous dinosaurs, mammals and now to omnivorous humans.

It is the humans who, unintentionally and dangerously, have now reversed some of that stratospheric ozone accumulation. To our great surprise, various industrial halogenated chemicals such as the chlorofluorocarbons (CFCs, used in refrigeration, insulated packaging and spray-can propellants), inert at ambient temperatures, react aggressively with ozone in the extreme cold of the polar stratospheric late winter and early spring. This season combines cold stratospheric temperatures with the 'polar dawn' as solar ultraviolet radiation begins to reach the polar stratosphere. This high-energy radiation causes photolytic destruction of human-made gases in the stratosphere, such as the CFCs, methylbromide and nitrous oxide. This, in turn, generates reactive 'free radicals' which destroy stratospheric ozone.

Spectacular colour-enhanced pictures of the winter–spring polar 'ozone hole' on the US NASA web-site depict an overall loss which, by the late 1990s, had crept up to around one-third of total Antarctic ozone relative to the pre-1975 figure. Winter-spring losses in the Arctic region are smaller because local stratospheric temperatures are less cold than in the Antarctic. Over the past two decades, at northern mid-latitudes (such as in Europe), the average year-round ozone concentration has declined by around 4% per decade, while over the southern regions of Australia, New Zealand, Argentina and South Africa the figure has approximated 6–7%.[27] Estimating the resultant changes in actual ground-level ultraviolet radiation remains technically complex. However, the exposures at these mid-latitudes are expected to peak during the early years of the twenty-first century, resulting in an estimated 12–15% increase in ground-level ultraviolet radiation relative to 1970s levels.

Governments responded with alacrity in the mid-1980s to the emerging problem of ozone destruction. The Montreal Protocol of 1987 was widely ratified and the phasing out of major ozone-destroying gases began. The protocol was further tightened in the 1990s. Yet our self-congratulation must be qualified. First, the solution to this particular global environmental change is unusually simple; it entails a substitution of certain industrial and agricultural gases for others. Second, the range of human-made ozone-destroying gases is larger than we initially thought. Third, compliance with the international agreement remains patchy. In the late 1990s there were indications that Russia was still manufacturing and selling CFCs on the black market, that China was hugely accelerating its production of halon-1211, and that some parts of the US military were still secretively using halocarbons. And fourth, and most worrying, scientists did not foresee the interplay between a warming lower atmosphere and an ozone-depleted stratosphere. As more of Earth's radiant heat is trapped in the lower atmosphere, the stratosphere cools further, enhancing the catalytic destruction of ozone.[28] Further, that loss of ozone itself augments the cooling of the stratosphere.

We hope that there will be slow but near-complete recovery of stratospheric ozone during the middle third of the twenty-first century. For the reasons just mentioned, however, this is not yet assured. For at least the first half of the twenty-first century, according to the UN Environment Programme (and subject to changes in individual behaviours), we can expect that the additional ultraviolet radiation exposure will augment the severity of sunburn, the incidence of skin cancer and the occurrence of various disorders of the eye (especially some types of cataract and 'snow blindness').[29] With ozone destruction due to decline from early in the twenty-first century, a 'European' population living at around 45 degrees North will experience, around mid-century, an approximate 5% excess of total skin cancer incidence – and higher if population ageing is allowed for.[30] The equivalent estimation for the US population predicts a 10% peak increase in skin cancer incidence by around 2050.

Since ultraviolet radiation exposure also suppresses some aspects of the human immune system (discussed in chapter 3), an increase in susceptibility to infectious diseases could occur. However, for this there is no direct evidence yet available. More fortuitously, the increased ultraviolet radiation exposure may well reduce the incidence and severity of various autoimmune disorders. The damping down of the antibody-based ('Th1') component of the immune system may alleviate diseases such as multiple sclerosis, rheumatoid arthritis and insulin-dependent (Type 1) diabetes. Partly in response to these questions about the biological impacts of stratospheric ozone depletion there is new interest among scientists in assessing the influence of ultraviolet radiation upon immune system function, vitamin D metabolism and the consequences for human disease risks.

Finally, there is an important, larger, ecological dimension to consider. Ultraviolet radiation impairs the molecular chemistry of photosynthesis both on land (terrestrial plants) and at sea (phytoplankton). This could reduce the world's food production, at least marginally, thereby contributing to nutritional and health problems in food-insecure populations. As yet we have insufficient information to estimate the health risks posed by this impact pathway.

Disruption of nitrogen and sulphur cycles

Over the past half-century we have greatly altered the biogeochemical circulation of nitrogen and sulphur.[31] These are two of the world's great elemental cycles, important to the functioning of many ecosystems. Since the 1940s there has been a spectacular upturn in the human 'fixation' of nitrogen, converted from the inert form (which abounds in the atmosphere) to biologically active nitrate and ammonium ions. Remarkably, humans now fix more nitrogen than does nature via lightning and the action of the nitrogen-fixing bacteria on the roots of leguminous plants. This we do primarily by synthesising nitrogenous fertiliser, by burning fossil fuel and by cultivating soybeans, alfalfa and other legume crops. Similarly, our annual release of 160 million tonnes of sulphur dioxide, by coal and oil burning, is more than twice the sum of all naturally occurring emissions of sulphur compounds.

Recent estimates indicate that by 2025 industrial agriculture and fossil fuel combustion will both double their nitrogen emissions, comprising mainly nitrous oxide (N_2O) and nitric oxide (NO). Nitrous oxide is increasing in the atmosphere at around 0.25% per year. It comes from many sources: synthetic fertilisers, burning of grasses and forests, and the manufacture of nylon. It is both a greenhouse gas and an ozone-destroying gas. Nitric oxide plays a key role in creating the photochemical ('summer smog') air pollutant ozone, harmful to humans and vegetation. Atmospheric nitric oxide forms nitric acid, a key component of the acid rain that has damaged forests in Canada, the US and Europe. Fossil fuel combustion is the main source of nitric oxide, followed by biomass burning. In recent decades, both these and other nitrogen compounds have replaced sulphur compounds as the main acidifying air pollutant. Because of these various contributions of fixed nitrogen to the atmosphere, biologically active nitrogen is being deposited back on land and oceans at an increased rate. In the United States, nitrogen deposition from atmosphere to land is now ten times greater than the natural rate, while in parts of northern Europe it is elevated 100-fold. The nitrate content of soil and waterways will increase as nitrogenous fertiliser use increases, particularly in Latin America and (if it can afford it) Africa.

Nitrates in soil and water have various ecological and public health consequences. The buildup of soil nitrates reduces the biodiversity of plant species by fertilising the growth of rapid-growing 'weed' species at the expense of slower-growing species. The nitrate-induced acidification of soil also leaches out calcium, magnesium and, eventually, aluminium – elements which, in turn, adversely affect aquatic ecosystems. The increasingly high nitrate levels in ground water pose a direct public health problem. They are a known cause of 'blue baby syndrome' (due to the disruption of oxygen transport by haemoglobin), and a probable cause of stomach cancer and congenital anomalies. In much of China, for example, water nitrate levels are already well above the WHO public health standard, and these may well double over the coming half-century. Nitrogen compounds are also a major cause of algal blooms which contribute to fish kills (as has happened in Chesapeake Bay, the Black Sea and the Baltic Sea) and which, as mentioned earlier, may facilitate the spread of cholera along coasts and estuaries.

Human economic activity has also greatly changed the biosphere's cycling of sulphur, via the use of modern chemical fertilisers (sulphate of ammonia) and the massive remobilisation of 'fossil sulphur'. China's increasing emissions of sulphur dioxide from coal-burning are likely to cause widespread acidification of soils and waterways by 2020 in eastern China, Korea and Japan. These human-made increases in the circulation of sulphur, as with activated nitrogen, are thus widely affecting the acidity and nutrient balances of the world's soils, and may thereby be impairing food production. This is another of those complex multivariate relationships that is only now attracting intensified scientific research.

Loss of biodiversity

We are living through what some have called the Sixth Extinction. There have been five great natural extinctions over the past half billion years, since the emergence of vertebrate life forms. These events, when upwards of two-thirds of all species have disappeared, have been caused by massive geological changes, continental drift and associated climatic reversals.[32] The current, human-induced, extinction is proceeding much more rapidly than did those earlier events. Through our spectacular reproductive 'success' and our energy-intensive economic activities, we have occupied, damaged or eliminated the natural habitat of many other species. The rate at which mammals went extinct in the twentieth century was about 40 times faster than the 'normal' – and the corresponding figure for bird species was around 1,000. Although our cataloguing of the world's species is still very incomplete, it seems likely that in the past several centuries we have lost 10–20% of all the species that existed around 1800, particularly tiny species such as insects, fungi and small plants. Although expert opinion varies, ecologists forecast that, on current trends, we may lose between a quarter and a half of the remaining species within the coming century.[33]

Climate change presents a further pressure on biodiversity. Many species and local populations may be threatened by regional climate changes that accompany the anticipated mean global temperature increase of 2–3 °C over the coming century.[26] These include various already endangered species, species with small ranges and low population densities, species with restricted habitat requirements, and species for which suitable habitat is limited and patchy, particularly if also under pressure from human land use activities. Examples include: forest birds in Tanzania, the mountain gorilla in Africa, amphibians endemic to tropical cloud forests, and sensitive plant species endemic to the Cape floral kingdom of South Africa. Natural systems under threat include coral reefs, mangroves, coastal wetlands, prairie wetlands, ecosystems on high mountainous slopes, remnant grasslands, ecosystems that overlie permafrost and ice-edge ecosystems which provide habitat for polar bears and penguins. In the late 1990s, marine biologists reported that three-quarters of the coral reefs in the Indian Ocean had recently died apparently as a result of rising sea temperatures. In the Arctic, sea ice diminished during the 1980s and 1990s, losing an area larger than the Netherlands each year. The southern edges of Greenland's ice sheet are now thinning rapidly, contributing an estimated 5–10% of the yearly rise in global sea level. As the arctic ice has melted, polar bear and seal populations have declined.[18]

The loss of biodiversity poses hazards to human health in three ways. Two of these are well known: the forfeiture of useful phenotypic and genetic material. Both these losses could restrict our supplies of food and pharmaceuticals. In particular, our major cultivated 'food' plants are selectively enhanced descendants of wild strains. To maintain their hybrid vigour and environmental resilience, a rich diversity of wild plants needs to be preserved as a source of genetic additives. Among the many valuable phenotypic materials from a bio-diverse world, about one quarter of all Western medicines and pharmaceuticals come from plants and another quarter from animals and microorganisms. These include analgesics, antibiotics, tranquillisers, diuretics, steroid contraceptives and anti-cancer drugs.

Worldwide, traditional indigenous medicines use substances from around 25,000 species of plants. An early success story was that of the anti-malarial, quinine, from the bark of the South American cinchona tree. In the seventeenth century, Amazon Indians introduced Jesuit missionaries to this miraculous life-saving substance. Subsequently, 'Jesuit powder' reportedly saved the lives of many bishops, cardinals and a pope or two. Many of these natural medicinals defy synthesis in the laboratory. The environmental scientist Norman Myers estimates that the usual hit rate in the bioprospecting of tropical plant extracts for new medicinal drugs is around 10^{-5} to 10^{-6}.[34] Therefore, the as-yet unprospected extracts – estimated at 750,000, each of which could be screened about 500 ways for different properties – should yield at least 375 new drugs. This compares with the 48 plant-derived drugs in current use, including curare, quinine, codeine, pilocarpine and the life-saving cancer drugs vincristine and vinblastine. This simple arithmetic suggests that the great majority of nature's vegetative medicinal goods have yet to be recruited for human benefit. Yet nature's medicine chest is larger still than that. From the animal kingdom come many promising compounds, secreted by frogs (antimicrobials and potent painkillers), sea-urchins, crustaceans, barnacles and others. Benefits to human wellbeing flow via other pathways too. The soil-dwelling bacterium *Bacillus thuringiensis* produces a distinctive toxin, used to control other pest organisms in agriculture. Indeed, the relevant *Bt* gene has now been spliced into genetically modified maize, potatoes and cotton, to increase their resistance to pests.[35]

The third way in which biodiversity loss can affect human health is much less appreciated, but potentially more damaging. The loss of biodiversity can lead to the unravelling of functional ecosystems. In particular, the loss of 'keystone species' can lead to the collapse of a whole ecosystem. The loss of pollinators reduces crop yields.[36] The decline in particular migratory birds in the Americas because of habitat loss in the tropics has lessened the natural control of the spruce budworm in the eastern boreal forests of Canada, resulting in damage to those forests. The chemicalisation of much agricultural topsoil has depleted it of vitality-restoring microbial, insect and earthworm life.

Invasive species and risks to health

To lose something is worse than merely to misplace it. Hence our justifiable widespread concern about the disappearance of species, from charismatic blue whales, elephants and Bengal tigers, to humbler local companions (backyard songsters, red squirrels and various earthworms) and species that are economically important (blue-fin tuna and pollinating insects). Yet, we are also misplacing species. Alongside the loss of species is another major problem: the accelerating introduction of 'alien' (or invasive) species into distant ecosystems, via the escalation in human mobility and trade.[37] Biological invasion occurs naturally – as was the case when humans radiated out of Africa. However, as with species extinction, human activity has increased its rate by orders of magnitude. On many islands, over half the plant species are introduced, and in several continental regions the figure approximates one quarter.[1] The list of introduced animal species is long: cane toads and rabbits in Australia, rats in the Pacific islands, possums in New Zealand, gypsy moths in North America, zebra mussels in the Great Lakes, and goats nearly everywhere.

Invasive species may eliminate other species, and they can disrupt indigenous ecosystems. This can affect human health in several ways. Introduced species can reduce or contaminate food supplies. This they do by impairing food yields (pests, pathogens, weed competitors, or herbivores such as rabbits in Australia) and food storage (fungi, moulds, and pests such as rodents and sparrows), or by producing foodborne toxins (various species of aquatic algae and toxin-producing moulds). They thereby jeopardise human health and nutrition. The other major hazard is the spread of infectious agents into new populations. This long-distance spread of infectious diseases is, as we saw in chapter 4, an age-old process: we humans have long been compulsive travellers, traders and tourists. However, the transporting of alien infectious agents has recently intensified. Indeed, the apparent generalised increase in the lability and spread of human infectious disease indicates that, for microbes, dissemination pathways and new ecological opportunities are increasing in today's world. Intercontinental trade has introduced various pathogens into distant populations: witness the reintroduction in 1991, via ship's ballast water, of the long-absent cholera bacterium to South America.

This problem has a long history. In recent centuries, European civilisation has played a central role in creating this modern global problem. The historian Alfred Crosby calls this the 'ecological imperialism' of Europe: a massive process of unintentional and intentional dissemination of alien species.[38] Initially, these invaders were the supporting, disease-inducing microbial agents that accompanied European military and commercial expansionism. They were followed later by the weeds, pests, predators, food-plants and land-pulverising hooved animals that European settlers took with them. In a few short centuries the fabric of local ecosystems was seriously damaged. This occurred at a time of general ignorance about the workings of the natural world; before Darwin's ideas about evolution and the early ecologists' ideas about complex interdependence between species were generally understood. Today, despite our greater knowledge, there is a globalised spread of alien species as trade and human mobility intensify.

Land degradation, ocean fisheries and food yields

Of the 30% of Earth's surface that is land, one tenth (approximately 1.5 billion hectares) is arable. That is, it is suitable for agriculture. Another one-tenth might be useable, if we could learn to manage the thin soils and could provide irrigation. With that, plus the pastoral land and the oceans, we must feed 6–9 billion people. We are getting by with an average of 0.3 hectares (one-eighth of an acre) of arable land per person – whereas many experts think that 0.5 hectares is the ecologically sustainable minimum for an adequate diet (largely vegetarian, with modest meat intake). Because we have been over-working the world's land in recent decades, it is not surprising that around 20–30% of all arable land (depending on the criteria used) has been seriously damaged or lost over the past half-century. Indeed, almost two-thirds of the world's agricultural land has been degraded to some degree, via compaction, erosion, salination, chemicalisation and loss of organic material. The average loss of organic humus from soil during recent decades has been about 30 times greater than over the preceding 10,000 years.[39] Even in the United States, with its modern soil conservation programmes, erosion occurs about ten times faster than the rate of new soil formation.

Whether we do the arithmetic in terms of arable land or pastoral land (and ignoring the water criterion), it looks as if we are now exceeding the long-term carrying capacity of the land by about 25–35%. Further, as dietary preferences shift towards increased meat consumption, more productive land per person will be required. The tensions in this situation are clear. As discussed in chapter 5, around one-eighth of the world population is malnourished to an extent that impairs function and health. In large part this is a consequence of inequitable and inefficient distribution, but this, regrettably, is likely to persist over the next several decades. Meanwhile, the world's cereal grain harvest, which accounts for two-thirds of world food energy, is no longer growing faster than the world population. As was discussed in chapter 5, the reasons for this seemingly precarious trend-line are complex and debatable. We will return to the arithmetic of land, water, food production and sustainable population health in chapter 12.

Many of the world's great fisheries are on the brink of overexploitation.[40] Yet by 2025 demand for fish and other aquatic foods is expected to rise by around 50%. Most of this, as foreshadowed in chapter 5, will have to come from aquaculture. Although yields from aquaculture are increasing it faces some unusual ecological difficulties, particularly with problems of water pollution, infectious disease in farmed fish, energy inefficiency and the genetic consequences of escape of domesticated species into the wild. The intensification of aquatic food production illustrates the more general hazards of intensified food production. Bovine spongiform encephalopathy (BSE, or 'mad cow disease') is a prime recent example. In the ten years after this apparently new disease of cattle was first described in the United Kingdom in November 1986, approximately 160,000 cattle were infected on over 25,000 farms. The epidemic in British cattle has now dwindled, following dramatic and expensive intervention. However, sporadic cases keep appearing in several other European countries and the numbers, while small, have been increasing for several years in France.

BSE is related to the group of 'scrapie-like' diseases which affect the brain and spinal cord. Scrapie is a long-established neurological disease of sheep that induces them to scrape their sides against poles and fences. The 'infectious' agent that causes the spongiform (swiss cheese-like) lesions in the brain in both scrapie and BSE is a 'prion', a mysterious proteinaceous molecular entity (devoid of DNA or RNA).[41] The transmission of BSE in Britain occurred because the recycled scraps of cows and sheep, used as protein supplement for cattle, were apparently contaminated with a scrapie-like agent, presumably the original pioneer prion. This contamination resulted from a basic change in the factory method of rendering meat-and-bone meal, coinciding with a Conservative government which insisted that self-regulation was ideologically preferable to governmental regulation. The change also reflected a naivety about the biological world and the readiness with which new niches can be created for novel infectious agents.

There are larger lessons to be learnt from this dramatic episode. Our modern intensive farming methods reflect increasingly the tension between food supply and demand. The mass expectation of cheap meat, often assisted by government subsidy, is spreading through the world's middle classes. The resultant intensification in meat production requires heightened inputs of energy, chemicals, water and protein-feed. As we saw in chapter 5, it also entails the widespread use of antibiotics as growth-enhancers in commercial livestock and poultry production – and the resultant risk of consumers acquiring antibiotic-resistant strains of enterococci, *Escherichia coli*, campylobacter and streptococci.[42] To what extent does meat production now depend on unsustainable resource inputs? Can we sufficiently boost production with genetically engineered plant, animal and marine foods? The answers will bear strongly on the long-term prospects for human health.

Systems, thermodynamic imperatives and sustainability

The continuing expansion of the human enterprise has depended on gains in technological efficiency – especially the efficiency of energy use as technologies have evolved from 'renewables' such as biomass combustion, oxygen, wind and water, through to the extractive sources: coal, oil, gas and uranium. The resultant gains in agricultural and industrial productivity, multiplied by increasing human numbers and rising consumer expectations, have exponentially increased the amount of energy and material flowing through the human economy.

According to the laws of thermodynamics, this surge in the mobilisation of materials and the use of energy must increase the level of entropy (disorder) in the 'host' system, the ecosphere. This increased entropy is evident today in declining natural ecological resources (forests, soils, fish-stocks and water-tables) and in the overflow of nature's sinks (greenhouse gases in the lower atmosphere and contaminated ground and surface waters). Clearly, then, efficiency gains cannot on their own achieve sustainability. The total throughput of our global economy must be much reduced. Note that this does *not* necessarily mean a reduction in the material standards and security of life. Rather, it means that we must achieve an economy based on circular metabolism rather than one that is based on linear-throughput metabolism. That is, we must become re-users rather than consumers and waste producers. Like all other species, we would then be living within the limits of the biosphere – rather than being the only species that generates non-useable, accumulating, wastes.

James Lovelock's 'Gaia Hypothesis' views the Earth and all life on it as an interdependent self-regulating system that maintains optimal conditions for life.[43] This radical idea, first proposed in the early 1970s, was initially treated with some disdain. Three decades later, however, science is recognising that the real world is indeed characterised by complex, dynamic, non-equilibrial systems – and that such systems have a self-organizing capacity that confers higher-order properties not predictable from reductionist knowledge about the system components. Lovelock reminds us that, despite the allegations of critics, his thesis does not assume purpose or planning. Rather, he says, this collective self-organising phenomenon is an emergent property of the complex system that is life on Earth. In the words of the eminent microbiologist Lynn Margulis, the Gaia hypothesis states 'that the surface of the Earth, which we've always considered to be the *environment* of life is really *part* of life ... When scientists tell us that life adapts to an essentially passive environment of chemistry, physics and rocks, they perpetuate a severely distorted view. Life actually makes and forms and changes the environment to which it adapts. Then that "environment" feeds back on the life that is changing and acting and growing in it.'[44]

Conclusion

> The beginning of a new millennium finds the planet Earth poised between two conflicting trends. A wasteful and invasive consumer society, coupled with continued population growth, is threatening to destroy the resources on which human life is based. At the same time, society is locked in a struggle against time to reverse these trends and introduce sustainable practices that will ensure the welfare of future generations. (UN Environment Programme, 1999)[45]

Throughout most of human history, the environment – fresh water, the local atmosphere, soils and the various food species – has been treated as a 'free good', as nature's bounty. Human communities have depleted natural resources and degraded local ecosystems, sometimes with adverse local consequences for nutrition, health and social viability. In general, this approach made sense since local civilisations exploited most resources on a modest enough scale for them to be replenishable. However, during the twentieth century the rate of consumption increasingly exceeded the rate of replenishment. Global economic activity increased twenty-fold during the century. Consequently, today our environmental capital is dwindling rapidly. Indeed, on various expert assessments we are now clearly operating in 'the red'.

In the past the familiar localised symptoms of human environmental impact have been urban-industrial air pollution, chemically polluted waterways and the manifestations of urban squalor in rich and poor countries. These local health hazards are now being supplemented with those due to changes to some of the planet's great biophysical and ecological systems. We have begun to alter the conditions of life on Earth – even as we remain largely ignorant of the long-term consequences. We must now extend our environmental health concerns, and research, to include the sustaining of natural systems that are the prerequisite to human survival, health and wellbeing.

11

Health and disease: an ecological perspective

Western cultures are underwritten by views of human nature that deny connection and dependence. They are, let us say, atomistic. . . . We believe the basic social unit is an autonomous individual working out his or her self-interest under the watchful eye of the state. This is the heritage of the Enlightenment. We believe our species is separate from and superior to other species; we are, as we say, God's Children, and the rest of creation is, and should be, subject to our whims. This is the heritage of Christianity.

Jack Turner, 1996[1]

During the twentieth century we humans doubled our average life expectancy, quadrupled the size of our population, increased the global food yield sixfold, water consumption sixfold, the production of carbon dioxide twelvefold and the overall level of economic activity twentyfold. In so doing we had, by the turn of the century, exceeded the planet's carrying capacity by approximately 30%.[2] That is, we are now operating in ecological deficit. These rates of change in human demography, economic activity and environmental conditions are unprecedented in history. This is why there is a need to seek an understanding, in ecological terms, of the underlying determinants of human population health. This is Big Picture stuff.

There are now serious questions about how we can reorient our social and economic priorities so that we conserve and reuse, rather than consume and despoil. And there are serious questions about the future risks to population health if life-support systems continue to weaken. The need, then, is for a more integrative approach that addresses the patterns of population health and disease in terms of our interactions with the natural world, with other species and their complex ecosystems, and within and between human societies. This, however, raises an important tension between the classical precepts of experimental science, which reduces complex realities to manageable and specifiable parts, and the recognition that the whole is usually greater than, and often very different from, the sum of its parts. The tension is the familiar one between reductionism and holism.

The empirical power and specificity of the germ theory dominated ideas about health and disease in the early twentieth century. Individuals got infected by agent X and duly contracted disease Y. That theory brought a type of simple determinism which, 100 years on, underlies the precepts of the human genome project – and the commercially fortified search for genes that 'cause' each type of disorder. It helped spawn the century-long dominance of the so-called biomedical model, with its emphasis on specificity of both agent and effect and its expectation of mathematically compliant relationships. It is no surprise that the inheritors of that intellectual legacy find monocausal models attractive. Indeed, we have a long history of seeking explanations in terms of single specific agencies: divine wrath, witches, sorcery, the conjunction of the planets, germs, carcinogens and genes.

In mid-twentieth century there were early stirrings towards an 'ecology of health' in both North America and Europe. This followed the enrichment of the germ theory in the 1930s and 1940s by the idea that there was a critical three-way interaction between the infectious agent, the host individual and the environment in which the encounter was occurring. To this perspective was added – perhaps in the wake of the soul-searching that followed World War II – a realisation that communities, indeed whole populations, shared experiences, outcomes and fates. Along with the talk about human ecology and health arose the idea of 'social medicine', seeking to understand the origins of disease within a social context and to tackle health problems at the community level and via social remediation.[3] These early ideas, however, were soon overwhelmed by the energy of the new post-war prosperity and the technical advances of biomedicine. Antibiotics, new vaccines, organ transplantation, cancer-arresting drugs and coronary artery repairs moved to centre-stage. Cancer research became focused on cellular and molecular mechanisms; gene sequencing became possible; the secrets and complexity of the immune system were reduced to a myriad measurable parts. Within this same frame, epidemiological studies of disease causation sought to estimate the health risks associated with specific itemised factors. This approach is what epidemiologist Nancy Krieger calls the study of 'decontextualised lifestyles'.[4]

At century's end there was a growing appreciation of the need to give greater emphasis to the study of human health and disease within an ecological perspective. This perspective recognises the interaction of human populations with their natural and social environments; it understands how ways-of-life vary as a function of time, culture, technology and economic change, and it views each population as an integrated entity with internal structures and relations, a history, and a shared core value system.[4] Needless to say, approaching human health from this larger perspective poses conceptual and methodological challenges to researchers. Studying disaggregated individual units is easier and tidier than studying how the more complex ecology of whole populations affects rates of disease.

The ancient disease cholera provides an interesting example of this larger dimension. Currently, the seventh cholera pandemic since 1817 is occurring widely around the world. This pandemic began in 1961, and it is by far the longest lasting of those seven pandemics.[5] It also has attained true worldwide spread – Asia, Europe, Africa, North America and Latin America. The strain of cholera bacterium is the familiar El Tor strain, so the explanation for this record-breaking pandemic lies not in bacterial biology. Rather, it is likely that the spread and persistence of cholera in this pandemic reflects the greatly increased volume of human movement between continents, the greater rapidity and distance of modern trade, the escalation in nutrient enrichment of coastal and estuarine waters by phosphates and nitrates in run-off waste-water, and the proliferation of urban slum and squatter settlements without access to safe drinking water. As a culture medium, the world today is more conducive to the spread and circulation of this infectious agent than in the past.

Evolution of ideas about health and disease

Much of this chapter will explore the notion of the 'ecological perspective'. But first let us recapture some of the main ideas about health and disease from earlier chapters.

In nature, health is a means to reproductive success, not an end in itself. Every population of animal and plant species displays a gradation of goodness of biological functioning. This gradation results, in part, from the continued genetic shuffling and random mutation that generates biological variation within a population – the variation within which the process of natural selection dispassionately sifts and discards. The rest of the within-population gradation in health reflects the differing life-course experiences of individuals and subgroups. Viewed from the perspective of nature, the health and fate of the individual organism is not important. What matters in the short term is that biological conditions enable the population at large to reproduce itself, while, in the longer term, natural selection exercises its preference for innately 'fitter' strains of individuals. As discussed in chapter 7, the health of an individual organism after the age of reproduction is largely irrelevant to the natural selection process (although this is less for that most cerebral primate *Homo sapiens*), and it may be for that reason that disease risks escalate progressively thereafter.

Human societies, of course, imbue 'health' with layers of additional meaning. Good health is both a desirable state of being, an end, for individuals, while it is a means to various social and economic ends for society. In thinking about the determinants of good health we modern urbanised humans, increasingly insulated from nature's rhythms and constraints, are tempted to assume that social management and technological advances are sufficient to confer future health gains. Population health status (commonly measured as average life expectancy) is, on this view, an index of our material standard-of-living, our health-care system and our personal health-related behaviours. This view, though, is seriously defective in that it ignores the relationship of population health to the quality and functioning of the wider natural world. This is not surprising since, up until now, we have not been much worried by the issues of longer-term ecological 'sustainability'.

TRADITIONAL BELIEFS ABOUT health and disease, especially in pre-literate societies, have typically invoked a super-natural explanation.[6] Often, when whole communities were not apparently being smitten by the Hand of God, an explanation was sought in terms of the goodness or badness of the individual. In pre-modern societies, health and illness have long seemed to be part of the natural currency of the gods, evil spirits and sorcerers. Personal physical injuries may have been perceived differently: the immediacy of an injury is readily understood in terms of simple causes such as falling, drowning or being attacked by predators. However, much sickness and death was visited wholesale upon humans by famine, pestilence, war, and life in subjugation. As malign external agencies, these 'Four Horsemen of the Apocalypse' have seemed to be beyond the control of hapless human communities. In an age before infectious microbes could be imagined, or the vicissitudes of seasons could be understood, much of this illness and early death was accepted as the result of either divine wrath or the cunning of one's enemies. Therefore, it was necessary to placate, through prayer, repentance or sacrificial offering, these potent and ubiquitous forces in order to stay their dreadful hand. In part these traditional philosophies displayed a type of pre-scientific ecological perspective, seeing human health and disease as beholden to the forces of nature; as being dependent upon the wellbeing of all living and non-living things with which humans share their habitat. In many religions and cultures, human life has been seen as a continuous thread, its great cycles transcending generations.

Classical Greek ideas about health and disease laid the foundations for long-enduring concepts in Western medicine. In Greek mythology, Hygeia and Asclepius represented the two polarities in approach to health and disease: prevention and cure. The goddess Hygeia was the guardian of (Athenian) health, not the healer of the sick. She symbolised the prevention of disease, the virtues of a sane life in a pleasant environment (as later reflected in the Roman *mens sana in corpore sano*), and the lofty hope of achieving an harmonious state with the surrounding world. Hygeia thus stood in contrast to the Greeks' god of healing, Asclepius. From the fifth century BC, as rational ideas about human biology, health and disease evolved and, later, as Hippocratic medicine emerged, Asclepius eclipsed Hygeia. She and Panakeia (representing the all-healing universal remedy) became his handmaidens. Then as now, the political reality was that an effective cure was more impressive, more tangible and more personal than effective prevention.

Hippocrates, however, was much more than a pioneering clinical 'father of medicine'. He sought a balance between prevention and cure. Emphasising the preventive perspective, Hippocrates explored the relations between the social and physical environment – the 'airs, waters and places' – and the occurrence of disease.[7] He regarded disease as due to the infringement of natural laws. His emphasis on the Hygeian goal of living in harmony with the natural world countered earlier primitive beliefs about the supernatural origins of disease. Disease, he argued, was due to an unbalanced or injudicious way of living, not due to a visitation from a hostile god or other capricious cosmic force as retribution for wrongdoing. Hippocratic medicine was able to address particular diseases in relation to particular environmental circumstances because Greek philosophy was evolving from pre-Socratic *mythos* to a more naturalistic post-Socratic *logos*. Hippocratic medicine also recognised the particularities of the real world, and employed a more empirical approach to observation and description, and thus to deducing associations. Indeed, the Hippocratic school of thought fostered an early awareness that humans both changed and interacted with their environment.

The theme of individualism, too, has deep roots in Western culture. Socrates, Plato and followers had little interest in ideas of egalitarian relations and community-wide collective effort. Theirs was a world of social stratification, in which each individual had a duty to reason correctly, to attain virtue and to contribute to civic life appropriately. The individualism theme remains evident throughout the Classical, Dark and Middle Ages in Europe. In the pre-classical era, monotheistic Judaism viewed the individual's soul as the focal point of value and salvation. The pantheistic Greeks extolled competitive individualism and personal betterment. Eight centuries later, the Christianisation of the eastern Roman Empire resulted in the eclipse of these classical ideas of individual striving and civic self-improvement. Christianity, instead, emphasised personal rectitude, the need for personal transactions with a jealous God, and the displacement of personal fulfilment to the after-life. For devout Christians, an earthly utopia was not on the agenda; Heaven was the Utopia. Christianity, however, brought a philosophical tension: there was also a premium on the work ethic and on investing one's talents – the values that the historian Lyn White pointed to in his influential essay of 1967 on the contribution of Christianity to the idea of 'progress' and to the environmental crisis in the modern developed world.[8]

Later, after the depopulating shock of the Black Death and the associated collapse of feudalism, the secularising Renaissance and the rise of merchant city-states reawakened interest in the diversity and independence of ideas. This interest drew on aspects of the long-archived intellectual heritage of classical thought. The novel assumption of continued 'progress' arose, and began to replace the theologically prescribed fatalism that foresaw apocalypse or Armageddon. The Enlightenment of the late seventeenth and eighteenth centuries proclaimed rational human societies, mastery over nature, material progress, individual initiative and a cornucopian future.

Today, after two centuries of industrialism, ideological turmoil, and the partial replacement of social democracy with an inflated reliance on the private sector and market forces, the non-sustainability of this way of living is becoming apparent. Environmentalism, reinforced by the evidence of serious large-scale environmental change, is beginning to influence mainstream political decision-making. In its more radical form, this movement seeks to replace the hard-edged, self-seeking individualism of late twentieth-century Western society with a more pliant and holistic view of humans as an integral part of the natural landscape. Can this latter view enrich our understanding of human health and disease?

Beyond individualism: ecological perspectives

There are many examples of how patterns of human health reflect ecological processes. Beyond those already discussed, consider these four examples:

First, after several decades of widespread beneficial use of antibiotics we now face an escalating problem of antibiotic resistance in infectious organisms, including several that are of great public health significance: tuberculosis, malaria and staphylococcal infections. With hindsight, and had we taken notice of early evidence, this problem could have been foreseen and attenuated. The development of resistance is, after all, an expression of the ancient evolutionary imperative. When exposed to environmental toxins, including antibiotics, only the 'fit' bacteria survive to reproduce. In dealing with microbes we are not confronting an eradicable alien invader. We are dealing with what, in simple numerical terms, is evolution's most successful category of living organism, with well-honed genetic adaptive capacities.

Second, an intriguing example comes from research done in a rural population in The Gambia, West Africa. An historical survival analysis of children born around mid-century revealed that those children born during the harvest season experienced distinctly better survival in adulthood than those born in the non-harvest season.[9] By the fifth decade of life, and with no survival difference apparent before age 15 years, the proportions surviving in each of the two groups were approximately 65% and 45% respectively. Something to do with perinatal nutrition has profoundly affected long-term biological robustness – most probably immune system functioning. Other survey data show that the average weight of adult women in that population fluctuates seasonally, being 5–7% greater in the harvest season than in the non-harvest season. Perhaps the level of maternal nutrition influences the early maturation of the immune system? Further research on this topic is proceeding.

Third, there is the enigma of asthma. For several decades epidemiologists have searched for the environmental causes impinging on individual children who suffer asthma attacks. Particular attention has been paid to outdoor air pollutants, environmental tobacco smoke and aeroallergens. Yet such exposures probably only trigger attacks in persons who are already susceptible. The more important question is why has asthma increased several-fold in Western populations over the last 25 years? Why, in ecological terms, are we producing successive generations of children with increasing susceptibility to asthma? Some scientists think that this may largely reflect changes in family size and domestic environments that, in turn, have reduced early-life exposures to microbial antigens. There would thus have been a generation-based change in the usual pattern of early-life maturation of the immune system. In particular, the traditional load of intestinal worms in childhood normally damps down the immune system's allergic response (IgE) system via an adaptive response acquired by those parasites during their co-evolution with primates. As discussed in chapter 4, the fact that modern children in wealthy societies no longer undergo that suppressive process may explain an increasing allergic, or Th2, tendency that predisposes to asthma and other allergic disorders. Dietary changes may also contribute. The reduced consumption of immune-suppressive n-3 fatty acids (see chapter 2), from fish, plant and lean meat sources, during much of the second half of the twentieth century may also have influenced the pattern of allergic response in generations of children born in the 1960s through to the 1980s.

Fourth, the incidence of food poisoning, especially due to infective agents such as salmonella, campylobacter, rotavirus and 'small round structured virus', has been rising widely in Western populations over the past two decades. In part, this is because the surveillance and reporting systems have improved. However, much of the increase is real. The contributory factors are many and complex. They include the lengthening of supply lines (the increase in 'food-miles'), the intensification of production processes (highlighted by the increasing salmonella contamination of battery-produced chickens and eggs – with tens of thousands of birds per hen-house, in stacked layers of cages), and changes in consumer behaviours (more frequent 'eating out' and, perhaps relatedly, less folk-wisdom about basic kitchen hygiene). The recent liberalisation of trade has contributed some further food-borne hazards – for example, in the lax labour standards that characterise the Central American agricultural production of strawberries and raspberries for the US market. It is hardly surprising that salmonella food poisoning escalated rapidly in both Europe and the United States during the 1980s and 1990s.

Each of these four examples illustrates how population-level processes influence patterns of disease. Now, here arises something of a predicament for epidemiologists, whose task is to describe and explain the occurrence of human disease in populations. On the one hand, the quality of the evidence – including the opportunity for controlled experimental studies – is usually greatest at the individual level. It is at that level that the specific causal factors for particular diseases are best identified. For example, epidemiologists have identified the causal link between cigarette smoking and lung cancer primarily by comparing groups of smoking individuals with groups of non-smoking individuals, and not by comparing populations with high and low proportions of smokers.

Yet, on the other hand, many of the important questions about human health and disease are about influences that arise and operate at the population level. Hence the salience of the various examples in earlier chapters: of how urban design influences the mortality excess during heatwaves; of how income distribution influences a population's social capital, cohesiveness, and its members' perceptions of fairness in ways that, via material and psychological paths, affect the overall level of health; and of how the modern patterns of trade, migration, urban poverty and non-availability of safe drinking water have potentiated the continuing pandemic of cholera.

The epidemiologist's perspective

Early in the nineteenth century, pioneering European epidemiologists gave much attention to the health disparities between rich and poor, between urban and rural populations, between factory worker, merchant and aristocrat. Occasional investigations of the specific causes of particular diseases were overshadowed by this more general interest in the health consequences of socioeconomic deprivation and exposure to airborne miasmas. During the 1820s and 1830s the more specific 'contagium vivum' idea, vying with the prevailing miasma theory, had been weakened by observations that typhus occurred widely and perennially among the poor, displaced and underfed, and by the failure of quarantine to preclude cholera from English shores. Clearly there were pervasive vapours at work. Eminent French doctors, investigating an outbreak of yellow fever in Spain in 1820, declared that 'contagion' was not plausible; the cause was clearly a miasma. For another half century the theory of pervasive miasmas continued to hold sway. Patterns of disease were understood to be primarily a manifestation of social and environmental conditions impinging on whole communities.

Concepts changed radically in the wake of the germ theory, formulated in the 1880s. Epidemiologists were now able to track down specific causal microbes for each infectious disease. Diagnoses could be made at the individual level; treatment could be applied at that level – and the causal explanation could be framed in terms of infectious contacts that the individual had made. In the twentieth century, epidemiologists extended this idea of specific causation to nutritional deficiencies, various occupational diseases, and subsequently to chronic non-infectious diseases such as heart disease and diabetes. Specific exogenous causal factors, such as vitamin deficiency, asbestos exposure, cigarette smoking and specific urban air pollutants, have thus been implicated as causes of these conditions. From mid-century, reinforced by the continued retreat of infectious diseases, public health research in Western countries has concentrated increasingly on the newly ascendant diseases of older age: coronary heart disease, stroke, cancers, diabetes, dementias and musculoskeletal disorders. Causal explanations have been sought primarily in terms of what *individuals* do – what they eat, smoke and drink; how they exercise; whether they use oral contraceptives or post-menopausal hormone replacement therapy; and so on. A whole generation of epidemiologists has therefore been imbued with the idea that their primary research task is to explain why disease occurs in some individuals but not in others. This perspective, not surprisingly, sits comfortably with the individualist orientation that characterises Western ideas and philosophy and which is therefore embedded in Western scientific thought.

This individual-oriented perspective is, of course, compelling. First, it is obviously true that individual choices and actions influence one's personal health prospects. Second, it is a biological fact that it is individuals, not entire populations, who get sick and die. Third, we in Western society have been living through an era that celebrates individualism and individual rights and freedoms, while traditional social and family structures have been weakening. It is not surprising, then, that populations are typically viewed by epidemiologists as aggregates of free-range consumers each exercising free individual choices, rather than as a collective body of citizens sharing values, experiences, social relations and history. As I have pointed out in earlier chapters, this type of epidemiological research is very valuable and has greatly advanced our knowledge of the specific, often avoidable, individual-level risks to health. However, we should not forget that the population's health is a public good, achievable by creating social and environmental conditions conducive to good health.

Within that larger frame, a full understanding of the determinants of population health requires consideration of how social and economic conditions influence patterns of knowledge, opportunity and behaviour within a population. Furthermore, the basic inputs to good population health derive not just from literacy, material assets, autonomy and equitable access to the health-care system. There are many other inputs from the wider natural environment, be it clean air, safe drinking water, stable climatic patterns, secure and wholesome food supplies, constraints on infectious agents, and a sufficient capacity of environmental 'sinks' to absorb society's wastes. Whether we are addressing the background socioeconomic and environmental conditions or the more specific foreground exposures, such as exposures to infectious disease agents, excessive alcohol consumption or traffic trauma, a priority for epidemiologists should be to undertake a 'reality check' of their research findings. Do they significantly help to explain the observed disease patterns and trends in the population at large? If, within a population, the coronary heart disease rate has halved since the 1970s while the prevalence of obesity has doubled, then the manifest association between an individual's relative weight and his/her risk of heart disease cannot be the explanation for that population's experience.

Within this larger frame, population health can be understood as a criterion of the population's social, cultural and economic performance, and of its stewardship of the natural environment. Its use for this purpose is not straightforward, however, since politically and economically powerful populations are able to subsidise themselves – and their health – at the expenses of weaker, often distant, populations. If that consideration can be allowed for, then, over time, a population's level of attained health serves as an important criterion of the sustainability of its way of life.

The 'sustainability' of population health

We conventionally measure a population's health status in terms of recent trends and current health-outcome indicators. Such indices include gains in life expectancy, or current levels of infant mortality or of HIV seropositivity. These, though, are measures of *achieved* health; they have no intrinsic predictive power. They resemble the way we conventionally measure society's economic performance, via indices of accrued wealth, financial turnover and overall domestic product. We have not yet devised an index of sustainable economic productivity – and, similarly, our measures of current health attainment within populations tell us little about the probability of sustaining or improving upon those achieved levels in the future.

There is, meanwhile, a myopic aspect to how we interpret some of our current population health trends. To argue that environmental conditions overall must actually be getting better simply because life expectancies have recently been increasing is to misconstrue the significance of incipient global environmental changes. In the natural world, gains in life expectancy (heavily influenced by the probability of early life survival) occur in circumstances conducive to rapid population growth. That is, they occur when the *immediate* carrying capacity (supply) of the environment exceeds the number of dependent individuals (demand). In an immediate sense, then, the recent generalised gains in human life expectancy indicate that the 'bottom-line' life-support capacity of the human-modified environment has been increasing.

It is likely, however, that these health gains have been achieved at some *future* cost to population health. Typically, there is a time lag between the weakening of environmental carrying capacity (especially if it is initially buffered by social and technical adaptation) and the eventual impact on population health. History has shown us countless examples of this at local and regional levels. For example, the population of Mesopotamia expanded as agricultural yields increased, even as the seeds of subsequent agroecosystem collapse – salination and erosion – were germinating.

Inevitably, there are great difficulties in dissecting out these relationships, even in well-documented modern society. Apportioning the recent gains in population health between the strengthening of social institutions, the spread of knowledge, the development of low-impact medical interventions and the trickle-down effects from wealth creation and health technologies with high environmental impact is a formidable task. Indeed, it has not yet been tackled in those terms. However, we know that the widespread gains in longevity over the past century have depended largely on reductions in early-life infectious disease mortality. These in turn depended on gains in food security, sanitation, housing and community literacy, supplemented by subsequent advances in vaccination, antibiotic treatment and oral rehydration therapy.

Typically, these health-enhancing physical, technical and social improvements have been closely associated with the processes of urbanisation, industrialisation and increasing material consumption. Thus, the resultant gains in life expectancy have proceeded in parallel with increasing levels of physical disruption and chemical contamination of our ambient environment. But we do not know to what extent this 'proceeding in parallel' represents an actual dependence by the health-improving factors on the extraction of resources from nature and the attendant impact upon the environment.

Therefore questions like: 'For how long can we expect to maintain these parallel increasing trends in consumption, life expectancy and environmental impact?' and 'When might depletion of the world's ecological and biophysical capital rebound against human health?' are still very difficult for scientists to answer. In principle, the answers will reflect the extent to which the ongoing health gains are achieved via increases in stocks of human and social capital, as opposed to the depletion of stocks of natural capital.[10]

Dealing with uncertainty and complexity

Modern Western science depends predominantly upon empirical evidence. We observe the world as it is: we compare, and we explain differences. From this process theories emerge, and these are used to predict future outcomes. If the evidence indicates that cigarette smoking causes lung cancer, then we predict that giving up smoking will be associated with a reduction in risk of lung cancer. If such predictions are testable, well and good. If they refer to something that is not amenable to empirical testing, such as the existence of black holes, then we must depend on the coherence of our theories of subatomic physics, fundamental forces and the supporting mathematics. However, if the task is to forecast the potential health consequences of the anticipated but uncertain future changes in complex global environmental systems, then the task exceeds the easy grasp of conventional science. Scientific methods must adjust and evolve accordingly.[11]

The nettle must be grasped. As the rate of social and technological change accelerates, and as evidence emerges of unexpected large-scale changes to global environmental systems, our society wants estimations from scientists about the likely future consequences. The issues of complexity and uncertainty must be faced by scientists. Policy-makers, too, must adjust to working with incomplete information and with making 'uncertainty-based' policy decisions. They must jettison any misplaced assumptions that white-coated scientists can tell them final and precise truths. Society at large must learn how and when to apply the Precautionary Principle, in order to minimise the chance of low-probability but potentially devastating outcomes. In other words, when the outcome of a course of action is uncertain, but potentially disastrous, then preventive action is the prudent option. Better to be safe than sorry.

Much of the uncertainty reflects the complexity of the processes and systems under consideration. Assessing the health impacts of climate change cannot possibly be the province of a single scientific discipline. And yet we have an historical legacy in the architecture of science. The many different, separate, scientific disciplines reflect the reductionist intellectual style of our immediate predecessors. In contrast, in classical Greece in the days of the Ionian Enchantment,[12] scientists such as Aristotle and Pythagoras studied everything – mathematics, logic, philosophy, natural science, political science and so on. Of course, in those times there was very much less to know. Today, knowledge about the complex real world is rendered manageable by differentiating the task between specialised disciplines. Both between and within these disciplines, the underlying assumption is that the whole is merely the sum of its parts. With this Newtonian reductionism we have made many great scientific advances. Without it we could not have landed a man on the Moon. Today, however, the logically precise clockwork world of Newton, Liebnitz and

Descartes, disturbed early in the twentieth century by the uncertainties of Einstein, Heisenberg and others, is now under further challenge by chaos, complexity theory and the ideas of self-ordering.

These ideas of complexity and self-ordering are best appraised in relation to the Second Law of Thermodynamics, to which we have referred earlier. This law consigns all ordered matter to a tendency to undergo decay and disintegration, to gain in entropy. Order is lost; heat is generated. This loss of order has been understood for several centuries, but we have been ignorant of the source of the initial 'order'. Today, complexity theory is beginning to shed some light on this question.[13] A process of *collective catalytic convergence* is evident in both experimental and mathematical models of evolving complexity. For example, in an initially limited cocktail of disparate chemical molecules, the variety of ensuing chemical reactions becomes mutually catalytic. Eventually a 'take-off' process occurs, with a rapid increase in the self-generated diversity and complexity of the chemical cocktail. An evolving interactive system has arisen. Such a process may have underlain the origins of self-replicating 'vital' chemistry, of life on Earth. This theory of self-ordering in nature, however, is not yet well understood. Complex systems appear to evolve towards the dynamic region that lies between stable, rather rigid, order on the one hand and chaos on the other. Within this region, the options for internal optimisation are greatest. The resultant 'self-organisation' is an entropy-defying process, bestowing a higher level of order, and guided by 'attractors' (stable nodes within the system's state cycles) that impart internal coherence. Complexity theorists propose that it is within this region, at 'the edge of chaos', that evolution occurs, that embryological differentiation occurs and that abstract thought occurs.

While theoreticians debate complexity, we can at least recognise that there is great complexity, dynamic change, and a self-ordering capacity within Earth's ecosystems. These are the systems – climatic, hydrological, ecological – which create the limiting conditions for levels of human population health. It is becoming clear that our conventional monodisciplinary science is incapable of addressing many of today's larger-scale environmental problems. Within the health sciences similar challenges have arisen: we must find how to study the complex ways in which global environmental changes impinge on human health.

The idiom of science is thus changing. The word 'complexity' is rapidly entering the lexicon. Although we have identified the apparently fundamental particles of matter (quarks, gluons, etc.) and we have recently seen, via microwave radiation, to within 300 light-years of the edge of the known universe, yet in between are the life-size problems that dominate today's agenda. They entail complex, non-linear, dynamic systems – including ecosystems, the climate, the workings of the human brain, urban transport systems and the economy. These phenomena are not susceptible to precise mathematical description. Often, as with climate change, the important question refers to plausible future conditions, not actual current conditions. This summons up an emergent branch of science that some have referred to as 'post-normal science' – that is, a type of science that must accommodate complexity, multiple layers of systems-based uncertainties, a high level of decision stakes, and a diversity of interested-party perspectives.[14] For those who like their science to be empirically verifiable, precise and mathematically compliant, this talk of post-normal science, complexity and a plurality of perspectives is unsettling.

Land use patterns and infectious diseases: ecological case-studies

Clearing a rain forest to plant annuals is like stripping an animal first of its fur, then its skin. The land howls. Annual crops fly on a wing and a prayer. And even if you manage to get a harvest, why, you need roads to take it out! Take one trip overland here and you'll know forever that a road in the jungle is a sweet, flat, impossible dream. The soil falls apart. The earth melts into red gashes like the mouths of whales. Fungi and vines throw a blanket over the face of the dead land. It's simple, really. Central Africa is a rowdy society of flora and fauna that have managed to balance together on a trembling geologic plate for ten million years: when you clear off part of the plate, the whole slides into ruin. Stop clearing, and the balance returns. (Barbara Kingsolver, *The Poisonwood Bible*)[15]

The microbiologist René Dubos, in the 1950s, oriented us towards thinking in 'systems' terms about environmental change and human health.[16] He pointed out that all human technological innovation, whether agricultural, industrial or medical, altered our relations with the rest of the natural world. Often, he said, the resulting disturbances in ecological relationships would rebound against human health, although there were also instances of health gains from such interventions in nature. He illustrated his argument with examples of the relationship between land-use patterns, water engineering projects and patterns of infectious diseases. At about the same time, other scientists began pointing out that big-engineering development projects in Third World countries were doing much to spread familiar diseases such as African sleeping sickness, schistosomiasis and malaria.[17] Schistosomiasis is a particularly salutary example, having spread rapidly in Africa, parts of the Middle East, Asia, South

America and the Caribbean following water resource development that involved construction of high dams, reservoirs and irrigation canals.[18] We have unwittingly created ecological 'free zones' for the vector snails. Today up to 300 million people are infected with schistosomiasis.

The story of the ebb and flow of African sleeping sickness (caused by a trypanosome spread by the tsetse fly) over the past century illustrates the ecological complexity of the interplay between natural ecosystems, human economic activity and human beliefs. The introduction of the disease rinderpest in the 1890s, via cattle imported into Ethiopia, decimated both domesticated cattle and wild herds of deer, antelope, wildebeest and other bovids in eastern and central Africa. That, in turn, caused the deaths of one quarter of the Masai pastoralists from starvation. Scrub and brush (the habitat of the tsetse fly) then proliferated in vacated grazing lands – but the absence of bovid hosts led to a net downturn in human trypanosomiasis. With the subsequent recovery of herds, and the re-clearing of land, human exposure greatly increased. This was a typical 'forest edge' effect. The European colonial authorities devised programmes for controlling the tsetse breeding-grounds, particularly the elimination of brush growth in moist valleys. This practice, however, was often resisted or discontinued in post-colonial times, sometimes because it did not square with local beliefs about the source of the disease. In the benighted Democratic Republic of the Congo (previously Zaïre), the number of annual cases of sleeping sickness has escalated by 20-fold to 40-fold over the past four decades, compounded further by the disintegration of social infrastructure and the health care system.[19]

Intrusive patterns of land use are also a frequent source of new infectious agents. This has been well illustrated over the past few decades by the emergence of various new haemorrhagic fever viruses in rural settings in South America and elsewhere. These diseases, spread by rodents, mosquitoes or midges, have arisen in response to forest and grassland clearance, often in association with extensive agricultural mono-cropping.[20] Meanwhile, extensions of forest-edge malaria also occur whenever roads, tracks and clearings hugely multiply the amount of 'edge' to which humans are exposed. This forest edge is a likely site for encounters with infectious agents. A classical example is yellow fever. This vector-borne viral disease originates from high in the forest canopy of Eastern Africa, where the virus unobtrusively circulates, via the *Aedes africanus* mosquito, among several local monkey species. Most of the monkeys are infected; but they are not affected – having coevolved over many millions of years, monkey, mosquito and virus all do well.

However, the redtail monkeys are adventurers. They descend from the tree-tops to raid the food supplies of itinerant humans. At the forest's edge the red-tails encounter a low-flying mosquito, *Aedes simpsoni*, which bites both monkeys and humans. And so the virus passes to mosquito-bitten humans, in whom it causes yellow fever.

Land use also affects infectious disease patterns by eliminating and frag-menting natural habitat, thereby reducing biological diversity. The resultant weakened and disordered ecosystems are susceptible to colonisation or over-growth by opportunistic species, many of which transmit infectious agents. The loss of predators enables their prey species – such as rodents, insects and algae – to proliferate. For example, frogs, birds, spiders and bats naturally control mosquito populations, upon which they feed. If these predators are diminished then the enlarged mosquito populations are better able to transmit malaria, dengue, yellow fever, filariasis and several types of encephalitis. Birds, snakes and cats eat rodents; and rodents carry hantaviruses, various arenavi-ruses, Lyme disease-infected ticks, and the bacteria of human bubonic plague and leptospirosis. Hence, the clearing of forested land in Bolivia in the early 1960s and the accompanying blanket spraying of DDT to control malaria mos-quitoes led, respectively, to infestation of cropland by *Calomys* mice and the poisoning of the rodents' predators (village cats). This resulted in the appear-ance of a new viral fever, the Bolivian (Machupo) Haemorrhagic Fever, which killed around one-seventh of the local population.

The ways in which we manage water resources also affect the likelihood of infectious diseases. The building of large dams has affected various vector-borne infectious diseases. For example, outbreaks of Rift Valley Fever occurred in the Nile Valley in 1977 and in Mauritania in 1987 following the damming of major rivers. The building of the Aswan dam on the Nile River resulted also in a sevenfold increase in schistosomiasis. Lymphatic filariasis in the southern Nile Delta has undergone a 20-fold increase in prevalence since the 1960s, pri-marily due to an increase in breeding sites for the vector mosquito *Culex Pipiens* that followed the rise in the water table due to extensions of irrigation. The situation has been exacerbated by the evolution of pesticide resistance in mosquitoes due to the heavy use of pesticide by local farmers, and by rural-to-urban commuting among farm workers.[21]

The news has not been all bad. In parts of Southeast Asia, forest clearance eliminated the habitat of the mosquito *Anopheles dirus*, thus reducing the occurrence of malaria. In the Punjab, Northwest India, irrigation and rural development removed the conditions that had historically facilitated epidemic outbreaks of malaria whenever rainfall episodes punctuated that semi-arid landscape.

Rich and poor: the political ecology of health

The great disparities in wealth and health between the rich nations (the North) and the poor nations (the South) present a daunting challenge to both researcher and policy-maker. The 30-fold gap between the richest one-fifth and poorest one-fifth of the world's population in the 1960s had become a 75-fold gap by the late 1990s. Likewise, there is a health gap. True, the gap in life expectancies (as measured at the national level) has narrowed over recent decades. Indeed, this is what you would expect from the graph shown in Figure 9.2. As any pair of rich and poor countries moves by a fixed amount to the right on the income scale, the gap in life expectancy between them will decrease. Nevertheless, as discussed in chapter 7, in many African, Asian and Latin American countries, the average life expectancy is still one or more decades less than for wealthy Western countries – and, in many of those countries, it is now under siege from HIV/AIDS.

It is important, though potentially facile, to point out that poverty is *the* major cause of disease and premature death in the world.[22] The proposition attained particularly poignant significance in 2000 when the new president of South Africa, Thabo Mbeki, seemed to reactivate doubts about the fundamental role of a viral agent in HIV/AIDS. His stance was ill-informed and misguided, but it reminded us again, forcibly, that the reason that Africa has most of the world's HIV/AIDS is not because it is afflicted with a different viral strain. Nor is it a simple matter of traditional high-risk patterns of sexuality. No, much of the problem derives from the privations of widespread poverty and ignorance, inevitable sexual improvisation in and around labour camps (such as the gold mines), and a susceptibility arising from widespread malnutrition. The immediate cause of HIV in individuals is exposure to the virus. However, the cause of the epidemic in Africa is primarily the poverty that is exacerbated by an inequitable and uncompassionate global economy, compounded by political ineptness and by a culturally-reinforced denial.

How then should public health researchers and the health sector at large address this primordial causal factor, poverty? After all, the task of poverty alleviation requires that society takes actions that transcend policy sectors and scientific disciplines. Further, in the international arena, it requires actions that make restitution for historical inequities.[23] The task for epidemiologists is to collaborate with other researchers in elucidating the ways, both generic and specific, in which socioeconomic disadvantage and material deprivation impair health. The several levels and pathways of causation were discussed in several earlier chapters, especially chapter 9. Clarification of these causal relationships will further strengthen the case for poverty alleviation.

The international dimension of world poverty can be better understood by examining the main political and economic currents that flowed during the twentieth century. In the first half of that century, wealth creation in Western countries was hugely subsidised by the material resources of empire. After World War II, Europe's empires dissolved and newly independent nations appeared. The nascent empire of the Soviet Union presented a major cross-current to Western aspirations for standardised linear national economic development around the world. In the noncommunist world the Western powers had already laid the foundations of a market-based new world order, establishing the two great international financial institutions of the modern world. These were the World Bank, to fund postwar rebuilding in Europe and economic development everywhere, and the International Monetary Fund to oversee the fiscal solvency and stability of struggling nations. Liberal economic values were to be universalised; wealth and progress would be available for all. Western donor countries set the agenda.

During the 1960s and 1970s ideas of social democracy and welfare support in the Western world ensured that the energy of capitalism was, in part, directed to the needs of wider society. But priorities changed in the 1980s. The values of individual responsibility, economic deregulation and welfare constraints were promoted. Governments opted for privatisation of major utilities. Increasingly the West's great Development Project, seeking a convergence of national economies upon the Western model, was replaced by a globalised model of economic development, trade and investment.[24] By century's end, with the newly reconfigured World Trade Organization in place, an international economic system had evolved that promoted trade and investment irrespective of the impacts on social wellbeing, population health or environmental protection. Those three aspects are 'invisible' casualties of the market-place. They are the readily ignored 'externalities' that do not figure in market prices. (We have hardly begun to consider how we might assign prices to the *future sustainability* of ecological and social entities.)

The increasingly inter-connected nature of the contemporary world is perhaps most evident in the realms of economic systems, international trade and the sheer physical mobility of humans (and, via them, of other species). These are the hallmarks of current 'globalisation'.[25] Meanwhile, the globalisation of information, culture and technology is intensifying this process, hugely amplified by the phenomenal revolution in electronic communications. These processes have great implications for future patterns of health. There have undoubtedly been some benefits to health, as new wealth has accrued in some population segments of low-income countries. But much of the wealth has flowed to the richer countries and their expanding transnational corporations.[26] In large measure, the recent spread of slums and shanty towns around big cities reflects this widening economic inequality. It is a world in which the opportunities for local urban employment are affected increasingly by global market forces. Economic globalisation has spawned a new international division of labour. The manufacturing of 'low-end' products – footwear, garments, toys, electronic assembly – is increasingly outsourced by the rich Northern countries to poorer countries where labour is cheap and workplace standards are relatively unregulated. Those countries, with small internal markets, must strive to generate wealth by exporting these light manufactured goods to the developed world. There, their low price helps maintain low inflation rates and a consumers' paradise.

These globalising changes have a range of social and health consequences for the developing countries. First, socioeconomic stratifications are widened; those in favoured sectors (e.g., tourism) prosper; those working in export-led manufacturing earn a subsistence wage; and those remaining in sectors not keyed in to the global economy (e.g., many rural workers) suffer. Many rural societies are thus becoming globally and nationally marginalised. This causes an inevitable downward spiral of environmental degradation, increased poverty, food insecurity, stunting and infectious disease health risks.[25] The resultant tensions can erupt in so-called ethnic or tribal conflicts (as has occurred in many sub-Saharan African countries). Second, the fall of commodity prices and the low prices paid for low-end manufactured goods, in an open competitive global marketplace where trading loyalties no longer count, consigns those exporting countries to continued poverty. Third, there is heightened pressure upon developing countries to open up their economies to imports (and capital investment) from developed countries. This process tends to exacerbate further the international rich–poor gap, with all the usual adverse consequences for population health and standards of health care.

In light of this analysis, we can take a much enlarged view of the root causes of the health deficit in poor Third World countries. It became increasingly apparent during the 1990s that the globalised economy, ostensibly a source of generalised wealth creation, has been operating to the disadvantage of poor debt-burdened countries. The resultant exacerbation of land degradation, losses of biological and ecological resources, rural unemployment, food short-ages and urban crowding all contribute to health deficits for the rural dispos-sessed, the underfed and the slum-dweller. In some ways, today's situation is a replay, on a larger stage, of the experience of the nineteenth century, when unregulated competitive capitalism in Western countries, unmodulated by state regulation or the power of labour unions, caused much local environ-mental blight, poverty, disease and early death.

The importance of building up stocks of social and human resources in order to achieve gains in population health has become apparent in recent years. During the latter half of the twentieth century, the combined improve-ments within low- and middle-income countries in early-life mortality and in adult life expectancy were attributable, approximately, to increases in literacy (35% contribution), in the application of new knowledge, including public health technologies and medical interventions (45% contribution) – and in income (20% contribution).[27] Differences in the balance of these assets between countries accounts for some of the 'outlier' countries that do not conform to the general graphed relationship of national average life expec-tancy against per-person Gross National Product (GNP – see Figure 9.1). Some countries have much higher life expectancies than their modest economic indices would predict. This occurs in countries with above-average commit-ments to mass education and primary health care and with below-average gra-dients in individual income. In simple terms, those countries get more health for their per-person wealth. Four well-recognised examples are Sri Lanka, where life expectancy is expected to reach 74 years by 2000 (having been 60 years in 1950), Costa Rica, Kerala State (southwest India) and China. By con-trast, life expectancy figures in Hungary, Romania and certain of the oil-rich OPEC nations are clearly below their GNP-related expectations.

Conclusion

Medical students, when assessing a patient in hospital, are encouraged to ask: Why this person, and why now? The question recognises that the individual is not a random and isolated representative of a homogeneous community. The patient's illness has a context and a background. Likewise, we can ask of a change in the rate of a disease in a population: Why this population, and why at this time? Again, the search is for contextual understanding. It is not sufficient to propose, for example, that the reason for an increase in the incidence of coronary heart disease is that the population began to increase its intake of saturated fat four to five decades ago. We also want to know why that dietary change occurred – what were the cultural, economic and other reasons?

We want to know why such a dietary change might be detrimental to human biology. By thinking about this within an evolutionary ecological frame we can understand better. First, we understand that 'Pleistocene' human biology is not attuned to eating a lot of saturated animal fat (remember, wild animals contain mostly unsaturated fats). So we should not be surprised if there is biological harm done by such a diet. Second, we understand that sweet and fatty foods were instinctively sought 'survival' foods in hunter-gatherer days – difficult to acquire, but high in energy. Third, the selective breeding of livestock (affecting the fat content in meat and milk) and the modern processing of foods have increased our capacity to produce and concentrate fat in the diet. Fourth, the social changes associated with urbanism, and the increasing consumer reliance on fast foods, convenience foods and baked goods, have increased the fat content in the typical daily diet. Those evolutionary and population-level insights help us to understand and contextualise the problem, and thereby identify the ways in which dietary fat intake might most effectively be reduced.

That is a rather simple example. But it reminds us that there is social, historical and evolutionary depth to most human diseases. It also reminds us that changes in human culture, technology and environmental incursions nearly always have consequences for health and disease. In order to understand and foresee the likely health impacts of today's unfamiliar large-scale changes, both in the global environment and in the urban social environment, we must think within an ecological 'systems' framework. The ideas of ecology, of interactive interdependent systems, have begun to influence many areas of human endeavour and enquiry. There is now a need to consummate the mid-twentieth-century stirrings towards an 'ecology of health'.

The high consumption lifestyle of Western nations continues to depend greatly on continued access to inexpensive inputs from non-Western nations, often resulting in depletion of the latter's natural resources or the diversion of traditional agriculture into export crop production. Meanwhile, as developing countries pursue their own economic aspirations, there will be additional strains upon our globally shared ecosphere. This will contribute to increasing risks to population health around the world. After two centuries of rapidly increasing fossil fuel combustion by today's rich countries, further increases in East and Southeast Asia will contribute greatly to the accumulation of greenhouse gases and, hence, to the diverse risks to health. Continuing forest clearance brings exposure to new and potentially mobile infective organisms such as the haemorrhagic fever viruses in Latin America. The over-fishing of the oceans is reducing *per capita* supplies of seafood. Continued pressure on agroecosystems in food-insecure regions, coupled with land degradation and population growth, will increase regional malnutrition and exacerbate migratory pressures and their attendant health risks.

How, then, can we make the future safe for human wellbeing and health?

12

Footprints to the future: treading less heavily

Few ape species survived the prolonged period of climatic cooling and environmental change that began in the Miocene around 15–20 million years ago. Today there are just the orangutans, gorillas, chimpanzees and humans. The three non-human ape species are being rapidly depleted as the human population expands its numbers and intensifies its activities. That fourth ape species, *Homo sapiens*, is in many ways a product of the unusually cold world over the past several million years.

Five million years ago, a bipedal hominid with short legs and long arms shuffled out of the receding forest, and managed to survive by foraging for plant foods in the thinning woodland and by occasionally scavenging meat or killing small animals. That hominid's descendants, much later, used stone tools and fire, and acquired the ability to share ideas and plans. This was a larger-brained, meat-eating species that lived primarily on its wits, possessing neither brawn nor specialised anatomical armoury. Indeed, as hunter-gatherers, humans are distinguished by their non-specialisation; they can survive, opportunistically, eating a mix of plant foods and animal species. They could hunt a local population to the point of extinction, and then switch to another species. In this way, they probably contributed to the extinction of many of the megafauna soon after the end of the last glaciation, 15,000 years ago. We see the same thing happening today. With our sonar-assisted fishing fleets we over-fish the ocean's great fisheries, switching almost nonchalantly from one prey species to the next.

The centrepiece of human evolution over the past 2 million years has been the large and complex brain. This organ conferred consciousness, abstract thought, forward planning, language and fine motor control. From that cerebral efflorescence have flowed our complex culture and technology – and all of the departures by humans from nature's usual evolutionary script. That script decrees that the attributes and behaviours of a species must fit with the conditions of its formative local environment. For humans the equation seems to be somewhat different. We have found ways of living at one or more removes from the ecological constraints of the natural world that apply unbendingly to other species.

This unique capacity among species to keep on expanding the carrying capacity of the natural environment is evident in the succession of human achievements: tool-making, meat-eating, geographic spread, diversity of food sources, agriculture and animal husbandry, harnessing of external energy sources, industrialisation, near-certain survival of childhood, increased life expectancy, birth control, virtuoso biotechnology, high-speed electronic communications and so on. We have split the atom and unleashed prodigious amounts of energy, and we have begun to reengineer the molecular architecture of life. Such breakthroughs, if harnessed aright and applied within the framework of ecological sustainability, could make for greater human wellbeing and material comfort. Indeed, there is now some urgency about our doing just that. We cannot go on expanding the carrying capacity of a closed-system ecosphere. Various of the planet's limits are being reached – in some cases breached.

The long succession of changes in human ecology over many millennia has improved our material conditions, made human life and survival more secure, and, in recent times, has greatly extended the average human lifetime. New infectious diseases have come and, sometimes, gone. The grip of pestilence has been loosened in industrialised societies over much of the past century. Various noncommunicable diseases of middle and late adulthood have increased, many of them the result of suboptimal ways of living rather than the inevitable concomitants of older age. More recently, some noncommunicable diseases, especially coronary heart disease, have decreased in Western populations. Life expectancy has increased and fertility rates have fallen. Living longer and breeding less, we have further loosened the ancient grip of nature – a grip which over many millennia has typically carried off adults and their newborn at rather short notice via starvation, infection or traumatic death. We have thus also loosened the grip of natural selection.[1]

Meanwhile, as human ecology has changed, so various disparities have emerged between innate human biological needs and the conditions of our modified living environments. Within developed countries technological advances and modern consumerism have radically changed our diet, levels of physical activity, patterns of sexual activity and social relations in general. The consequences for heart disease, raised blood pressure, diabetes, various cancers, sexually transmitted diseases, mental health and anti-social behaviours are well documented. Social and technological changes have also introduced new types of public health hazard, including mass-produced cigarettes and car-based urban transport systems. As energy-dense processed foods, sedentariness and the other trappings of 'Westernism' encroach upon other cultures, so the adverse health consequences of these historically unfamiliar lifestyles become more prevalent. The rapid increase in obesity in urban populations everywhere is one obvious manifestation.

Those changes in patterns of health and disease have been very much in the foreground, readily visible to science, amenable to epidemiological research. Meanwhile, in the background, on a different scale, there are other forces abroad that will much influence the future of human health and disease. Global environmental changes are occurring. At the same time humankind is connecting up, globalising, on many different fronts. The consequences for human society and population health from both these processes have been discussed in earlier chapters. We must ensure that the globalising process will yet bring a more coordinated international approach to managing the global commons, such as the stratosphere, the world climate, freshwater, forests, fertile land and the stocks of biodiversity.

THOSE PRIMORDIAL AUSTRALOPITHECINE footprints in the Laetoli volcanic slurry, over 3 million years ago, pointed our ancestors towards many future paths of dispersal and cultural endeavour. We have left footprints on landscapes far and wide. Human adaptations to unfamiliar environments around the world are evident today in the molecular footprints imprinted on our genome. Over time we have trodden increasingly heavily, disturbing larger patches, disrupting the environment on an enlarging scale. Our ecological footprints have now become too large for the world to bear for long.

The task of achieving sustainability does not easily fit into our usual frame of social and political decision-making. It requires us to give as much weight to the future as to the present. Yet the very logic of biological evolution, of natural selection, militates against doing that. Life reaches the future by dealing with the present. We, however, must now modify the present so that we can safely reach the future.

There are many footprints behind us, on the path from past to present. Can we envisage, now, making safe footprints to the future? After all, the present is merely a way-station between past and future. It happens to be where we are currently standing. Part of what we need to know in order to render the future safe will come from studying our evolutionary history and our palaeoanthropological past. This elucidates how we fit into the web of life. The fossil trail has revealed much about human origins. Modern molecular biology has revealed our forebears' trails across continents and the complex intermixing of human populations. It is helping to elucidate the sources of variations in human biology and culture, and how these have arisen in response to environmental pressures. In recent decades, with the rise in importance of ecology and the earth sciences, we have learnt much about the workings of the Earth and its ecosystems. The integration of these new scientific insights is also confirming the dependence of human wellbeing and survival upon nature's 'goods and services'. Increasingly, we understand that the sustained good health of a population is an index of how well nature's local and, now, global life-support systems are being maintained. (This is something that any good veterinary scientist already knows: the health profile of an animal population reveals how well matched the environmental circumstances are to the population's biological needs.)

The word 'sustainability' is overused, indeed widely misused. Even if we wish to use it correctly, we cannot, of course, see far into the future. But we can understand what a *prolonged* time means. Sustaining means supporting for at least a prolonged time. The fundamental importance of ecological sustainability to humans is this: successful economies, access to natural amenities, the ethic of conservation and the aesthetics of the wondrously varied world around us are all important – but they will count for little if we cannot sustain the health and viability of our populations. In the short term we may be able to 'buy' good health by consuming natural capital. In the longer term, however, good health is sustained by good management of both natural and social environments.

We cannot now turn the clock back. All of Earth's ecosystems, whether exploited or protected, are now under human domination.[2] The tropical forests of Amazonia and Indonesia, the expanses of Antarctic ice, coral reefs everywhere, the slopes of the Himalayas – all are subject to occupancy, use or tourism. The foreseeable future of this planet will be human-dominated. The Holocene is rapidly becoming the 'Anthropocene'.[3] We may yet find ways of partitioning nature into wild and managed compartments; of keeping a sufficient quota of ecosystems intact and functional; and of maintaining natural preserves for other species great and small, animal and vegetable.[4] With genetically engineered food crops and with 'precision agriculture', applied within a fairer and cooperating world, we may yet boost the yield of the world's croplands without increasing the chemical and energy inputs. All of this will require co-ordinated planetary stewardship.

We thus face a formidable agenda. Against great odds we must reduce the size of our collective ecological footprint. There will be need for an economics

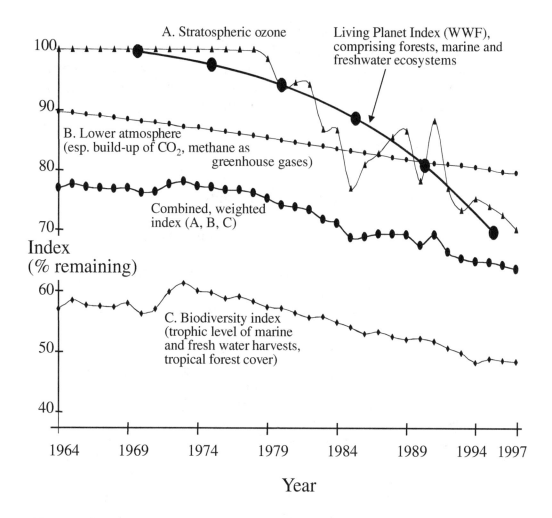

Figure 12.1 Time trends in depletion or disruption of major biophysical components of the ecosphere. The rate of change has generally increased since the 1970s. The initial values shown for three of the indices are below the figure of 100 because there had already been substantial change over preceding decades. The Living Planet Index (World-Wide Fund for Nature) is a composite of three different ecosystem indices. These graphs are broadly congruent with the several independent estimations made by other scientists showing that the total rate of resource use and waste generation is now well above the capacity of the planet to provide and absorb. On those calculations humankind's aggregate 'ecological footprint' now exceeds the capacity of Earth several-fold. These statistics, even if only approximately correct, provide a clear indication that, collectively, we are now generally on a non-sustainable path.

that assigns priority to social development, not to the consumption-driven throughput of energy and materials. However, we bring to this task a large and complex brain that can think about the future, imagine alternative scenarios, share and build ideas with other human brains, and make rational judgements about risks and benefits. Knowing a little about ourselves, we have some grounds for optimism. Sadly, we also know enough about our selfishness, competitiveness and short-termism to know that success is not assured.

Science and social policy: enlarging the frame

In the preceding chapters I have argued that it is changes in the social, economic, biological and ecological conditions of living that shape the patterns of health and disease in populations. These population-level relationships, entailing changes in cultural processes, social structures and environmental systems, are often not amenable to reductionist, itemised scientific analysis. Rather, they should be addressed within a systems context. Epidemiologists can easily 'miss seeing the woods because of the trees'. After all, the routine rewards in science are for specificity, precision, quantitation and crisp causal inference. Big questions often get side-stepped, or not even asked.

Those bigger questions do not get deliberately ignored. They simply do not 'fit' the template of orthodox research. Western science frames its questions in a particular way and, not surprisingly, some larger and more complex issues fall outside that frame. It was in this context that 'post-normal' science was described in chapter 11. 'Normal' reductionist science is, on its terms, extremely successful. Indeed, it is one of the later triumphs of the long human narrative. Yet it is also becoming clear that there is a lengthening list of complex, larger issues that require a more integrative systems-based type of science.[5]

The two great frontiers of challenge are at the extremes of scale. At one extreme is the need to achieve cooperative and equitable stewardship of the ecosphere.[6] At the other extreme, we are entering the 'post-genome' age. Evolutionary biologist Edward Wilson considers that the human species has reached the third stage of its relationship with its own genotype.[7] The first stage, spanning nearly all of human existence, entailed a total ignorance of natural selection and of genetic mechanisms. The second stage, seemingly ephemeral, occurred during the twentieth century when we sought to attenuate genetic disadvantage via eugenics and, later, by remedial treatment of single-gene disorders such as phenylketonuria and cystic fibrosis. We thus blurred the sorting function of natural selection. In the third stage, we are embarking on what he calls 'volitional evolution'. We are rapidly acquiring the technical power to direct genotypic change, to genetically engineer plants, animals, bacteria – and humans. We will have the power to usurp natural selection, to choose our own genetic future.

Each of these great frontiers pose enormous ethical dilemmas. Each will require us to reformulate our views of human social objectives. Each will have great consequences for the future patterns of health and disease.

THE TASK OF halting large-scale environmental change entails addressing issues that are global and intergenerational. We are, it seems, approaching the end of the era of essentially localised human activity with its immediate and small-scale environmental impacts and a need for local stewardship. We are, says the historian Lynton Caldwell, 'between two worlds'.[8]

This shift is happening at a time when we have embraced the values of free markets, open competition and deregulated economic activity. This has tipped the balance of economic and social power towards the private sector and its increasingly large transnational corporations. It has left governments and their elector-constituencies less able to control the social priorities and development directions of the modern world. This is in contrast to the middle third of the twentieth century when, in Western countries, there was a reasonable balance between capitalism and social democratic values. The former provided raw energy, creativity and risk-taking; the latter regulated the processes and socialised part of the profits. During the final decades of the twentieth century, however, we gave the private sector its head, dismantled barriers to trade and investment around the world, and declared that various essential utilities and services are better run by the private sector.

It is against this backdrop of free-wheeling market economics that we must now contemplate taking radical actions in order to sustain Earth's life-support systems. The problems will require supra-national policy-making and cooperation. We are moving to a world in which more and better global governance is essential.

Two problems arise. The first, the subject of growing public protest during 1999–2000, is that, to date, the evolution of global governance has been most active in relation to economic development, trade, investment and intellectual property rights. The World Trade Organization has, by design, neither interest in nor responsibility for the social, health and environmental consequences of economic activities. Its clear aim is to enhance the efficiency of global trade.

The second problem is that the meaningful implementation of many policies that are conducive to ecologically sustainable living (such as the development of environment-friendly transport systems, and the production of 'organic' food) will work best through local communities at a sub-national level. In between these two foci – global governance and community engagement – is the rather awkwardly meso-sized nation-state. It is, say some political scientists, a nineteenth-century political device with a twentieth-century morality, ill-equipped to tackle many of the problems of the twenty-first century.

Beyond efficiency: seeking a different economics

To a miser, a guinea is far more beautiful than a tree. (William Blake, 1799)

The idea that humanity is now pressing up against global limits not previously encountered is, by definition, new and unfamiliar. When the Heinz food company set up a turtle soup factory on Heron Island in Australia's Great Barrier Reef early in the twentieth century they rejoiced publicly in the fact that the supply of turtles was 'limitless'. The idea that, one day, the continuing exploitation of nesting turtles (slaughtered before they laid their eggs!) could cause their extinction was simply not conceivable. Unfortunately, it remains similarly inconceivable to many in the developed world today that we are increasingly overloading the ecosphere and jeopardising the future wellbeing and health of human populations everywhere.

Various traditional human cultures, now displaced to the sidelines of the modern world, have a more humble, participatory and dependent view of the role of humans within the natural world. They too were exploitative of their environment, and often changed its biotic profile. But there was a clear difference in ethic and, of course, in scale. In Australia, the latter-day European arrivals have only recently begun to understand that the Australian Aborigines, during 60,000 years of occupancy of that continent, maintained a spiritual continuity with the land and its animals; an intimate involvement without ownership. However, such cultures, from the jungles of Sarawak and South America to the Khoi and the San of southern Africa, have little impact in today's globalising world.

It is important that we understand that the human economy is actually a dependent subset of the ecosphere. As a human-made cultural device, the economy 'adds value' to nature. The true producer is the natural world – the source of food, fibre, timber, metals, fossil fuels and fresh water. Humans are modifiers, processors and consumers. Indeed, by imposing structure and by directing chemical reactions, we imbue the 'product' of our economic activity (e.g., dehusked cereal grains, a wooden chair, or a plastic bowl) with order, while disorder and degraded energy (heat) are released to the environment. Our economic activity thus adds wastes to the environment and increases entropy. Increasingly, those environmental consequences are matters of concern to us, and yet they are outside the calculus of conventional economics.

The science of economics is about the allocation of limited resources: commodities, labour and expertise. The marketplace is an important social device for achieving that allocation efficiently, thereby maximising the usefulness ('utility') of the exchanged resources to the two transacting individuals. The monetised 'value' of the transacted resource is expressed in its market price. The early proponents of market economics 200 years ago, at the dawn of modern capitalism, spoke of the satisfaction of mutual self-interest. In practice, while markets are efficient, in the absence of social intervention they tend to be unfair. The marketplace, by its nature, amplifies differentials in wealth and power. This is not by design; it is simply a property of unregulated markets. So, while we might welcome the efficiency of the market, we need to find a way of achieving greater fairness.

One of the key insights of the sub-discipline of ecological economics is that the concept of fairness includes all those currently, or in future, who are at risk from the environmental 'externalities' of the marketplace. This would include, for example, all those populations whose safety, health and viability is endangered by the consequences of global climate change. The price paid for petrol at the pump does not include the full environmental and health costs, to current and future populations, of its combustion. Taking this larger view of economic systems, our objective is implicitly to achieve ecological sustainability: that is, we want nature to continue to produce in order that we might continue to harvest. The threefold goal, therefore, must be to develop a type of economics that gives equal weighting to efficiency, fairness and sustainability.[9]

Costing the externalities, however, poses a major problem for market-based economics. There are many things that are important to human societies, including aspects of the world's natural resources, that cannot sensibly be assigned a market price. Consider two examples. Recognising that there once was the possibility of indefinite harvesting of a well-managed Grand Banks cod fishery, what was the *real* economic value of each cod in the last 10 tonnes that were landed before the fishery effectively collapsed in the early 1990s? And, in contemplating policy decisions about the preservation of biodiversity, how would we know the *real* economic value of a species of insect (such as a pollinating bee) that is at risk of extinction? According to Edward Wilson: 'So important are insects and other land-dwelling arthropods that if all were to disappear, humanity could not last more than a few months. Most of the amphibians, reptiles, birds and mammals would crash to extinction about the same time.'[10] Can markets assign meaningful money values to the residual cod stocks or to the disappearing pollinator insects?

That final example, about insects, illustrates another aspect of the problem. Market transactions are only possible if there is a seller who 'owns' the saleable item. No-one owns a species of insect. It is part of our natural heritage; it is 'common property'. So is the air, the stratospheric ozone, all wild species and the human genotype. In Garrett Hardin's famous essay on 'the tragedy of the commons', written in 1968, he pointed out that it is because they are collectively owned that many commons become overused and damaged.[11] The gain to the individual villager of putting another grazing cow on the village's common pasture is greater than his/her share of the 'cost' due to diminished viability of that overgrazed common. The modern equivalent is driving a car and emitting yet more carbon dioxide into the already overloaded lower atmosphere. The immediate gain in convenience or comfort to the motorist exceeds the cost occasioned by his/her share in the resultant damage to the global environment.

The essence of the problem, the private alienation of common property, is well captured in this old English rhyme:

The law locks up the man or woman
Who steals the goose from off the common
But lets the greater villain loose
Who steals the common from the goose.

The type of economics that we use in future must come to terms with the dependence of human economic activity on the natural world. It must come to terms with the need for fairness for its own sake *and* in order to enable social and economic systems to function and progress. Most importantly, it must treat common property such that the vital functions of the ecosphere can be sustained.

Fairness and sustainability

The world is currently becoming more unequal. The dimensions of poverty in the world were discussed in chapter 11. Part of the problem lies with the global machinery of economic aid and trade. For example, when development banks assist many different poor countries to produce, say, coffee, then the resultant oversupply causes the price to drop, and, while the rich importers get cheap cups of coffee, the producers receive little. Meanwhile, there are other more basic impediments to reducing the world's income inequality. United Nations figures show that over 250 million children of primary school age, especially girls, have either never attended school, or have had to drop out. In many poor countries educational facilities and standards have fallen in the 1990s. Poverty and lack of education create a downwards spiral. During a visit to South Africa early in 2000 I saw school buildings on the urban outskirts whose roofs had been removed by impoverished shanty-town dwellers desperate for materials with which to build their own one-room dwellings.

The alleviation of poverty, especially in the Third World, requires a broad agenda of social change. It requires improved access to land and (especially in urban environments) to other productive assets, including financial credit. It requires the provision of basic social services; the full and educated participation of women; and equitable and voluntary participation in networks of trade. It requires, somehow, the alleviation of political tension and militarism that squanders precious national assets. India currently spends twice as much on arms and defence as it does on education; Pakistan spends six times as much. Most basic of all, it is clear that the world's poorest nations cannot break free of the cycle of continuing and worsening poverty so long as up to one-third of their national earnings must be spent in paying the interest on their international debts. That indebtedness was not incurred via ineptness in the global marketplace; it is the legacy of a long history, in which powerful Western societies over the past several centuries have exploited the resources of weaker countries.

Land reform in poor countries is central to social progress and equity. Much of the recent formalisation of land holdings, re-orientation of agriculture to export crops, and introduction of new local technologies has typically benefited men, not women.[12] In much of the world, developed and developing, females are disproportionately poor, uneducated, ill and exploited. Yet, the success of women – as workers, food producers, family health providers, teachers of children, managers of natural resources, and participants in a democratic society – is essential to successful social development. The provision of small-scale credit to women, as has been provided by the Grameen Bank in Bangladesh, has a powerful multiplier effect in empowering women, banishing poverty, constraining fertility and fuelling local social and economic development.[13]

The social and economic reshaping of the South by the North is a fact of recent history.[8] This process not only diminishes cultural diversity; it also erodes the capacity for food security and material sufficiency on a local and environmentally friendly scale. Traditional lifestyles and local economies have been dissolving for a century or two. The rise of large consumer-oriented middle classes in much of Asia and Latin America has been under way for several decades. East Asia is rapidly emerging as a new centre of economic gravity in the world. The southern cone of South America may soon follow suit. The genie of global development is thus out of the bottle, and the challenge is now to achieve control over its direction to ensure ecological sustainability.

THE MODERN DEBATE on 'sustainable development' has been much influenced by the definition popularised in 1987 by the UN's World Commission on Environment and Development: 'meeting the needs of today's generation without compromising the needs of the future generations'.[14] The Commission was explicit about the formidable structural, political and ideological impediments to taking action on behalf of the distant future.

Our natural focus is the present, our own lifetime. We invent, we build, we manufacture and we decorate primarily to satisfy the needs and aspirations of the present. Pharoahs may have planned their mausolea for eternity; and Europe's bishops, masons and townsfolk may have hoped that their mighty Gothic cathedrals would inspire future believers. But mostly we act on behalf of the present and the immediate future. The ice-age artists of Chauvet Cave in southern France were not recording their symbolic ideas and fears for future generations of archaeologists; they were expressing their reverence, dependence, and, perhaps, totemic identity with the animals upon which they fed. Mozart was not writing music for unimagined music-lovers of the twenty-first century. Likewise, most of our social policy-making is seemingly indifferent to the distant future. Democratic politicians generally have shorter time-frames than autocrats. God may sit in judgement in the distant and ineffable future; but electors will make their choice next year. To many politicians, then, there can be no serious future beyond the next election. To economists who discount future costs and benefits at a compounded 5% per year, there is no real future beyond about 30 years.

Resolution of this constrained time horizon could come from two quarters. First, the public at large may become more aware of, and more concerned about, the risks to the long-term future of the world. In this they may merely be being selfish, worrying about their own descendants – or they may be concerned about future human populations and the world in general. No matter which, their concern would reorient the priorities of vote-hungry politicians. Second, there are many potential win-win situations. Some actions taken now, such as curbing the burning of fossil fuels, will achieve immediate environmental and health benefits as well as mitigating long-term environmental changes. Likewise, the alleviation of world poverty (via international debt relief and the control of exploitative trade) would reduce misery and illness immediately, while also reducing the desperate need to clear land, burn cheap coal and kill saleable endangered species.

We are beginning to see beyond the narrow orthodoxies of market-based economics, and envisage a fairer and more far-sighted approach to managing the needs of human societies and of the natural world. Efficiency, fairness and sustainability should become the joint and interdependent goals of our social and economic policies.

Preparing for a post-genome world

Gregor Mendel deduced the essence of genetic inheritance over a century ago. The basic genetic code, the double helix of complementary nucleotides, was cracked a half-century ago. Today we stand on the brink of a 'post-genome' age in which we know the molecular geography of the genes and have the techniques to induce specific mutations in those genes. We, the product of natural selection, are about to become the controllers of artificial selection.

Over a brief half-decade we have catalogued the human genome, with its 3 billion nucleotides. We are learning how to modify the molecular structure of genes, how to insert genes from one species into another thereby producing transgenic organisms, and how to clone. By combining those last two techniques, we anticipate mass-producing transgenic organisms such as cows that make vaccine proteins in their milk, to immunise young milk-consuming humans. We look forward to successful gene therapy for diseases with simple genetic causation. We recognise, nervously, the possibilities of genetically modified designer babies.

Biology has thus been transformed. Today the gene is the centrepiece of biotechnology and has become a cultural icon. Within the health sciences it proclaims an alternative view of the nature and causation of disease. Molecular genetics, say its proponents, will transform the preventive and curative dimensions of medicine. So, is the main payoff from the Human Genome Project to be a directory of disease determinism? A manual for the personalised management of genetically based risks of disease? Or is the human genome, in reality, a complex interactive system not reducible to a simple, itemised button-pushing approach?

This idea of biological determinism remains very contentious. Its critics argue that we cannot understand the behaviour, the dynamics, of complex wholes from the analysis of disaggregated parts. The champions of molecular genetics disagree, arguing that if we can 'reduce' finely enough then we can achieve causal exactitude. Epidemiologists, for their part, cannot ignore this debate. There is a need to keep genes in perspective relative to the many non-genetic determinants of human disease. There is a need to explore the interaction between genetic susceptibility and environmental triggers. As discussed in chapter 3, in the absence of obesity any population differences in inherited patterns of insulin sensitivity have little impact on the occurrence of diabetes.

The quest for somatic gene therapy has begun, albeit with adverse consequences in its initial trials in the United States. The prospect of germ-line gene therapy is also becoming more plausible. Where somatic gene therapy does running repairs on selected body cells of an extant individual, germline gene therapy changes the heritability of genes between generations. The fertilised egg is the likely target of germline therapy. Indeed, technically, it may be easier to achieve germline therapy, on just the one primordial cell, than to attempt to alter genes in a large number of somatic cells within a particular organ or tissue.

We must be quite clear about the implications of germline therapy. It would be a way of altering, permanently, the human genetic code. With this technique we could take direct control of the genetic inheritance of the human species. Humans, too, would become genetically modified organisms. For the moment, our society rejects the idea of 'designer babies'. But it is only a quarter-century since we rejected the unsettling, even shocking, idea of in vitro fertilisation – and that procedure is now common. I expect that we will readily agree to use gene therapy to eliminate genetically based disease. However, we may well choose not to programme body height and shape, not to modulate personality and intelligence, and not to converge upon an idealised set of 'perfect' genes. I think that the better we understand our evolutionary origins and our interdependence with the natural world, and the importance of genetic diversity as the population's insurance policy against future environmental change, the more likely it is that we will opt, collectively, for continued human genetic and phenotypic diversity. We would thus retain the essence of being a species. Peter Medawar encapsulated the argument well in 1960, stating that 'genetic diversity is part of our heritage, and part of the heritage of most other free-living and outbreeding organisms'.[15]

The Sustainability Transition

We enter the new millennium with unprecedented stocks of new knowledge and material resources. However, there is an imbalance in this knowledge. We have not yet, I think, become wise enough to understand that humans are not free agents on a cornucopian planet without limits. The exemptionalists are wrong: *Homo sapiens* does not exist apart from the natural world; we are a part of that natural world.

Over the past two centuries, our societies have already experienced, or in some countries are still experiencing, the demographic transition and the epidemiological transition. These have occurred in response to changes in ways of life, technologies and patterns of risk to health. Those inter-related transitions have shifted our populations to increased life expectancies and new age structures, to a greater proportional weight of the diseases of later adulthood, and to an amplified risk of various of those diseases because of social, material, environmental and lifestyle changes.

Meanwhile, the aggregate weight of human numbers and patterns of consumption has created an industrial metabolism that exceeds the absorptive and regenerative capacity of the ecosphere. We must therefore seek to achieve the Sustainability Transition. A guiding criterion must be to avert the anticipated risks to human wellbeing and health from the overloading of this planet's biophysical and ecological systems. A central task is to manage our natural and social environments in ways that will sustain the wellbeing and health of present and future generations. The achievement and maintenance of good population health is not a sideshow to the main policy event.

Now, as noted in the opening chapter, the optimists are probably thinking: 'Yes, but here we are at the beginning of the twenty-first century, living through what is, historically, a spectacular improvement in human health. There have been broad gains in life expectancy over the past half-century. Fertility rates are now declining widely – albeit less fast in many low-income countries than is desirable. The profile of major causes of death and disease is being transformed. The age-old scourge of infectious diseases, notwithstanding some local setbacks, seems to be in gradual retreat. So what can the matter be?' Well, all these encouraging things are true. And yet there is manifestly widespread and increasing environmental stress and disruption around the world. Is there a paradox here?

We noted earlier the two possible explanations. Either humans, with their remarkable cultural and technological achievements, have become independent of the life-support systems of the ecosphere. Or there may be a lag-period between our depleting the stocks of natural capital and experiencing the full population health consequences. The first answer cannot be true. As our consumer economies intensify we become more, not less, dependent on the natural world. People in high-income countries today each require 10–20 times as much of Earth's surface to provide the materials for their lifestyle and to absorb their wastes as do people in poor countries. On this basis we are already in ecological deficit, even as the numbers of people and their levels of consumption increase. The second answer, then, is much more plausible. We can subsidise ourselves for a while by living off nature's capital, by consuming stocks of natural physical and ecological resources. But that situation is not sustainable.

India provides a pointer to the nature of this problem. During the last half-century, living standards have risen and life expectancy has doubled, while the proportion of poor people fell (although not the absolute numbers). Food production, buoyed by the Green Revolution, kept up – even surpassed – population growth. The last serious famine in this historically famine-ridden country was in 1943. Meanwhile, India's environment has deteriorated markedly.[16] Common property resources such as forests, water supplies and natural habitats have receded under population pressures. Many rivers have been so grossly polluted that long stretches are biologically 'dead' and may not be capable of natural recovery. Air pollution in large cities is often now of biblical proportions. Arable farmland, particularly in the fertile Punjabi plains, has been widely eroded, salinated and waterlogged. Underground aquifers in that region, which take centuries or longer to refill, have been seriously depleted. These are unsustainable trends for India.

Estimating an optimum population size

We inevitably come up against the question: How many people can Earth support?[17] As discussed in chapter 1, the answer depends crucially on the average person's presumed way of life – the level of consumption and the types of technology. We assume also that the question refers to supporting *sustainably*, by keeping intact the stocks of essential natural resources. The question is not a mere conceit. We are not mediaeval scholastics estimating how many angels can stand on the end of a pin. Without some agreed approximate answer to this question, the ongoing debates about birth rates, immigration and the desirability of extending life expectancy by another decade or two are conducted in a vacuum.[18]

The task is daunting. There is no simple arithmetic here; no exact answer. The demographer Joel Cohen has summarised approximately 60 estimates published over the past 220 years. The figures he presents are nearly all within the range of 2 billion to 200 billion.[17] The dozen or so serious estimates made since 1980 are mostly within the range 3–12 billion, with the more recent estimates tending to be the lowest. Ecologists' estimates are consistently lower than those of demographers and economists.

The main determinants of the environmental carrying capacity for humankind are these: food production, the availability of fresh water, energy supplies and biodiversity. A more integrative type of determinant is the availability of ecologically productive land. For each of these criteria we can apply a two-step logic:

(1) What is the maximum level of consumption that the ecosphere can stand?
(2) What is an adequate share of that consumption per person?

Dividing the first answer by the second answer gives an estimate of the sustainable population. If we assume that the consumption of resources will be shared equally throughout the world – as unrealistic as that might be – then the answer will tend to be surprisingly low. Today we are 6 billion, going on 9 billion by 2050. But for the moment three-quarters of that total population consumes very little. If consumption were equal, we could certainly not support 6 billion at the level of modern Western society with its current technologies. To do that would require an estimated two extra planet Earths. To do so for 10 billion would require four extra Earths.[19]

Consider the first of the above criteria, food. As discussed in chapter 10, the increase in land degradation and the decline in groundwater supplies indicate that our recent methods of land use are not sustainable. But we are not sure what continuing level of food production the ecosphere can stand. So let us assume, here, that we can find a sustainable way of producing food at today's volume. Based on calculations published by several commentators, the world's current primary food supply could support around 7 billion on a basic, principally vegetarian, diet; 4 billion people on a modest diet with about 15% of calories from animal foods; and 3 billion people on a full but healthy diet with about 25% of calories from animal foods. Thus, in a fair and nutritionally healthy world it looks as if current food production capacity and methods would support around 4 billion people.

Now, since sustainable food production depends on land, water, energy and biodiversity, let us look at the arithmetic for each of those criteria. In so doing, bear in mind that we cannot foresee future technological advances that may confer an increase in global environmental carrying capacity. Malthus, 200 years ago, could not foresee the impending agricultural revolution that subsequently alleviated Europe's struggle with malnutrition and sporadic famine. Our arithmetic is therefore necessarily conservative, but prudent. There are no guarantees that humankind will achieve substantial gains in Earth's carrying capacity – that is, ecologically sustainable gains; not (as in the past) short-term gains.

Biodiversity is the most elusive of the four criteria. We have insufficient knowledge to do any direct calculation. Yet the seriousness of the criterion is apparent in Edward Wilson's statement about the fundamental importance of insects and other land-dwelling arthropods. In a myriad ways that we are beginning to document, but cannot quantify, the other species with whom we cohabit provide most of nature's 'goods and services'.[20] They regulate the climate, cleanse the water, enrich the soil, dispose of 'wastes', recycle essential nutrients, keep pest species under control, limit the spread of infectious diseases and pollinate flowering plants.

Water is widely becoming a limiting resource for local populations. Assuming that 1,000 cubic metres of water per person per year is a population benchmark for actual water scarcity, then the countries of North Africa and the Middle East, with a combined current population of around 200 million and a projected population of around 380 million in 2025, can actually carry only around 140 million without importing fresh water or doing without. Globally, if we are to continue to feed an extra 80 million people each year at the current annual average of 300 kilogrammes of grain, then the world must produce an extra 25 million tonnes of grain annually. That will require much more water. Yet already we are over-pumping aquifers and diverting river flows excessively to produce today's food. Assuming an individual quota of 3,500 calories of wheat energy daily (as food, animal feed and seed-stock), Cohen calculates that the global sustainable population supportable by mixed rain-fed and irrigated agriculture is less than 5 billion.

Energy is a complex criterion, since there are diverse energy sources and its use has multiple environmental consequences. The total energy throughput that the ecosphere can stand without causing degradation of natural systems and exhaustion of energy sources is not known. The total rate of annual world energy use by humans was around 17 billion kiloWatts (kW) in 1999, which included approximately 35% oil, 25% coal, 25% gas and 5% nuclear.[18] The present average per-person use is around 7.5 kW in high-income countries and 1 kW in low-income countries. The currently most serious consequence of energy use is the emission of carbon dioxide and other greenhouse gases from fossil fuel combustion. As we saw in chapter 10, worldwide fossil fuel combustion is already three times greater than would allow stabilisation of atmospheric carbon dioxide concentration at an ecologically tolerable level. If we assume that fossil fuels will remain the dominant source of energy for at least the next quarter-century, then, allowing for a doubling in energy efficiency and assuming a more equitable sharing of energy use, a population of approximately 4 billion could be supported sustainably. The advent of renewable energy technologies (via the harnessing of solar, wind and tidal power – and, perhaps, the eventual taming of nuclear power) will loosen this constraint on human numbers.

Finally we come to land, which some consider to be the best single criterion for estimating human carrying capacity.[18] In earlier chapters, the important idea of the 'ecological footprint' has been discussed. It is defined as: 'the total area of productive land and water required on a continuous basis to produce all the resources consumed, and to assimilate all the wastes produced, by that population, wherever on Earth that land is located'.[21] This leads us to the concept of 'ecologically productive land' comprising arable land, pasture land, forest land, and energy land. Those land components make up most of humanity's ecological footprint. Currently, terrestrial footprint sizes are very unequal. Those of Australians, American and Canadians occupy approximately 10 hectares per person, while those of India, China and Bangladesh are about one-tenth of that size. If the 9 billion hectares of Earth's ecologically productive land were divided equally so as to provide, say, 2.5 hectares per person – sufficient for a satisfactory standard of living if used efficiently and with reasonably forseeable technologies[22] – then a population of around 3.5 billion people would be supportable. Advances in coastal and freshwater aquaculture could well expand that figure to 4 billion.

During the 1990s, several scientific organisations and individual scientists tackled this question.[17,18] Although different approaches and assumptions were used, most estimates were within the range of 3–5 billion people. This figure may surprise us, since we are already well over that number and heading to higher levels. Again, we must remind ourselves that the fact that we have recently attained such a large population size, and have managed also to increase the average life span, proves little in terms of the sustainability of human numbers and ways of living. After all, the count of 4 billion was reached only a little less than three decades ago.

Managing the future

These momentous issues of the early twenty-first century are attracting increasing, and urgent, attention from international organisations, such as the UN agencies, the World Bank, various large NGOs, and the scientific research community. Early in 2000 the World Health Organization set up a Commission on Macroeconomics and Health and an advisory committee on Globalisation and Health. The World Bank, despite the enormous conservative momentum embedded in its ranks of conventional development economists, has become increasingly oriented to seeking national development that fosters education, the strengthening of civil institutions, health protection and environmental conservation. The UN's Intergovernmental Panel on Climate Change has paid increasing attention to assessing how global climate change is likely to affect social wellbeing and population health and to identifying the economic and situational determinants of population vulnerability.

These initiatives and explorations are all part of a counter-balancing of the undue emphasis previously given to improving conventional growth-oriented economic performance, building physical infrastructure, boosting export production, promoting unfettered freedom of trade and investment, and extending the security of intellectual property rights during the 1980s and 1990s. They thus prefigure a move towards more cooperative forms of global governance. This is likely to be a future world in which there is a balance between global institutions empowered to take decisions according to criteria that are integral to ecological sustainability, and local government that reflects community values, needs and stewardship of local environment. A likely configuration would be global management of the 'commons', and interdependent local communities confederated within regional political and trading blocs. This would allow for the maintenance of local traditions and community life, and their evident health-promoting influences. In such a world we can hope to see the following:
• international debt alleviation
• an expanded provision of education and training

- more equal income distribution within and between countries
- increased international transfer of environment-friendly technology
- enhancement of the role of the state as a modern, efficient and transparent institution, collaborating in global governance
- international commitment to sharing the world's common property resources (such as the lower atmosphere) via a targeted convergence, over time, towards an equal per capita access.

THERE IS NOT space here to embark upon a more detailed discussion of how humans should organise and govern themselves in future. That is a huge topic in itself, and one on which there are much more expert commentators. The main objective of this book has been to make the case that human biology and human society have arisen, and belong, within an ecological framework. The essence of the political task, then, is to maintain those natural life-support systems, if for no other reason than that they are the necessary foundation for enhancing and sustaining the health of human populations.

Earlier chapters have shown that the health of human populations is never static. Not only do environmental circumstances fluctuate, but human cultures evolve and ways of living change. Patterns of health and disease change accordingly. Several such changes are already clearly visible:
- Obesity is rising in urban populations; diabetes will follow.
- The prevalence of mental health disorders, particularly depression, appears to be rising around the world. In part this is because of population ageing.
- Lung cancer will escalate markedly in the developing world over the coming quarter-century.
- Road deaths will continue to decline in developed countries, but will increase in other countries.
- The use of hard drugs is increasing, especially among young adults in urban populations. In part this reflects aspects of the urban social environment, the structural unemployment in many countries, and the predations of an increasingly sophisticated and globalised international drug trade. The consequences – addiction, crime and transmission of bloodborne infections – will increase.
- As the proportion of elderly people increases so the dementias of old age will tend to increase in prevalence.

Other future shifts in health risks are less certain. Rates of coronary heart disease and stroke will continue to decline in developed countries, especially as fetal and child nutrition improve and as lifelong diets incorporate more fruits and vegetables and a lesser level of saturated fat intake. Those cardiovascular diseases will, however, continue to increase over coming decades in low-income countries as they 'Westernise' their diets, take up smoking, and reduce their physical activity levels. Subsequently, a decline can be expected (even though epidemiologists are not yet sure why the decline has occurred in Western countries!). Other likely shifts include increased risks of breast cancer in women because of changes in reproductive behaviour, especially the deferral of child-bearing (although new forms of hormonal supplementation may offset this), and a continuing increase in allergic disorders such as asthma and hay fever (even though we are not yet sure of the underlying ecological explanation for this shift).

The future for infectious disease is unclear. As diseases of poverty in low-income countries, many infectious diseases *could* be greatly reduced. That task still confronts us. HIV/AIDS will almost certainly continue to increase in poorer countries, and will increasingly erode population growth rates and economic performance. Some new infections can be expected as we continue to clear forests, change our sexual practices and intensify commercial food production. Various vector-borne infections, such as malaria, dengue and schistosomiasis, could yet be reined in by new and better coordinated methods of control – thereby countering new tendencies to increase as our environmental incursions intensify, as urban-fringe populations expand in poor countries and as the world's climate changes. The continuing emergence of antimicrobial resistance will present a problem. On the plus side, the advent of DNA vaccines and of designer antimicrobials based on new molecular biological knowledge should assist in preventing and treating infectious diseases. Other as yet unimagined molecular biotechnologies may come to our assistance also.

The main gains in life expectancy will presumably be in poorer countries as they close the current gap between themselves and the developed world. We certainly have the knowledge and assets to achieve this, but the recent substantial declines in life expectancy in sub-Saharan Africa because of HIV/AIDS must qualify our optimism. Life-lengthening clinical treatments are proliferating, but access to them is limited to societies and individuals able to pay. The richer stratum of the world may soon have access to gene therapy for some disease processes. Indeed, if the world were to continue to be driven by naked market forces, and if no environmental crises intervened, then a world divided between a rich genetic elite and an impoverished genetically average underclass could yet emerge. At first sight this may seem fantastic. Yet the world has a way of surprising us. Could our forebears just one century ago have foreseen the loss of stratospheric ozone or human-induced climate change? In the optimistic days of social democracy, four decades ago, we would not have anticipated a threefold steepening of the world's income inequality gradient. These novel changes arise without intent, without malice and without overt wickedness. The future is always uncertain.

Conclusion

History has shown more than once that the fates of the greatest empires have been decided by the health of their peoples or their armies, and there is no longer any doubt that the history of epidemic diseases must form an inseparable part of the cultural history of mankind. Epidemics correspond to large signs of warning which tell the true statesman that a disturbance has occurred in the development of his people which even a policy of unconcern can no longer overlook. (Rudolph Virchow, 1848)[23]

The early chapters in this book looked back in time, not just because there is a fascinating story to tell, but to enable us to see our future more clearly. Human biology has been shaped by long slow evolutionary pressures, stretching back through millions of years of hominid adaptation in a changing environment. Human society, especially over the past 10,000 years, has likewise been shaped by environmental conditions, interacting with human cerebral and cultural facilities. The constant struggle with infectious agents, dietary deficiencies and environmental toxins has left a range of imprints on our genetic makeup. Cultural evolution, too, has had major consequences for human biology, social wellbeing and health. However, the cultural assets of modern societies have buffered us against direct accountability to the wider ecological realm, and have diminished our awareness of it.

The scale of today's environmental problems requires us to seek sustainable ways of living. Time is relatively short, the issues are complex, communities are naturally conservative, and politicians in democratic systems have limited horizons. We may find technologically clever ways of lessening our environmental impact and thus preserving our natural resource base. The application of biotechnology, the use of precision farming and water management, the development of radical new materials via nanotechnology, and the use of alternative energy sources may all be part of the solution. However, we will need more than technological ingenuity. We will need to reform our social priorities and economic systems. We will need to constrain both human numbers and levels of waste-generating consumption in order to protect the life-supporting systems of the natural environment. Meanwhile, we must strive to reshape the social environment in order to achieve greater equity and conviviality, enhanced child development and adult health, and, above all, sustainability.

To achieve the Sustainability Transition, we must understand the ecological frame within which we exist. The essential two strategies, I suggest, are these:

(1) To consume nature's flows while conserving the stocks (that is, live off the 'interest' while conserving natural capital)

(2) To increase society's stocks (human resources, civil institutions) and limit the flow of materials and energy

We cannot continue to grow in number and appetite, and to commandeer an increasing proportion of available food energy, without damaging the ecosphere. The human species now accounts for approximately 40% of the total terrestrial photosynthetic product – by growing plants for food, by clearing land and forest, by degrading land (both arable and pastoral), and by building over the land.[24] If human numbers double, then, this arithmetic indicates that we would not leave much for other species.

That, then, is the dilemma for the human species as we complete our tenth millennium since the advent of agrarian living. The twenty-first century will pose a mighty challenge. Demographic stresses due to ageing populations, social stresses in large cities, ethnic fragmentation as nation-states falter, and conflicts over scarcity may all increase. Optimists predict that, as the world economy globalises, as geographic regions connect, as trade liberalises and as transnational corporations assume greater control over international consumerism, gains in material wealth will bring social progress and improved health. Others, however, foresee an amplification of the rich–poor divide, an indifference to environmental management, and a deterioration in health and life expectancy. A widening rich–poor divide would create the conditions in which acts of desperation and terrorism increase – the conditions in which modern civilisation could begin to unravel. Hopefully, the Darwinian self-interested logic of altruism (discussed in chapter 2) will intervene, since 'altruism' by the world's rich, to alleviate poverty and avert ensuing environmental crises, would be in their long-term interests.

We humans have responded to many new challenges before with adaptability, versatility, improvisation and invention. Further, we alone among species can imagine distant futures and intervene in ways that shape long-term environmental outcomes. That recent wild card of evolution, the human brain, has created a magnificent, diverse pageant of human culture and technology. However, in the late twentieth century, the pageant – ever larger, ever louder –

has encountered unexpected problems, particularly the incurring of an ecological deficit at the global level.

The human brain, source of the problem, could yet provide the solution. The ongoing story of evolution on Earth is about testing new biological and behavioural formulations when facing new environmental challenges, and thereby maintaining good health. *Homo sapiens* is about to take the next part of that test.

Notes

Preface

1 *Holy Bible* (King James version). The Revelation of St John the Divine. Chapter 6 (esp. verses 1–8). This graphic text was written while St John was in political exile on the Greek island of Patmos during 95–97 AD. It contains a vivid fantasy-like account of the opening of the Seven Seals, which give an account of the apocalyptic destiny of mankind: 'And I saw in the right hand of him that sat on the [heavenly] throne a book written within, and on the backside, sealed with seven seals.' The seven-horned seven-eyed Lamb of God takes the book and breaks open the seals. The first four seals reveal four terrible horsemen astride coloured horses: white (conquest), red (warfare), black (famine), and pale (death, or pestilence). 'And I looked, and behold a pale horse: and his name that sat on him was Death . . . And power was given unto them . . . to kill with sword, and with hunger, and with death, and with the beasts of the earth.' The fifth seal reveals the souls of the dead; the sixth seal reveals the repertoire of cosmic and earthly violence of a wrathful God: 'and the sun became black as sackcloth of hair, and the moon became as blood'. The dreadful seventh seal reveals the subsequent cataclysmic destruction of much of earth and its peoples by the seven fearsome trumpet-sounding angels who stood before God.

2 Beaglehole R, Bonita R. *Public Health at the Crossroads*. Cambridge: Cambridge University Press, 1997.

3 McMichael AJ, Beaglehole R. The changing global context of public health. *Lancet* 2000; 356: 495–9.

4 Flannery T. *The Future Eaters*. Chatswood, NSW: Reed Books, 1994.

5 Rees W. Revisiting carrying capacity: area-based indicators of sustainability. *Population and Environment* 1996; 17: 195–215.

6 McNeill J. *Something New Under the Sun: An Environmental History of the Twentieth Century*. London: Allen Lane, 2000.

1 Disease patterns in human biohistory

1 Murray CJL, Lopez AD. *The Global Burden of Disease: A Comprehensive Assessment of the Mortality and Disability from Diseases, Injuries, and Risk Factors in 1990 and Projected to 2020*. Boston: Harvard School of Public Health, 1996. By the year 1990, the noncommunicable disease death rate in adults aged 15–70 years was estimated to be as great in sub-

Saharan Africa as in Western countries (see p. 177 of above reference). Approximately two-thirds of all cardiovascular disease deaths below age 70 years are now occurring in developing countries. WHO has described this as 'the hidden epidemic of cardiovascular disease'.

2 This assumption has its counterpart in traditional societies, where individual disease was often attributed to specific local agents – witches, sorcery or the 'evil eye' – or to the individual having transgressed a social taboo. See also 'Evolution of ideas about health and disease' in chapter 11.

3 Carson R. *Silent Spring*. New York: Houghton-Mifflin, 1962.

4 Meadows D, et al. *The Limits to Growth*. London: Earth Island, 1972; The Ecologist. *Blueprint for Survival*. London: Penguin, 1972; Commoner B. *The Closing Circle*. New York: Bantam, 1972; Ehrlich P, Ehrlich A. *Population, Resources, Environment: Issues in Human Ecology*. San Francisco: W.H. Freeman, 1970.

5 Tainter JA. *The Collapse of Complex Societies*. Cambridge: Cambridge University Press, 1988; Diamond J. *Guns, Germs and Steel. The Fates of Human Societies*. New York: Norton, 1997.

6 Erik the Red's son, Leif Eriksson, later explored the icy northern American Atlantic coast and, amidst 'salmon and wild vines', established a tiny short-lived colony near the mouth of the St Lawrence river. Archaeological remnants appear to corroborate the written records of settlement dating from that time.

7 Barlow LK, Sadler JP, Ogilvie AEJ, et al. Interdisciplinary investigations of the end of the Norse western settlement in Greenland. *The Holocene* 1997; 7: 489–99. This paper cites in particular the palaeo-anthropological studies of Tom McGovern and colleagues of the western settlement.

8 Fisher DA, et al., 1996 – cited in Barlow et al. (1997) above. They examined data from ice cores for the past 3,500 years in Canada and Greenland. (Ratios of oxygen isotopes indicate the temperature.)

9 Fagan B. *Floods, Famines and Emperors. El Niño and the Fate of Civilisations*. New York: Basic Books, 1999.

10 Vitousek P, Ehrlich P, Ehrlich A, Matson P. Human appropriation of the products of photosynthesis. *Science* 1986; 36: 368–73.

11 East Asians also have low tolerance for alcohol, because of their genetically determined low level of alcohol dehydrogenase enzyme. These and other examples are discussed further in chapter 3.

12 Rees W. A human ecological assessment of economic and population health. In: Crabbé P, Westra L, Holland A (eds.) *Implementing Ecological Integrity*. Dordrecht: Kluwer, 2000, pp. 399–418.

13 Meyer WB. *Human Impact on the Earth*. Cambridge: Cambridge University Press, 1996; Vitousek P, Mooney HA, Lubchenco J, Melillo JM. Human domination of Earth's ecosystems. *Science* 1997; 277: 494–9.

14 The British evolutionary biologist, William Hamilton, showed in the 1960s that apparently cooperative behaviour has its basis in 'kin selection'. As part of the natural selection process, genetically driven self-denying behaviour by an individual will be selected for if it succeeds

in protecting related family members who then survive to transmit that individual's 'altruistic' gene. Reproductive success is about propagating genes, not preserving individuals.

15 See Strickland S, Tuffrey VR. *Form and Function. A Study of Nutrition, Adaptation and Social Inequality in Three Gurung Villages of the Nepal Himalyas.* London: Smith-Gordon, 1997 (see especially chapter 16).

16 Indeed, rogue individuals genetically disposed to noncooperation often prosper at the expense of the larger group. As population geneticists point out: selfish mutants invade. Tantalisingly, however, if cooperation is in an individual's interest then the 'cooperation gene' will spread within that population. Hence the population will acquire a greater collective cooperative behaviour – as an emergent property of the population at large. However, this property will be subject to erosion by any other genes that specify self-seeking individual behaviours at the expense of the group.

17 Rapport D, Costanza R, McMichael AJ. Assessing Ecosystem Health. *Trends in Ecology and Evolution* 1998; 13: 397–402.

18 Dubos R. *Man Adapting.* New Haven: Yale University Press, 1965.

19 Dubos R. *Mirage of Health. Utopias, Progress and Biological Change.* New York: Harper and Row, 1959.

20 Daily GC (ed.) *Nature's Services. Societal Dependence on Natural Ecosystems.* Washington, DC: Island Press, 1997.

21 *Holy Bible* (King James version). Genesis 1: 28.

22 Lloyd G. *Adversaries and Authorities.* Cambridge: Cambridge University Press, 1996. In Classical Greece, the Stoics and Epicureans fiercely debated free will and determinism.

23 Capra F. *The Web of Life.* New York: Anchor, 1996; Kaufman S. *At Home in the Universe. The Search for Laws of Complexity.* London: Viking, 1995.

24 Three decades later evolutionary psychologists such as Stephen Pinker are building upon this idea. See Pinker S. *The Language Instinct.* New York: Morrow, 1994.

25 Shepard P, McKinley D. *The Subversive Science. Essays Toward an Ecology of Man.* Boston: Houghton Mifflin, 1969. This book reprints the widely discussed essay of Lyn White: The historical roots of our ecological crisis. *Science* 1967; 155: 1203–7.

26 The important arguments about the adverse trends emerging in human numbers and environmental impacts were forcefully presented in the writings of Paul and Anne Ehrlich, as in their book *Population, Resources and Environment* (1970) – see n. 4 above. At about that same time Barry Commoner, in *The Closing Circle* (1972 – see n. 4), was packaging the new ecological awareness for a wider public with his four folksy laws: (i) everything is connected to everything else; (ii) there is no 'away'; (iii) nature knows best; and (iv) there is no such thing as a free lunch.

27 Rose G. Sick individuals and sick populations. *International Journal of Epidemiology* 1985; 14: 32–8.

28 Wilkinson R. *Unhealthy Societies. The Afflictions of Inequality.* London: Routledge, 1996.

29 Giovanucci E. Dietary influences of 1,25(OH)$_2$ vitamin D in relation to prostate cancer. *Cancer Causes and Control* 1998; 9: 567–82. However, it is also possible that the gradient, in

Europe, reflects certain cancer-protective effects of the southern European (Mediterranean) diet – see *Cancer Causes and Control* 2000; 7: 609–15.

30 Hetzel BS. *The Story of Iodine Deficiency*. Oxford: Oxford University Press, 1989.

31 Feachem R. Health decline in Eastern Europe. *Nature* 1994; 367: 313–14; Bobak M, Marmot M. East–West mortality divide and its potential explanations: proposed research agenda. *British Medical Journal* 1996; 312: 421–5. These and other papers have pointed out that basic differences between countries in social structure, economic relationships and political processes underlay these divergent national trends in life expectancy.

32 Leon D, Chenet L, Shkolnikov VM, et al. Huge variations in Russian mortality rates 1984–94: artefact, alcohol, or what? *Lancet* 1997; 350: 383–8.

33 I use the word 'race' in a non-categorical sense that recognises our species' long history of intermixing and the resultant continuous (versus discontinuous) genetic gradients. (See also chapter 3.) Population geneticists estimate that around 90% of all genetic variation in humans is between individuals within populations, about 5% is between subgroups within populations, and about 5% is between the major regional populations.

34 Rees W. Revisiting carrying capacity: area-based indicators of sustainability. *Population and Environment* 1996; 17: 195–215. This 'ecological footprint' metaphor is both instructive and evocative. I have been pleased to use variants of it throughout this book.

2 Human biology: the Pleistocence inheritance

1 The icy death of Otzi, the freeze-dried hunter-gatherer who perished in the Austrian Alps a brief 5,300 years ago and was rediscovered in the 1990s, attests to the physical hazards of the hunter-gatherer life. His skin bears the marks and scars of assorted wounds.

2 Ehrlich PR. *Human Natures. Genes, Cultures and the Human Prospect*. Washington, DC: Island Press, 2000.

3 Shepard P. *Traces of an Omnivore*. Washington, DC: Island Press, 1996.

4 Strassman BI, Dunbar RIM. Human evolution and disease: putting the Stone Age in perspective. In: Stearns SC (ed.) *Evolution in Health and Disease*. Oxford: Oxford University Press, 1999: pp. 91–101.

5 Kaufman S. *At Home in the Universe. The Search for Laws of Complexity*. London: Viking, 1995.

6 The germ-line cells produce the gene-bearing gametes – in animal species, the sperm and ova – each of which contains a random 'haploid' half-set of the full 'diploid' set of that parent's paired alleles.

7 The usual convention is to use the word 'gene' to refer to 'specific' alleles. Hence to say that an individual has the gene for sickle cell anaemia means, strictly, that he/she has the 'sickling' allele at that particular gene locus.

8 See notes 14 and 16 from chapter 1.

9 James Lovelock's 'Gaia Hypothesis' views the Earth and all life on it as an interdependent self-regulating (but 'non-purposeful') system that maintains optimal conditions for life

(Lovelock J. *Gaia*. New York: Oxford University Press, 1979). This radical idea, initially treated with disdain, has gained recent support and some scientific corroboration. (See also chapter 10.)

10 Clark JGD.*World Prehistory in New Perspective*. Cambridge: Cambridge University Press, 1961.

11 This also includes high-grade information about interregional genetic variation on the male's Y chromosome. Unlike the other 22 pairs of chromosomes, the 'pair' of X and Y chromosomes do not undergo recombination at meiosis. Hence, the genes on the Y chromosome are transmitted exclusively down the male line. It therefore provides a simpler record of human migration and mutation over the millennia than do studies of genes on the other chromosomes. Further, mutations of the Y chromosome occur at a slower rate than in the mitochondrial genome.

12 McElwain JC, Beerling DJ, Woodward FI. Fossil Plants and Global Warming at the Triassic–Jurassic Boundary. *Science* 1999; 285: 1386–90.

13 By quantifying mutational differences between species in the molecular structure of their DNA, scientists estimate the time elapsed since the species shared a common ancestry. The technique presumes a constant background mutation rate, as an analogue of time. Note, also, the special power of this approach in revealing the evolutionary past. Fossils point forwards from the past; extant molecules point backwards from the present. Therefore, any particular fossil bone may or may not be ancestral; it may be a dead end. The molecular approach entails the comforting certainty that today's genes *did* have ancestors. What is less certain, though, is the speed at which the molecular clock 'ticks', and whether that speed might have differed between species. Once clock-speed is agreed, it is possible to back-project to the time when the compared species last shared a common ancestor. (See also n. 11.)

14 Diamond J. *The Rise and Fall of the Third Chimpanzee*. London: Vintage, 1991.

15 Cavalli-Sforza L, Cavalli-Sforza F. *The Great Human Diaspora*. New York: Addison Wesley, 1995.

16 Such holes could also be due to the talons of large aerial raptors. Colin Tudge (*The Day Before Yesterday*. London: Jonathan Cape, 1995, p.198) judges that the australopithecines, with chimp-like hunting rituals, were unlikely to become any mega-predator's main meat meal. Obligate predators, such as leopards and lions, tend to be specialised hunters. 'These hyperactive [hominid] hordes', he says, 'would have been outside their ken: too unpredictable; too weird . . . they would have been creatures to leave alone. Better stick to antelope.'

17 Asfaw B, White T, Lovejoy O, et al. *Australopithecus garhi:* A new species of early hominid from Ethiopia. *Science* 2000; 284: 629–33; De Heinizelin J, Clark JD, White T, et al. Environment and behaviour of 2.5 million-year-old Bouri hominids. *Science* 2000; 284: 626–9.

18 Although we refer to these early hominids as 'hunter-gatherers', debate persists as to when hunting replacing the scavenging of meat. Evidence from at least the past half-million years shows that early humans were using wooden spears and were butchering animals *before*

other carnivores arrived at the kill site. Electron microscopic evidence from that era shows carnivore tooth marks superimposed over the preceding human butchery marks, made by sharp stone cutters.

19 Dart RA. *Australopithecus africanus*: The man-ape of South Africa. *Nature* 1925; 115: 195–9.

20 On a visit to this museum my reverent viewing of Turkana Boy was punctured by a boisterous crowd of secondary school students, viewing the panoramic life-size display of two family groups of *A. africanus* and *H. habilis* in the African savannah. First, came a group of teenage female *H. sapiens* who, giggling, tried to see behind the well-placed foliage that shielded the australopithecine penis from casual view. Then came the males, watchful of their teacher's roving eye, crouching down to peer between the legs of the squatting australopithecine mother. Perhaps Turkana Boy, in his time, would have sneaked a look also.

21 Foley R. *Humans Before Humanity*. Oxford: Blackwell, 1995. See also: Williams MAJ, Dunkerley DL, de Deckker P, et al. *Quaternary Environments*. London: Edward Arnold, 1993.

22 Among otherwise closely related species of primates the brain:body ratio is highest in those with more diverse diets. The ratio in omnivorous chimps is twice that of leaf-eating gorillas. See: Foley R. *Humans Before Humanity*. Oxford: Blackwell, 1995, p. 166. Foley also argues for the importance of increased meat intake as a 'release' for evolutionary expansion of a metabolically expensive organ, the brain (pp. 191–2). See also n. 27 below.

23 This is the same painful condition that the ill-fated members of Scott's Antarctic exploration team suffered when forced, out of survival desperation, to eat the livers of their sled-dogs.

24 Evidence of dependence on plant foods is the distinctive inability of humans (along with guinea pigs and carp) to synthesise vitamin C. Evidence of dependence on animal foods is the inability to synthesise the essential amino acid taurine.

25 Steven Pinker suggests that the first traces of language could have appeared in the Lucy australopithecines around 4 million years ago. See: Pinker S. *The Language Instinct*. Morrow: New York, 1994.

26 Stanley SM. *Children of the Ice Age. How a Global Catastrophe Allowed Humans to Evolve*. New York: Harmony Books, 1996.

27 Wheeler PE, Aiello LC. The expensive tissue hypothesis. *Current Anthropology* 1995; 36: 199–222.

28 Brand Miller JC, Colagiuri S. The carnivore connection: dietary carbohydrate in the evolution of NIDDM. *Diabetologia* 1994; 37: 1280–6.

29 The evolutionary story-line may be more complex. Because of the 50% discordance in their genotypes there is unavoidable 'genetic conflict' between mother and fetus. This is well described in: Haig D. Genetic conflicts of pregnancy and childhood. In: Stearns SC ed. *Evolution in Health and Disease*. Oxford: Oxford University Press, 1999: pp. 77–90. In this situation, natural selection is torn between the competing interests of mother and fetus. The mother's 'genetic' interest lies in conserving biological resources to maximise the future number of babies born. However, the fetal 'genetic' interest is in appropriating maternal nutrients. Hence, the fetal-placental unit secretes a hormone (human placental lactogen) which boosts the fetus' access to maternal glucose by increasing the mother's insulin resistance. The

mother counters by releasing more insulin to increase deposition of blood glucose in her own energy storage tissues. The fetus responds by increasing the enzymatic destruction of that insulin as the maternal blood passes through the placenta. An uneasy balance between competing interests is thereby achieved.

30 British Nutrition Foundation. *n-3 Fatty Acids and Health*. Briefing Paper. London: British Nutrition Foundation, 1999.

31 Wendorf M. Diabetes, the ice-free corridor, and the Paleoindian settlement of North America. *American Journal of Physical Anthropology* 1989; 79: 503–20.

32 Neel JV. Diabetes mellitus: a thrifty genotype rendered detrimental by 'progress'? *American Journal of Human Genetics* 1962; 14: 353–62.

33 Neel JV. The thrifty genotype revisited. In: Kobberling J, Tatersall R (eds.) *The Genetics of Diabetes Mellitus*. London: Academic Press, 1982, pp. 283–93. See also: Neel JV, Weder AB, Julius S. The 'thrifty genotype' hypothesis enters the 21st century. *Perspectives in Biology and Medicine* 1998; 42: 44–51.

34 'Neander' is German for 'new man', but its inclusion in the word 'Neanderthal' is merely coincidence. The valley, or Thal, in which the fossil bones were found in the nineteenth century had been named after a German poet, Joachim Neander. So the bones, like the valley, were labelled 'Neanderthal'.

3 Adapting to diversity: climate, food and infection

1 Strassman BI, Dunbar RIM. Human evolution and disease: putting the Stone Age in perspective. In: Stearns SC, ed. *Evolution in Health and Disease*. Oxford: Oxford University Press, 1999: pp. 91–101.

2 Haldane JBS. Disease and evolution. *La richercha scientifica* 1949; 19 (suppl): 68–76.

3 Kingdon J. *Self-Made Man and His Undoing*. London: Jonathan Cape, 1993.

4 Diamond J. *The Rise and Fall of the Third Chimpanzee*. London: Vintage, 1991.

5 Africans have a relatively high bone calcium content, despite having low levels of dietary calcium. The reasons for this are currently the subject of research.

6 Steinbock T. Rickets and osteomalacia. In: Kiple KF (ed.) *The Cambridge World History of Human Disease*. Cambridge: Cambridge University Press, 1993, pp. 978–81.

7 In men, recent epidemiological evidence suggests that a reduction in bloodborne vitamin D level, as occurs with darker skin pigmentation, increases the risk of prostate cancer – presumably by lessening the stabilising effect of vitamin D on prostate cells. See: Giovanucci E. Dietary influences of $1,25(OH)_2$ vitamin D in relation to prostate cancer. *Cancer Causes and Control* 1998; 9: 567–82. This, as another late-life cancer, would not have exerted any significant selection pressure on skin pigmentation.

8 McMichael AJ, Hall AJ. Does immunosuppressive ultraviolet radiation explain the latitude gradient for multiple sclerosis? *Epidemiology* 1997; 8: 642–5.

9 Cavalli-Sforza LL, Piazza A, Menozzi P. Demic expansions and human evolution. *Science* 1993; 259: 639–46. A wider-ranging account of genetic, linguistic and archaeological evidence

is given in: Cavalli-Sforza L, Cavalli-Sforza F. *The Great Human Diaspora*. New York: Addison Wesley, 1995.

10 Other genetic vectors in Europe indicate a southerly drift of Uralic–Finnish genes and a westerly drift of 'Aryan' genes from the Asian steppes from around 5,000 year ago.

11 Richards M, Corte-Real H, Forster P, et al. Paleolithic and neolithic lineages in the European mitochondrial gene pool. *American Journal of Human Genetics* 1996; 59: 185–203. This analysis indicates that only 15% of the genetic variation in Europe is due to the subsequent in-migration of farming groups. However, reliance on mitochondrial DNA entails several risks. First, the mutational rate may be faster than is thought. Second, only women transmit mitochondrial genes (the male sperm cell contains only nuclear genes) – and perhaps women, as acquired brides, migrated faster than did men. See also a more general discussion in: Lewin R. Ancestral Echoes. *New Scientist* 1997; 2089: 32–7.

12 Abdominal (or central) obesity, which is characterised by a high ratio of waist circumference to hip circumference, must be distinguished from peripheral (hips-and-thighs) obesity. The abnormal metabolic activity of the abdominal fat deposits tends to increase the levels of cardiovascular disease risk factors.

13 O'Dea K. Westernisation, insulin resistance and diabetes in Australian Aborigines. *Medical Journal of Australia* 1991; 155: 258–64.

14 Zimmet P, Alberti K. The changing face of macrovascular disease in non-insulin dependent diabetes mellitus: an epidemic in progress. *Lancet* 1997; 350 (Suppl 1): SI1–4.

15 Hales CN, Barker DJP. Type 2 (non-insulin-dependent) diabetes mellitus: the thrifty phenotype hypothesis. *Diabetologia* 1992; 35: 595–601. For a more general account of the thesis regarding the fetal origins of adult disease, see: Barker DJP. *Mothers, Babies and Disease in Later Life*. London: BMJ Publishing, 1994.

16 McKeigue P. Diabetes and insulin action. In: Kuh D, Ben-Shlomo Y. (eds.) *A Life Course Approach to Chronic Disease Epidemiology*. Oxford: Oxford University Press, 1997, pp. 78–100. (Recently, several genes with this type of dual action have been provisionally identified.)

17 Clausen JO, Hansen T, Bjorbaek C, et al. Insulin resistance: interactions between obesity and a common variant of insulin receptor substrate-1. *Lancet* 1995; 346: 397–402.

18 Stern MP. Primary prevention of type II diabetes mellitus. *Diabetes Care* 1991; 14: 399–410.

19 Brand Miller JC, Colagiuri S. The carnivore connection: dietary carbohydrate in the evolution of NIDDM. *Diabetologia* 1994; 37: 1280–6.

20 Kretchmer N. Lactose intolerance and malabsorption. In: Kiple KF (ed.) *The Cambridge World History of Human Disease*. Cambridge: Cambridge University Press, 1993, pp. 813–17.

21 Stearns SC. Introducing evolutionary thinking. In: Stearns SC (ed.) *Evolution in Health and Disease*. Oxford: Oxford University Press, 1999: see p. 9.

22 Allen JS, Cheer SM. 'Civilisation' and the thrifty genotype. *Asia-Pacific Journal of Clinical Nutrition* 1995; 4: 341–2.

23 The future diabetes rates in Papua New Guinea highlanders will provide a good test of this hypothesis. They have been agrarians for almost as long as Europeans, eating a moderately

glycaemic diet that includes taro, yams and bananas – but *not* dairy foods. If the onset of urbanisation and increased obesity induces a diabetes rate similar to that already evident in their lowland compatriates, this would support the idea that dairy foods conferred a critical further reduction in diabetes susceptibility in proto-Europeans.

24 Recent anthropological research indicates that the Pacific colonisation by island-hopping seafarers, originating from East Asian shores, entailed prudent eastwards 'latitude sailing'. This risk-minimising strategy allowed near-certain, faster return to home-base, assisted by the westerly trades winds if no land was found before half the on-board food ran out. Therefore, the Pacific islanders would not have experienced unusual feast-or-famine selection pressures during their actual migrations – but may have done so for several years after first settling on a new island.

25 Meyer UA. Medically relevant genetic variation of drug effects. In: Stearns SC ed. *Evolution in Health and Disease*. Oxford: Oxford University Press, 1999, pp. 41–9.

26 Risch A, Wallace D, Bathers S, Dim E. Slow *N*-acetylation genotype is a susceptibility factor in occupation and smoking related bladder cancer. *Human Molecular Genetics* 1995; 4: 231–6; Vineis P, McMichael AJ. Interplay between heterocyclic amines in cooked meat and metabolic phenotype in the aetiology of colon cancer. *Cancer Causes and Control* 1996; 7: 479–86.

27 Garnham PCC. *Malaria Parasites and Other Haemosporidia*. Oxford: Blackwell, 1966.

28 See for example: Dawkins R. *The Blind Watchmaker*. London: Longman, 1986.

29 Bruce-Chwatt LJ. History of malaria from prehistory to eradication. In: Wernsdorfer WH, McGregor I (eds.) *Malaria. Principles and Practice of Malariology (Vol. 2)*. Edinburgh: Churchill Livingstone, 1988, pp. 1–59.

30 Falciparum malaria is also less well adapted to the anopheline mosquito, since most bird malarias are transmitted by culicine mosquitoes. Studies show that the anopheline mosquito is a reluctant host for falciparum malaria. The mosquito, no less than the human, is disadvantaged by infection by the plasmodium, and has acquired some, as yet unelucidated, defences.

31 Angel JL. Health as a crucial factor in the changes from hunting to developed farming in the Eastern Mediterranean. In: Cohen MN, Armelagos GJ (eds.) *Paleopathology at the Origins of Agriculture*. London: Academic Press, 1984, pp. 51–73.

32 This is due to the absence of the Duffy antigen on the red blood cell surface, which the plasmodium requires for its entry into the cell.

33 Dobson M. *Contours of Death and Disease in Early Modern England*. Cambridge: Cambridge University Press, 1997.

34 Reiter P. From Shakespeare to Defoe: malaria in England in the Little Ice Age. *Emerging Infectious Diseases* 2000; 6: 1–11.

35 Hill AVS, Motulsky AG. Genetic variation and human disease. In: Stearns SC (ed.) *Evolution in Health and Disease*. Oxford: Oxford University Press, 1999: pp. 50–61.

36 The 'Duffy negative' mutation has apparently arisen in response to vivax specifically, since the falciparum parasite can gain entry to red cells via another membrane protein – the glycophorin B receptor.

37 The French nobleman, Count Arthur de Gobineau, argued, in his *Essay on the Inequality of*

the Human Races (1855), that civilisations rose and fell in relation to the purity of their Aryan blood. He fancied, remarkably, that the ten great civilisations in history had arisen because Aryans had infused into local populations their superior knowledge and culture! Such arguments laid a direct foundation for the turn-of-century popularity of eugenics in both Europe and North America.

38 The Romani Gypsies present a tragic experience of persecution and discrimination. In the 1970s they were subjected to an unofficial campaign of racial eugenics in Czechoslovakia via enforced sterilisations. The Roma are distinctive in appearance, culture and language. Nazi Germany regarded Roma and Jews as the dominant alien blood in Europe (the politically inconvenient Aryan connection of the Roma was discounted because of its alleged long 'contamination' by interbreeding outside Europe). The Roma came to Europe 500 years ago from northern India, not from 'little Egypt' (hence 'gyp-sy') as was commonly believed. Their original tracks through the Middle East are discernible via linguistic and molecular genetic analyses.

39 In the United States, the hereditarian view has been controversially advanced in the book Herrnstein RJ, Murray C. *The Bell Curve. Internal and Class Structure in American Life.* New York: Free Press, 1994. Those authors described intelligence gradients across major racial groups in the United States with reference to the *g score*, a postulated measure of general intelligence. There have been many strong critiques of this book. Edward Wilson, in his book *Consilience* (New York: Alfred Knopf, 1998), points out (p. 140) that *The Bell Curve* overlooks the 'genotype–environment correlation' which amplifies human diversity beyond its biological origins. The debate about race and biology in the United States is, of course, an old one. In the mid-nineteenth century, most whites attributed the poor health of black Americans to innate biological inferiority, whereas several (black) physicians argued that it was because of their enslavement. (See Krieger N. Shades of difference: theoretical underpinnings of the medical controversy on black–white differences, 1830–1870. *International Journal of Health Services* 1987; 7: 258–79.)

4 Infectious disease: humans and microbes coevolving

1 In 1954, the Royal Society of Medicine, in London, celebrated the advent of anti-tuberculosis drugs with public anticipation of 'the last tubercle bacillus'. In 1972 two eminent infectious disease scientists, Macfarlane Burnet (Nobel laureate) and David White, wrote: 'If for the present we retain a basic optimism . . . the most likely forecast about the future of infectious disease is that it will be very dull. There may be some wholly unexpected emergence of a new and dangerous infectious disease, but nothing of the sort has marked the past fifty years' (Burnet M, White D. *Natural History of Infectious Disease.* 4th edn. Cambridge: Cambridge University Press, 1972 p. 263).

2 Pigs have cell-surface receptors for both avian and human strains of influenza virus. Hence their special ability to effect recombination between strains of the virus from those two different sources.

3 Snow's reasoning also posed a threat to Britain's prevailing *laisser-faire* ethos, by suggesting that trade, human mobility and local entrepreneurial practice (e.g., the private water companies) influenced the probabilities of 'contagion'. The alternative, prevailing, view was that diseases arose from pervasive miasmas. Even after the exposition of the germ theory, ambiguity persisted about these competing explanations. For instance, in December 1899, the president of the Royal Meteorological Society noted that 'while it is admitted that plague is due to a specific microbe, it cannot spread except under certain meteorological conditions associated with the conditions of the ground, which must be in such a state as to exhale what is necessary for the propagation and spread of this particular disease'.

4 Colwell R. Global climate and infectious disease: the cholera paradigm. *Science* 1996; 274: 2025–31.

5 Snow J. *On the Mode of Communication of Cholera*. London: Churchill, 1855, p. 2.

6 This topic is explored by Paul Ewald in *Evolution of Infectious Disease* (New York: Oxford University Press, 1994). He concludes that there is no general tendency for infectious agents to evolve towards lesser virulence, via some sort of coevolutionary truce with the host. After all, biological evolution favours increasing 'fitness', and each infectious agent faces a particular configuration of obstacles to successful transmission between persons. The HIV/AIDS virus needs a seemingly healthy and sexually active host for many years, whereas the malarial parasite – which relies on mosquitoes for transmission – can afford to debilitate.

7 The presence of tuberculosis in Peru several thousand years ago raises an interesting question as to its origin. Could 'tuberculosis' have arisen twice, in Eurasia and in the Americas? If it had a shared ancestry with the European tuberculosis bacterium it must have migrated overland, eastwards through Asia, and made the Beringian crossing – unless it came via coastal migrations later.

8 Prions – proteinaceous infectious agents – are a newly identified, still controversial, form of 'infection'. They do not replicate by multiplying *de novo*; they pseudo-replicate by recruiting erstwhile normal protein molecules to adopt their own abnormal shape and behaviour. They practise molecular origami.

9 Bloom BR, Small PM. The evolving relation between humans and *Mycobacterium tuberculosis*. *New England Journal of Medicine* 1998; 338: 677–8. An example in European populations is the defect in cellular uptake of vitamin D by some individuals, which may reflect an earlier successful coevolutionary adaptation that denied the tuberculosis bacterium entry into host cells. Vitamin D and the bacterium both use the same receptor to gain cell entry.

10 Farmer P. *Infections and Inequalities. The Modern Plagues*. Berkeley: University of California Press, 1999.

11 An extraordinary 90% of all the 10^{14} cells in and within a human body are single-celled bacteria. However, since they are so much smaller than the host body's 10^{13} cells they account for only around 10% of total body weight.

12 Anderson RM, May RM. *Infectious Diseases of Humans: Dynamics and Control*. Oxford: Oxford University Press, 1991. When the infecting agent and the host are relatively new acquaintances, evolutionarily, and have not yet fully come to terms with one another the

resultant disease tends to be more severe because of greater 'virulence' of the infecting agent. However, it is often (though not always) to the advantage of the micro-organism to damage the host less, and it is always to the advantage of the host to acquire some additional resistance. In the 1950s, Australian scientists deliberately introduced viral myxomatosis into the rabbit population. The disease eliminated a very high proportion of rabbits, killing over 98% of all those infected. This created an intense selection pressure in favour of genetically resistant rabbits – and in favour of less lethal strains of virus that were more likely to pass on viral progeny. Myxomatosis-resistant rabbits and the less virulent strain of myxomatosis virus now predominate in Australia. (See: Fenner F. Myxomatosis in Australian wild rabbits: evolutionary changes in an infectious disease. *Harvey Lecture* 1957; 53: 25–55.)

13 McNeill WH. *Plagues and Peoples*. Middlesex, England: Penguin, 1976. This book provides the classic historical account of infectious disease as an ecological entity, evolving in human populations in response to changes in environment, culture and patterns of contact.

14 Karlen A. *Plague's Progress. A Social History of Disease*. London: Gollancz, 1995.

15 Mathews J, personal communication. For example, a strain of ear-nose-throat bacteria that persists for an average of four months may be sustained by a group of only 70 persons, while one that persists for only one month may require up to 500 persons if continuing transmission is to be achieved.

16 Cohen MN, Armelagos GJ (eds.) *Paleopathology at the Origins of Agriculture*. London: Academic Press, 1984.

17 Cockburn A. Where did our infectious diseases come from? The evolution of infectious disease. *CIBA Foundation Symposium 49*. London: CIBA Foundation, 1977 p.103. See also McNeill (1976, n. 13 above).

18 There must be an interesting story to tell about the ancient travels of the African trypanosome, as an enzootic infection in herbivores migrating via Asia and the episodic Beringian land bridge to the American continent sometime during the past several million years – or perhaps even dating from a much earlier time tens of millions of years ago when South America and Africa were still in tectonic contact, and when early monkeys could spread westwards and thereby bequeath to us today the Old World monkeys in Eurasia and New World monkeys in the Americas.

19 Crosby A. *Ecological Imperialism. The Biological Expansion of Europe, 900–1900*. Cambridge: Cambridge University Press (Canto edn), 1986, p. 30.

20 This curiously familiar word fascinates young English-speaking children. It derives from the Arabic word 'mummia', for pitch or bitumen, a natural preservative and medicinal substance that flowed down the Mummy Mountain in Persia. Mummia was used by the Egyptians to preserve their dead.

21 Sandison AT, Tapp E. Disease in Ancient Egypt. In: Cockburn A, et al. (eds.) *Mummies, Disease and Ancient Cultures*. Cambridge: Cambridge University Press, 1998, pp. 38–58.

22 Holy Bible. *Book of Samuel*, chapters 5 and 6.

23 Parmenter RR, Yadav EP, Parmenter CA, et al. Incidence of plague associated with increase winter-spring precipitation in New Mexico. *American Journal of Tropical Medicine and*

Hygiene 1999; 61; 814–21. Many other studies have shown that periods of increased rainfall are followed by proliferating rodent populations. Interestingly, the two major historical outbreaks of plague in Europe, in the fourteenth and seventeenth centuries, were associated with decadal periods of falling temperatures and unusual cold.

24 McNeill (1976, see n. 13 above) speculates that plague may have reached China by sea-trading routes, via the Southeast Asian region. However, some commentators doubt that the great epidemic in seventh-century China was bubonic plague.

25 Ziegler P. *The Black Death*. London: Penguin, 1982.

26 Recent evidence of genetically based variation in the capacity to survive infection has been reported. See, for example, Westendorp R, et al. Genetic influence on cytokine production and fatal meningococcal disease. *Lancet* 1997; 349: 170–3.

27 Diamond J. *Guns, Germs and Steel. The Fates of Human Societies*. New York: Norton, 1997.

28 This story has been told in several of the sources mentioned elsewhere in these notes: Dubos (1959), Crosby (1972, see n. 29 below), McNeill (1976), Karlen (1994) and Diamond (1997).

29 Crosby A. *The Columbian Exchange*. Westport, CT: Greenwood, 1972.

30 Zinsser H. *Rats, Lice and History. A Chronicle of Pestilence and Plagues*. Boston: Little Brown, 1935, p. 272.

31 A detailed and engaging account of this debacle is to be found in Zinsser (1935), see n. 30 above.

32 Kiple KF. *The Carribean Slave Trade: A Biological History*. Cambridge: Cambridge University Press, 1984. The less deadly vivax malaria had already been introduced to the Americas by Europeans in the sixteenth century. The enslaved West Africans were refractory to vivax malaria (see chapter 3), but they were the vehicles by which falciparum malaria and yellow fever were introduced to the western hemisphere. Those two diseases killed many native Americans and European settlers. Tragically for Africans, their lesser susceptibility to those diseases then became a major reason for their being the preferred source of labour in the Americas and the Caribbean. Thus was the slave trade reinforced.

33 Kunitz S. *Disease and Social Diversity: The European Impact on the Health of Non-Europeans*. New York: Oxford University Press, 1994.

34 Flannery T. *The Future Eaters*. Chatswood, NSW: Reed Books, 1994, p. 321.

35 WHO. *Fighting Disease, Fostering Development*. Geneva: WHO, 1996.

36 Barthold S. Globalisation of Lyme borreliosis. *Lancet* 1996; 348: 1603–4. See also Karlen A. *The Biography of a Germ*. New York: Victor Gollancz, 2000.

37 Note, again, this recurring feature in science – as also in the story of Raymond Dart and *Australopithecus africanus* in chapter 2. Western science represents our best-yet attempt to reveal truths about the world in objective and verifiable fashion. In this it has largely supplanted both rationalism (as in Aristotelian science and philosophy) and revelation (the essence of religious belief). But, unavoidably, science is prey to the distortions of prevailing theories, intellectual fashion and prejudice.

38 Pyper JM. Does Borna disease virus infect humans? *Nature Medicine* 1995; 1: 209–10; Bode

L, Zimmermann W, Ferszt R, et al. Borna disease virus genome transcribed and expressed in psychiatric patients. *Nature Medicine* 1995; 1: 232–6.

5 The Third Horseman: food, farming and famines

1 Flannery T. *The Future Eaters*. Chatswood, NSW: Reed Books, 1994.

2 Maurice King, in particular, has developed this concept of 'demographic entrapment'. He argues that certain poor countries, because of their continuing substantial population growth (resulting from a chronically incomplete 'demographic transition'), will soon face an inevitable and tragic choice: (i) starvation; (ii) fratricide (e.g., Rwanda); (iii) out-migration; or (iv) chronic dependency on international hand-outs. See King M. The demographic trap. *Lancet* 1991; 337: 307–8. The term has not gained acceptance among demographers (see also King and Elliott, 1997, in n. 8 below).

3 Malthus TR. *An Essay on the Principle of Population*. London, 1798 (London: Penguin Classics, 1985).

4 Boserup E. *Population and Technological Change. A Study of Long-Term Trends*. Chicago: Aldine, 1981; Simon J. *The Ultimate Resource*. Princeton: Princeton University Press, 1981.

5 Arrow K, Bolin B, Costanza R, et al. Economic growth, carrying capacity, and the environment. *Science* 1995; 268: 520–1; Costanza R, Daly H, Folke C, et al. Managing our environmental portfolio. *BioScience* 2000; 50: 149–55.

6 Fogel RW. Economic Growth, population theory, and physiology: the bearing of long-term processes on the making of economic policy. *American Economic Review* 1994; 84: 369–95.

7 Although the Netherlands can grow only enough food to feed one-third of its population, it easily buys in the rest of its needs. Similarly, Hong Kong and Singapore import most of their food needs. Ethiopia and Somalia have coped with recent famine crises via air-lifted food aid. Sixty years ago, the Machakos District in Kenya was thought to have exceeded its carrying capacity as land became increasingly degraded. Subsequently, its population has increased sixfold while, concurrently, soil erosion has been arrested, reafforestation has occurred and agricultural output has risen fivefold (Tiffen M, Mortimore M. Environment, population growth and productivity in Kenya. *Development Policy Review* 1992; 10: 359–87). Machakos, however, has a favourable natural environment. In contrast, in the highlands of neighbouring Ethiopia, severe soil erosion spreads rapidly once the size of a rural population exceeds the population-supporting capacity of the region (Grepperud S. *Population-environment Links. Testing a Soil degradation Model for Ethiopia*. Divisional Working paper No. 1994–46, Environment Department. Washington, DC: World Bank, 1994).

8 King M. The demographic trap. *Lancet* 1991; 337: 307–8; King M, Elliott C. To the point of farce: a Martian view of the Hardinian taboo – the silence that surrounds population control. *British Medical Journal* 1997; 315: 1441–3.

9 Cassen R, Visaria P. India: looking ahead to one and a half billion people. *British Medical Journal* 1999; 319: 995–7; FAO. Food Insecurity Report 1999/2000.

10 Sen A. *Poverty and Famines. An Essay on Entitlement and Deprivation.* Oxford: 1981. Sen also makes the interesting point that no famine has ever occurred in a functioning democracy.

11 Bryson RA, Murray TJ. *Climates of Hunger: Mankind and the World's Changing Weather.* Madison, 1977. See also n.13.

12 The most recent famine in India occurred in 1943–44, during World War II, when rail services were disrupted and famine relief was inefficient. Otherwise during the twentieth century, the extensions of the national rail grid in India and the building of trunk roads enabled rapid food distribution to famine-afflicted areas. 'Famines' then became, officially, 'crises'.

13 Fagan B. *Floods, Famines and Emperors. El Niño and the Fate of Civilisations.* New York: Basic Books, 1999.

14 Ponting C. *A Green History of the World.* Harmondsworth: Penguin, 1991.

15 For a succinct and up-to-date review see: Nestle M. Paleolithic diets: a sceptical view. *Nutrition Bulletin* 2000; 25: 43–7.

16 Schmidt EB, et al. n-3 fatty acids from fish and coronary artery disease: implications for public health. *Public Health Nutrition* 2000; 3: 91–8. In addition to the experimental research evidence of beneficial effects of n-3 fatty acids on the heart and blood vessels, epidemiological studies have consistently shown that adding fish to the diet reduces the occurrence and recurrence of coronary heart disease.

17 Kingdon J. *Self-Made Man and His Undoing.* London: Jonathan Cape, 1993.

18 The establishment of endemic bacterial infections in early agrarian-herders would have coincided with a shift in the profile of dietary fatty acids, as domesticated meat began to replace wild meat. Presumably, cell-mediated immune activity also increased as the dietary intake of n-6 fatty acids increased and n-3 fatty acids decreased. (This, however, would not have conferred protection against viral diseases for which antibodies, not T cells, are the mode of immune defence.)

19 Cohen MN. *The Food Crisis in Prehistory. Overpopulation and the Origins of Agriculture.* New Haven: Yale University Press, 1977.

20 Diamond J. *Guns, Germs and Steel. The Fates of Human Societies.* New York: Norton, 1997.

21 Solbrig OT, Solbrig DJ. *So Shall You Reap.* Washington, DC, Island Press, 1994.

22 Cohen MN, Armelagos GJ (eds.) *Paleopathology at the Origins of Agriculture.* New York: Academic Press, 1984; Eaton SB, Konner MJ. Paleolithic nutrition: a consideraton of its nature and current implications. *New England Journal of Medicine*, 1985; 312: 283–9.

23 Angel JL. Health as a crucial factor in the changes from hunting to developed farming in the Eastern Mediterranean. In: Cohen MN, Armelagos GJ (eds.) *Paleopathology at the Origins of Agriculture.* New York: Academic Press, 1984, pp. 51–73.

24 The interpretation of these apparent disparities is not straightforward. Perhaps the capacity of agrarian societies to keep ailing members alive ensured that nutritional deficiency diseases could become chronic, and therefore more evident in skeletal remains. See Strassman and Dunbar, 1999 – n. 4, chapter 2.

25 Goodman AH, Lallo J, Armelagos GJ, Rose JC. Changes at Dickson Mounds, Illinois (AD

950–1300). In: Cohen MN, Armelagos GJ (eds.) *Paleopathology at the Origins of Agriculture*. New York: Academic Press, 1984, pp. 271–305.

26 Allison MJ. Palaeopathology in Peruvian and Chilean populations. In Cohen MN, Armelagos GJ (eds.) *Paleopathology at the Origins of Agriculture*. New York: Academic Press, 1984, pp. 515–29.

27 Mata LJ. *The Children of Santa Maria Cauque. A Prospective Field Study of Health and Growth*. Boston: MIT Press, 1978.

28 Taylor CE. Synergy among mass infections, famines and poverty. In: Rotberg RI, Rabb TK (eds.) *Hunger and History*. Cambridge: Cambridge University Press, 1983, pp. 285–303.

29 Carmichael AG. Infection, hidden hunger, and history. In: Rotberg RI, Rabb TK (eds.) *Hunger and History*. Cambridge: Cambridge University Press, 1983, pp. 51–66.

30 Hetzel BS, Pandav CS. *SOS For a Billion. The Conquest of Iodine Deficiency Disorders*. Oxford: Oxford University Press, 1994.

31 Dyson T. Prospects for feeding the world. *British Medical Journal* 1999; 319: 988–91. Dyson (usually an optimist about future food trends) comments thus: 'a worrying recent development is the increasing volatility of harvests in North America, which is possibly caused by climate change occurring as a result of carbon dioxide emissions'. And: 'Worryingly, sub-Saharan Africa is experiencing a similar trend.'

32 Repetto R. The 'Second India' revisited: population growth, poverty, and environment over two decades. In: Pachauri RK, Qureshy LF (eds.) *Population, Environment and Development*. New Delhi: TERI, 1997, pp. 153–75.

33 Food and Agricultural Organization. *World Food Insecurity Report*. Rome: FAO, 1999.

34 Greenland DJ, Gregory PJ, Nye PH. Land resources and constraints to crop production. In: Waterlow JC, et al. (eds.) *Feeding a World Population of More than Eight Billion People*. Oxford: Oxford University Press, 1998, pp. 39–55.

35 FAO, 1999 (n. 33 above). See also: Food and Agricultural Organization. *World Agriculture: Towards 2010*. Alexandratos N (ed.) Chichester: Wiley, 1987, p. 488.

36 The recent licensing by the US government of Olestra, as a non-caloric synthetic 'fat', has resulted in the distinctly unappealing side-effect of 'anal leakage'. On balance, the reliance by the Roman upper classes on self-induced vomiting during extravagant feasting seems preferable!

37 Potter JD, Chavez A, Chen JC, et al. *Diet, Nutrition and the Prevention of Cancer: A Global Perspective*. London: World Cancer Research Fund, 1997.

38 Food and Agricultural Organization. *The State of World Fisheries and Aquaculture 1998*. Rome: FAO, 1999; Naylor RL, Goldburg RJ, Primavera JH, et al. Effect of aquaculture on world fish supplies. *Nature* 2000; 405: 1017–24.

6 The industrial era: the Fifth Horseman?

1 *Holy Bible* (St James version). *The Revelation of St John the Divine*. Chapter 6. See also more detailed discussion in n. 1 in Preface.

2 McMichael AJ. *Planetary Overload. Global Environmental Change and the Health of the Human Species.* Cambridge: Cambridge University Press, 1993.

3 Newman P, Kenworthy JR. *Sustainability and Cities. Overcoming Automobile Dependence.* Washington, DC: Island Press, 1999.

4 Rees W. A human ecological assessment of economic and population health. In: Crabbé P, et al. (eds.) *Implementing Ecological Integrity.* Dordrecht: Kluwer, 2000, pp. 399–418.

5 Vitousek PM, Mooney HA, Lubchenco J, Melillo JM. Human domination of Earth's ecosystems. *Science* 1997; 277: 494–9. See also: Watson RT, Dixon JA, Hamburg SP, Janetos AC, Moss RH. *Protecting Our Planet. Securing our Future. Linkages Among Global Environmental Issues and Human Needs.* UNEP, USNASA, World Bank, 1998.

6 John Evelyn, quoted in: Dubos R. *Mirage of Health. Utopias, Progress and Biological Change.* New York: Harper and Row, 1959, p. 201. See also: Brimblecombe P. *The Big Smoke: A History of Air Pollution in London since Medieval Times.* London: Routledge, 1988.

7 The quotes attributed to Alcmaeon and Hippocrates are from Dubos 1959 (see n. 6), pp. 36–7.

8 Hippocrates. Airs, Waters and Places. An essay on the influence of climate, water supply and situation on health. In: Lloyd GER (ed.) *Hippocratic Writings.* Harmondsworth: Penguin, 1978, p. 148.

9 Appleton JD, Fuge R, McCall GJH (eds.) *Environmental Geochemistry and Health.* London: The Geological Society, 1996.

10 See also the discussion of the genetic evolution of metabolic polymorphisms (e.g., NAT2) in chapter 3.

11 The Minamata industrial disaster killed and neurologically crippled hundreds of villagers who were exposed to organic mercury in seafood. The London smog (a heavy mixture of smoke, sulphur dioxide and fog) of December 1952 killed several thousand extra people in the space of two weeks. (More details of those two events are given later in the chapter.) Seveso and Bhopal entailed industrial explosions, exposing adjacent communities to highly toxic dioxins and isothiocyanate, respectively.

12 LaDou J, Jeyaratnam J. Transfer of hazardous industries: issues and solutions. In: Jeyaratnam J, Chia KS (eds.) *Occupational Health in National Development.* River Edge, NJ: World Scientific Publications, 1994.

13 Riley JC. *The Eighteenth-Century Campaign to Avoid Disease.* New York: St. Martin's Press, 1987.

14 Engels F. *The Conditions of the Working Class In England* [1845]. London: Penguin, 1987, p. 130.

15 Ibid., pp. 129–30.

16 McMichael PD. *Development and Social Change. A Global Perspective,* 2nd edn. Thousand Oaks, CA: Pine Forge Press, 2000. In the past two decades the 'Development Project' vision has been superseded by a thrust for a globalised world economic system, shaped by the market needs and ambitions of transnational corporations. This globalisation reflects the integrating power of deregulated trade, mobile capital, electronic communications, mass

media and ease of long-distance travel. As discussed in the final three chapters, these developments – at least in the near term – are having many, and often adverse, impacts upon human health.

17 Carson R. *Silent Spring*. New York: Houghton Mifflin, 1962.

18 The Ecologist.*A Blueprint for Survival*. London: Penguin, 1972; Meadows DH, Meadows DL, Randers J, Behrens WW. *The Limits to Growth*. London: Pan, 1974.

19 Kaiser J. Acid rain's dirty business: stealing minerals from the soil. *Science* 1996; 272: 198.

20 Quoted in Carson. *Silent Spring*. 1988 (reprint) p. 169 (see n.17 above).

21 Sharpe RM, Skakkebaek N. Are oestrogens involved in falling sperm counts and disorders of the male reproductive tract? *Lancet* 1993; 341: 1392–5.

22 Colborn T, Clement C (eds.) *Chemically-Induced Alterations in Sexual and Functional Development: The Wildlife-Human Connection*. Princeton, NJ: Princeton Scientific Publishing, 1992.

23 It may be relevant that femaleness is the 'default' sex in humans and other mammals. The mammalian fetus is exposed to maternal oestrogens. Hence, for an XY fetus to become phenotypically male it must produce sufficient androgen to counteract the feminising influence of maternal hormones. Impairment of this balance by environmental hormone-mimicking chemicals may thus cause subtle shifts in human sexual function. (The situation is different in birds, reptiles and frogs, since they lay eggs.) Incidentally, the scientific uncertainty about recent trajectories in sperm counts did not deter the novelist, P.D. James, from telling the story in *The Children of Men* (London: Faber, 1992) of how the human species in the twenty-first century reaches the 'omega point' which, with dwindling sperm counts, unleashes a great drama around the last remaining fertile individuals.

24 World Resources Institute. *1998–99 World Resources. A Guide to the Global Environment. Environmental Change and Human Health*. Oxford: Oxford University Press, 1998.

25 Colborn T, Vom Saal F, Soto A. Developmental effects of endocrine-disrupting chemicals in wildlife and humans. *Environmental Health Perspectives* 1993; 101: 378–84.

26 Schmidt CW. Spheres of influence. *Environmental Health Perspectives* 1999; 107: A24–A25.

27 Smith KR. Environmental health – for the rich or for all? *Bulletin of the World Health Organization* 2000; 78: 1156–7.

28 Williams C. *Terminus Brain. The Environmental Threats to Human Intelligence*. London: Continuum, 1997. Feeley M, Brouwer A. Health risks to infants from exposure to PCBs, PCDDs and PCDFs. *Food Additives and Contaminants* 2000; 17: 325–33.

29 Smith D. Worldwide trends in DDT levels in human milk. *International Journal of Epidemiology* 1999; 28, 179–88.

30 McMichael AJ. From hazard to habitat. Rethinking environment and health. *Epidemiology* 1998; 10: 460–4.

31 Smith AH, Lingas EO, Rahman M. Contamination of drinking-water by arsenic in Bangladesh: a public health emergency. *Bulletin of the World Health Organization* 2000; 78: 1093–103.

32 The concept of a 'global public health good' is one that the UN Development Programme is

now promoting. This reflects a new awareness that there are various social and environmental 'commons' that are prerequisites for sustained good health in populations.

33 There have been many studies of urban air pollution levels and death rates. However, most of them have been confined to assessing the covariation in daily exposures and daily deaths. This is only part – probably a minor part – of the problem. The greater health impact appears to accrue from long-term exposure to elevated air pollutant levels. See: McMichael AJ, Anderson HR, Brunekreef B, Cohen A. Inappropriate use of daily mortality analyses for estimating the longer-term mortality effects of air pollution. *International Journal of Epidemiology* 1998; 27: 450–3. Note also that it has been difficult for epidemiologists to elucidate causal relationships, particularly at lower levels of exposure. The complexity of air pollution as an exposure, and its changeability over time make epidemiological research into causal relationships difficult. Nevertheless, increased understanding of underlying toxicological mechanisms in humans, the accrual of data from diverse community-based epidemiological studies, experimental breathing-chamber studies in humans, clinicopathological research and animal experiments have enhanced our understanding of the causal relationships between various air pollutants and health.

34 Wang X, Smith KR. Secondary benefits of greenhouse gas control: health impacts in China. *Environmental Science and Technology* 2000; 33: 3056–61.

35 World Health Organization. *Health and Environment in Sustainable Development. Five Years After the Earth Summit.* Geneva: WHO, 1997.

36 Mishra VK, Retherfore RD, Smith KR. Biomass cooking fuels and prevalence of tuberculosis in India. *International Journal of Infectious Diseases* 1999; 3: 119–29.

37 Bell JNB, McNeil S, Houlden G, et al. Atmosphere change: its effects on plant pests and diseases. *Parasitology* 1993; 106: S11–S22.

38 Gilfillan SC. Lead poisoning and the fall of Rome. *Journal of Occupational Medicine* 1965; 7: 53–60.

39 Tong S, von Schirnding YE, Prapamontol T. Environmental lead exposure: a public health problem of global dimensions. *Bulletin of World Health Organization* 2000; 78: 1068–77.

40 Here, again, Earth's source of geothermal energy – its internally generated energy – is from the 'sun'. But, unlike the incoming daily solar radiation, this particular energy is not from 'our' sun. Radioactive uranium derives from now-extinct stars within the same intra-galactic neighbourhood, and which preceded the formation of the solar system. In nuclear reactors or weapons, these uranium and thorium atoms can be made to split (fission) and thereby release more energy – a different process from the radioactive decay occurring in today's Earth.

41 Bassett M. Paper presented to *Epidemiological Society of South Africa*, annual scientific conference, East London, 23–25 February, 2000. See also: Loewenson R. Labour insecurity and health: an epidemiological study in Zimbabwe. *Social Science and Medicine* 1988; 27: 733–41.

42 The ratios of energy input:output in livestock production, of 2:1 to 8:1, contrast markedly with those of pre-industrial agriculture where the ratio reverses, and is approximately 1:10. Indeed, that favourable ratio applies to many other free-range creatures expending energy to

acquire food energy. (Several generations of budding young piano students have rote-learned the space notes in the bass clef, ACEG, via the mnemonic 'All Cows Eat Grass.' It may have been approximately true half a century ago, but it certainly is no longer true. In North America, parts of East Asia and elsewhere, feed-lot cattle are fed substantially on grain – along with sub-clinical doses of antibiotics to suppress intestinal bacterial diversion of food energy, and thus hasten growth.)

43 Care is needed with this argument. Anthropological studies have shown that various pre-industrial societies used fire extensively for hunting (e.g., Australian Aborigines) and for land management for food production (e.g., swidden agriculturalists), entailing very high per capita use of energy from this biomass burning.

44 Evans L. Greater crop production. Whence and whither? In: Waterlow JC, et al. (eds.) *Feeding a World Population of More than Eight Billion People.* Oxford: Oxford University Press, 1998, pp. 89–97.

45 Dawkins R. *The Selfish Gene.* Oxford: Oxford University Press, 1976.

46 Loh J, Randers J, MacGillivray A, Kapos V, Jenkins M, Groombridge B, Cox N. *Living Planet Report, 1998.* Gland, Switzerland: WWF International, Switzerland; New Economics Foundation, London; World Conservation Monitoring Centre, Cambridge; 1998; UN Environment Programme. *Global Environment Outlook 2000.* London: Earthscan, 1999.

7 Longer lives and lower birth rates

1 Kane P, Choi CY. China's one child family policy. *British Medical Journal* 1999; 319: 992–4.

2 Cohen JE. *How Many People Can the Earth Support?* New York: Norton, 1995, p. 28.

3 Wilson C, Airey P. How can a homeostatic perspective enhance demographic transition theory? *Population Studies* 1999; 53: 117–28.

4 For a succinct discussion of the inter-relationship between these two transitions see: Caldwell JC. Commentary on Abdel R Omran. The epidemiologic transition: a theory of the epidemiology of population change. *Bulletin of the World Health Organization* 2000; 79: 159–60.

5 Dasgupta P. Population, resources and welfare: an exploration into reproductive and environmental externalities. *Population and Development Review* 2000; 26: 643–89. According to some economic historians the health gains associated with these rapid modern transitions in Britain accounted for one-third of the increase in per capita income from the late eighteenth to late twentieth centuries; see: Fogel RW. New findings on secular trends in nutrition and mortality: some implications for population theory. In: Rosenzweig MR, Stark O (eds.) *Handbook of Population and Family Economics,* Vol. 1A. Amsterdam: Elsevier Science, 1997, pp. 433–81.

6 McMichael AJ, Corvalan C, Smith KR. The sustainability transition: a new challenge. *Bulletin of the World Health Organization* 2000; 78: 1067.

7 The word 'rate' is crucial here. It is to be distinguished from a simple proportion. While 100% of the population eventually dies, the *rate* of death per unit of time (e.g., per year) reflects the average duration of life. Shortened lives mean increased death rates.

8 Material advance and new wealth are not a prerequisite to the demographic transition. Sweden began its demographic transition before substantial industrialisation and urbanisation had occurred.

9 Leung AKC. Premodern period in China. In: Kiple KF (ed.) *The Cambridge World History of Human Disease.* Cambridge: Cambridge University Press, 1993, pp. 354–62.

10 McMichael PD. *Development and Social Change. A Global Perspective* (2nd edn). Thousand Oaks, CA: Pine Forge Press, 2000.

11 Wilkinson RG. The epidemiological transition: from material scarcity to social disadvantage? *Daedalus*; Fall 1994: 61–77.

12 Farmer P. Social inequalities and emerging infectious diseases. *Emerging Infectious Diseases* 1996; 2: 258–69. See also: Farmer P. *Infections and Inequalities. The Modern Plagues.* Berkeley: University of California Press, 1999.

13 Olshansky SJ, Ault AB. The fourth stage of the epidemiologic transition: the age of delayed degenerative diseases. *Milbank Memorial Quarterly* 1986; 64: 355–91.

14 This is why demographers often prefer to use life expectancy at, say, age 15 – since this gives a better indication of the force of mortality during adulthood.

15 Angel JL. Health as a crucial factor in the changes from hunting to developed farming in the Eastern Mediterranean. In: Cohen MN, Armelagos GJ (eds.) *Paleopathology at the Origins of Agriculture.* London: Academic Press, 1984, pp. 51–73.

16 Olshansky SJ, Carnes BA, Cassel C. In search of Methuselah: estimating the upper limits to human longevity. *Science* 1990; 250: 634–40.

17 Medawar PB. *An Unsolved Problem of Biology.* London: Lewis, 1952.

18 The Australian Nobel laureate immunologist, Macfarlane Burnet, noted that invertebrates have no humoral immunity (no antibody production). Instead they use basic cell-mediated defences to protect against infection, with white blood cells that destroy and scavenge. He suggested that antibodies arose in vertebrates several hundred million years ago initially as a means of maintaining tissue integrity (by eliminating aberrant cells) in more complex, longer-lived organisms. That capacity for making antibodies was later recruited into the immune system as a second line of defence against foreign invaders.

19 Livi-Bacci M. The nutrition–mortality link in past times: a comment. In: Rotberg RI, Rabb TK (eds.) *Hunger and History.* Cambridge: Cambridge University Press, 1983, pp. 95–100.

20 Wrigley EA, Schofield RS. *The Population History of England, 1541–1871. A Reconstruction.* London: Edward Arnold, 1981.

21 McKeown T. *The Modern Rise of Population.* New York: Academic Press, 1976.

22 See in particular: Szreter S. The importance of social intervention in Britain's mortality decline *c.* 1850–1914: a re-interpretation of the role of public health. *Social History of Medicine* 1988; 1: 1–37; Kunitz J. Making a long story short: a note on men's height and mortality in England from the first through the nineteenth centuries. *Medical History* 1987; 31: 269–80. Kunitz argues that the recession of plague (improved quarantine), smallpox (conversion to a disease of early childhood, and uptake of vaccination) and typhus (professionalisation of armies and recession of famines) all contributed to a mortality

decline that was not primarily dependent on nutritional status. See also: Wrigley EA, Davies RS, Oeppen JE, Schofield RS. *English Population History from Family Reconstitution 1580–1837*. Cambridge: Cambridge University Press; 1997, p. 202 ('The relationship between economic advance and mortality trends in the past is best regarded as uncertain and ambiguous.').

23 World Bank. *World Development Report. Development and the Environment*. Oxford University Press, Oxford, 1992.

24 Caldwell JC. Major new evidence on health transition and its interpretation. *Health Transition Review* 1991; 1(2): 221–9. John Powles (personal communication) has adduced recent evidence for the increasing insensitivity of national health indices to changes in average income levels. This has been particularly evident in the recent gains in infant survival and life expectancy in various low-income countries.

25 World Health Organization. *World Health Report 1999: Making a Difference*. Geneva: World Health Organization, 1999.

26 Caldwell JC. Routes to low mortality in poor countries. *Population and Development Review* 1986; 12, 171–220. Note that it is young girls, not young boys, who are at risk of becoming pregnant. There is, therefore, an obvious evolutionary dimension to the traditional conservative management of unmarried girls. Parents wish to ensure the best prospects ('reproductive fitness') for genes transmitted via daughters. This requires their combination with genes from a carefully selected male, to produce secure and biologically robust grandchildren. Political correctness aside, the corresponding 'reproductive fitness' argument for genes transmitted by sons is different. The more inseminations they achieve, the greater the probability of dissemination of those genes. (However, the argument must also accommodate the importance of parental stability for extended child-rearing. Pair-bonding and, therefore, stable marriage are valuable and valued. In this respect there is convergence of the biological interests of the young male and young female.)

27 Flinn MW. The stabilization of mortality in pre-industrial Western Europe. *Journal of European Economic History* 1974; 3: 285–318.

28 See, for example, Floud R, Gregory A, Wachter R. *Height, Health and History*. Cambridge: Cambridge University Press, 1990. This volume makes clear that there was actually a decline in height in England in the early 1800s. Thus, it seems unlikely that the gain in real wages from around the 1750s directly improved the standard of living. See also Wrigley et al., 1997, in n. 22 above.

29 Bunker JP, Frazier HS, Mosteller F. Improving health: measuring effects of medical care. *Milbank Memorial Quarterly* 1994; 72: 225–58.

30 Tunstall-Pedoe H, Vanuzzo D, Hobbs M, et al. Estimation of contribution of changes in coronary care to improving survival, event rates and coronary heart disease mortality across the WHO MONICA Project populations. *Lancet* 2000; 355: 688–700.

31 Kuh D, Davey Smith G. When is mortality risk determined? Historical insights into a current debate. *Social History of Medicine* 1993: 101–23.

32 Robine J-M. Extending human life: longevity and quality of life – can we hope for both long

life and good health? 2000 unpublished ms. Also: Robine J-M, Romieu I, Cambois E. Health expectancies and current research *Reviews in Clinical Gerontology* 1997; 7: 73–82.

33 Fries JF. Aging, natural death and the compression of morbidity. *New England Journal of Medicine* 1980; 303: 130–5.

34 Olshansky SJ, Carnes BA, Cassel C. In search of Methuselah: estimating the upper limits to human longevity. *Science* 1990; 250: 634–40. Bonneux L, Barendregt JJ, Van der Maas PJ. The expiry date of man: a synthesis of evolutionary biology and public health. *Journal of Epidemiology and Community Health* 1998; 52: 619–23.

35 Recent research has shown that the telomeres at the ends of chromosomes undergo progressive attrition as body cells go through successive divisions. Telomeres are somewhat like the little plastic tips on shoe-laces; they prevent the end of the chromosome from fraying. This finding suggests that there is an inbuilt limit to the number of successful divisions, since frayed chromosomes would cause some scrambling of the genetic code and resultant cellular dysfunction. The evolutionary process has evidently provided each of our body cells with a generous, but finite, sufficiency of telomere.

36 This is the 'disposable soma' theory propounded by Tom Kirkwood: so long as genes survive, the body is expendable. See: Kirkwood TBL. Evolution of aging. *Nature* 1977; 270: 301–4.

37 Medvedev counted over 300 theories of ageing. See: Medvedev ZA. An attempt at a rational classification of theories of ageing. *Biological Reviews* 1990; 65: 375–98. See also: Austad S. *Why We Age*. Chichester: John Wiley, 1997.

38 Williams GC. Pleiotropy, natural selection and the evolution of senescence. *Evolution* 1957; 11: 398–411.

39 UN Population Division. *World Population Prospects: The 1998 Revision*. New York: United Nations, 1998.

40 Bush A. Metals and neuroscience. *Current Opinion in Chemical Biology* 2000; 4: 184–9.

41 O'Connell JF, Hawkes K, Blurton Jones NG. Grandmothering and the evolution of *Homo erectus. J Human Evolution* 1999; 36: 461–85.

42 Strassman B, Dunbar R. Putting the Stone Age in perspective. In: Stearns SC (ed.) *Evolution in Health and Disease*. Oxford: Oxford University Press, 1999, pp. 96–107. See also: Early JD, Headland TN. *Population Dynamics of a Philippine Rain Forest People*. Gainesville: University Press of Florida, 1998. This contains summary vital statistics from forager and agrarian subgroups of traditional populations in East Asia, Africa and South America. It indicates considerable variation in fertility, as a function of culture and environment.

43 Moore SE, Cole TJ, Poskitt EM, et al. Season of birth predicts mortality in rural Gambia. *Nature* 1997; 388: 434–6.

44 This surge of infanticide in Europe included the overlying of babies by mothers, and their drowning, abandonment (half the babies in foundling hospitals perished within several months), and wet-nursing with either neglect or deliberate (paid) murder (typically induced by a slug of gin or other spirits).

45 Raleigh VS. World population and health in transition. *British Medical Journal* 1999; 319: 981–4.

46 Jack Caldwell and Pat Caldwell summarise the theory of evolutionary demography thus: 'evolution provided [humans with] only: (1) a unique brain among living things, (2) an urge to copulate, (3) an urge to survive and succeed. For hundreds of thousands of years this maximized the transmission of genes. But eventually the urge to succeed produced the modern world and the big brain invented contraception. The three factors still operated but they no longer worked to maximize the transmission of genes.' See: Caldwell JC, Caldwell P. Reactions to evolutionary demographers. *American Journal of Human Biology*, **in press.**

47 Vineis P, Miligi L, Crosignani P, et al. Delayed infection, family size and malignant lymphomas. *Journal of Epidemiology and Community Health* 2000; 54: 907–11.

48 These issues are well discussed in: Raleigh, 1999 (see n. 45).

49 Cassen R, Visaria P. India: looking ahead to one and a half billion people. *British Medical Journal* 1999; 319: 995–7.

50 This question has been tackled by various commentators. It is addressed further in chapter 12. For a thorough treatment of the issues (although not for a specific answer) see: Cohen J. *How Many People can Earth Support?* New York: Norton, 1995.

51 Caldwell JC. Rethinking the African AIDS epidemic. *Population and Development Review* 2000; 26: 117–35.

52 The reason that menstruation occurs in humans remains a puzzle. The equivalent shedding of the lining of the uterus, with visible bleeding, is rare among other mammals. The competing theories include the flushing out of sperm-borne pathogens, the conservation of energy (it is less expensive to rebuild the uterine lining once a month than to supply its metabolic needs on a continuing basis), and menstruation as a manifestation of a hair-trigger mechanism for expelling defective embryos. (See: Haig D. Genetic conflicts of pregnancy and childhood. In: Stearns SC (ed.) *Evolution in Health and Disease.* Oxford: Oxford University Press, 1999: pp. 77–90.)

8 Modern affluence: lands of milk and honey

1 Rose G. Sick individuals and sick populations. *International Journal of Epidemiology* 1985; 14: 32–8.

2 Popkin BM, Doak CM. The obesity epidemic is a worldwide phenomenon. *Nutrition Reviews* 1998; 56: 106–14; James WPT. The nutritional crisis to come. In: Koop E, Pearson CE, Schwartz MR (eds.) *Critical Issues in Global Health.* San Francisco: Jossey-Bass, 2000, pp. 238–50.

3 Boyden S. *Western Civilization in Biological Perspective. Patterns in Biohistory.* Oxford: Oxford University Press, 1987.

4 Jenner E. Quoted in Will C. *Plagues. Their Origin, History and Future.* London: Harper Collins, 1996, p. 29.

5 Walter Willett and colleagues have reported a substantial increase in risk of coronary heart disease in American women consuming above-average levels of trans fatty acids. See:

Ascherio A, Katan MB, Zock PL, Stampfer MJ, Willett WC. Trans fatty acids and coronary heart disease. *New England Journal of Medicine* 1999; 340: 1994–8.

6 Ulijszek S, Strickland S. *Nutritional Anthropology.* London: Smith Gordon, 1993, pp. 35–7.

7 Kushi LH, Lenart EB, Willett WC. Health implications of Mediterranean diets in light of contemporary knowledge. 1. Plant foods and dairy products. *American Journal of Clinical Nutrition* 1995; 61: 1407S–15S; Kushi LH, Lenart EB, Willett WC. Health implications of Mediterranean diets in light of contemporary knowledge. 2. Meat, wine, fats, and oils. *American Journal of Clinical Nutrition* 1995; 61: 1416S–27S. Note, however, that many of the apparently health-conferring components of the contemporary Mediterranean diet were introduced during the twentieth century, especially in poorer rural regions previously too poor to produce or acquire fresh green vegetables. Tomatoes were not introduced into the regional diet until the nineteenth century.

8 Murray C, Lopez A. Alternative projections of mortality and disability by cause 1990–2020: Global Burden of Disease Study. *Lancet* 1997; 349: 1498–504.

9 Powles JW, McMichael AJ. Human disease: effects of economic development. *Encyclopaedia of Life Sciences.* London: Macmillan, 2001 **in press.**

10 Barker DJP. Rise and fall of Western diseases. *Nature* 1989; 338: 371–2.

11 But see: Law M, Wald N. Why heart disease mortality is low in France: the time lag explanation. *British Medical Journal* 1999; 318: 1471–80. They argue that the gap will tend to close as heart disease rates rise in France in deferred response to the post-1970 increase in saturated and total fat consumption. The evidence for this, however, remains debatable.

12 Zatonski W, McMichael AJ, Powles JW. Ecological study of reasons for sharp decline in mortality from ischaemic heart disease in Poland since 1991. *British Medical Journal* 1998; 316: 1047–51.

13 Simopoulos AP. Genetic variation and nutritional requirements. *Bulletin of the Nutrition Foundation of India* 1999; 20: 6–8.

14 Trowell H, Burkitt D. *Western Diseases: Their Emergence and Prevention.* London: Edward Arnold, 1981.

15 Barker DJP. *Mothers, Babies and Disease in Later Life.* London: BMJ Publishing, 1994.

16 Kuh D, Ben-Shlomo Y. (eds.) *A Life Course Approach to Chronic Disease Epidemiology.* Oxford: Oxford University Press, 1997.

17 World Health Organization. *The World Health Report 1999.* Geneva: WHO, 1999.

18 Ebrahim S, Davey Smith G. Systematic review of randomised controlled trials of multiple risk factor interventions for preventing coronary heart disease. *British Medical Journal* 1997; 314: 1666–74.

19 International Obesity Task Force. *Obesity: Preventing and Managing the Global Epidemic.* Geneva: WHO, 1998.

20 Prentice AM, Jebb SA. Obesity in Britain: gluttony or sloth? *British Medical Journal* 1995; 311: 437–9.

21 Manson JE, Willett WC, Stampfer MJ, et al. Body weight and mortality among women. *New England Journal of Medicine* 1995; 333: 677–85. Body weight and all-cause mortality were

directly related within this large cohort of middle-aged American women, followed over a decade. The lowest mortality rate was in women who weighed at least 15% less than the US average for women of similar age and among those whose weight had been stable since early adulthood.

22 Nevertheless, various carved figurines from the late palaeolithic, 20,000 to 30,000 years ago, portray female figures of very ample buttocks, abdomens and breasts. Was this a rendition of unusually plump womanhood, idealised for high fertility?

23 Lean MEJ, Han TS, Seidell JC. Impairment of health and quality of life in people with large waist circumference. *Lancet* 1998; 351: 853–56.

24 McKeigue P. Cardiovascular disease and diabetes in migrants: interaction between nutritional changes and genetic background. In: Shetty P, McPherson K (eds.) *Diet, Nutrition and Chronic Disease. Lessons from Contrasting Worlds.* Chichester: John Wiley, 1997, pp. 59–70.

25 Field A.E, Camargo CA, Taylor CB, et al. Relation of peer and media influences to the development of purging behaviours among preadolescent and adolescent girls. *Archives of Pediatrics and Adolescent Medicine* 1999; 153: 1184–9; Monteath SA, McCabe MP. The influence of societal factors on female body image. *Journal of Social Psychology* 1997; 137: 708–27.

26 Key TJ, Fraser GE, Thorogood M, et al. Mortality in vegetarians and nonvegetarians: detailed findings from a collaborative analysis of 5 prospective studies. *American Journal of Clinical Nutrition* 1999; 70: 516S–24S; Appleby PN, Thorogood M, Mann JI, Kay TJA. The Oxford Vegetarian Study: an overview. *American Journal of Clinical Nutrition* 1999; 70: 525S–31S.

27 Parsonnet J (ed.) *Microbes and Malignancy: Infection as a Cause of Human Cancers.* New York: Oxford University Press, 1999.

28 Doll R, Peto R. *The Causes of Cancer.* Oxford: Oxford University Press, 1981.

29 Armstrong BK, Doll R. Environmental factors and cancer incidence and mortality in different countries with special reference to dietary practices. *International Journal of Cancer* 1975; 15: 617–31.

30 World Cancer Research Fund. *Diet, Nutrition and the Prevention of Cancer: A Global Perspective.* London: World Cancer Research Fund, 1997.

31 Franceschi S, Bidoli E, Baron AE, La Vecchia C. Maize and risk of cancers of the oral cavity, pharynx, and esophagus in northeastern Italy. *Journal of the National Cancer Institute* 1990; 82: 1407–11. See also: World Cancer Research Fund, 1997, n. 30 above.

32 van't Veer P, Jansen MC, Klerk M, Kok FJ. Fruits and vegetables in the prevention of cancer and cardiovascular disease. *Public Health Nutrition* 2000; 3: 103–7.

33 McMichael AJ, Beaglehole R. The changing global context of public health. *Lancet* 2000; 356: 495–9.

34 Saloojee Y, Dagli E. Tobacco industry tactics for resisting public policy on health. *Bulletin of the World Health Organization* 2000; 78: 902–10; Mackay J. Lessons from private statements of the tobacco industry. *Bulletin of the World Health Organization* 2000; 78: 911–12.

35 I thank George Davey Smith for historical information about the rise of cigarette smoking.

36 The World Trade Organization, in particular, has been a major vehicle of this mono-ocular vision. This, in turn, has contributed to the recent groundswell of public opposition to the

policies of the WTO and other international financial and investment agencies. The message about the need to assign high priority to protecting population health is apparently getting through. See, for example, Moore M. Global Health Policy. *Lancet* 2000; 356: 680.

37 Joossens L, Raw M. How can cigarette smuggling be reduced? *British Medical Journal* 2000; 321: 947–50.

9 Cities, social environments and synapses

1 Kostoff S. *The City Shaped: Urban Patterns and Meanings Through History.* London: Thames and Hudson, 1991.

2 Darwin C. *Journal of Researches into the Natural History and Geology of the Countries Visited during the Voyage of HMS 'Beagle' Round the World.* London: Ward Lock and Co., 1845/89, p. 166.

3 For gorillas and chimpanzees, the natural group size is measured in tens, not hundreds.

4 Several authors have drawn a more stark comparison of the health profile of the world's poor sub-populations with other better-off populations. See: Farmer P. *Infections and Inequalities. The Modern Plagues.* Berkeley: University of California Press, 1999; Gwatkin DR. Health inequalities and the health of the poor. *Bulletin of the World Health Organization* 2000; 78: 3–17.

5 UN Centre for Human Settlements (HABITAT). *An Urbanizing World: Global Report on Human Settlements, 1996.* Oxford: Oxford University Press, 1996.

6 Shepard P. *Traces of an Omnivore.* Washington, DC: Island Press, 1996.

7 Durkheim E. *The Rules of Sociological Method* [1895]. Glencoe, IL: Free Press, 1965.

8 Richardson's ideas, and their subsequent influence on North America, are discussed in: Hancock T. The evolution, impact and significance of the Healthy Cities/Communities movement. *Journal of Public Health Policy* 1993: Spring: 5–18.

9 Newman P, Kenworthy J. *Sustainability and Cities. Overcoming Automobile Dependence.* Washington, DC: Island Press, 1999.

10 Poulter NR, Khaw KT, Hopwood BE, et al. The Kenyan Luo migration study: observations on the initiation of a rise in blood pressure. *British Medical Journal* 1990; 300: 967–72.

11 Rooney C, McMichael AJ, Kovats S, Coleman MP. Excess mortality in England and Wales, and in Greater London, during the 1995 heatwave. *Journal of Epidemiology and Community Health* 1998; 52: 482–6.

12 Fletcher T, McMichael AJ. *Health at the Crossroads: Transport Policy and Urban Health.* Chichester: Wiley, 1997.

13 Desjjarlais R, Eisenberg L, Good B, Kleinman A. *World Mental Health. Problems and Priorities in Low-Income Countries.* New York: Oxford University Press, 1995.

14 Weller M. London's mental health problems. *Lancet* 1997; 349: 224.

15 Lewis G, David A, Andreasson S, Allebeck P. Schizophrenia and city life. *Lancet* 1992; 340: 137–40.

16 An alternative, more speculative thesis, supported by the higher rates of schizophrenia in

children born soon after the winter season, is that low levels of vitamin D are to blame. Levels of this vitamin, which forms in the skin under the action of solar ultraviolet radiation, are typically lower in urban than in rural populations. See: McGrath J, et al. Hypothesis: is low prenatal vitamin D a risk-modifying factor for schizophrenia? *Schizophrenia Research* 1999; 40: 173–7.

17 Nesse RM. Testing evolutionary hypotheses about mental disorders. In: Stearns SC (ed.) *Evolution in Health and Disease*. Oxford: Oxford University Press, 1999, pp. 260–6.

18 Rees W. Revisiting carrying capacity: area-based indicators of sustainability. *Population and Environment* 1996; 17: 195–215.

19 Folke C, Larsson J, Sweitzer J. Renewable resource appropriation. In: Costanza R, Segura O (eds.) *Getting Down to Earth*. Washington, DC: Island Press, 1996.

20 Rees W. Consuming the earth: the biophysics of sustainability. *Ecological Economics* 1999; 29: 23–7.

21 A metaphor to illustrate this difference between studying individuals and studying populations is that of a group of corks bobbing on the surface of a lake. We are readily fascinated by the pattern of movement of individual corks: some rise while others fall; several seem to be a little more submerged, a little less buoyant, than others. We are preoccupied by observing and comparing the individual corks. Meanwhile all the corks are slowly drifting to the left in response to deeper unseen currents. This happens slowly, and we do not notice – at least for a while – that the whole flotilla of corks has shifted to a new position along the shoreline of 'risk'. We have been preoccupied with watching the individual corks and noting the differences between them.

22 Krieger N, Zierler S. The need for epidemiologic theory. *Epidemiology* 1997; 8: 212–14; Pearce N. Traditional epidemiology, modern epidemiology, and public health. *American Journal of Public Health* 1996; 86: 678–83.

23 Durkheim E. *Suicide. A Study in Sociology* [Le Suicide. Etude de sociologie, 1897]. New York: Free Press, 1951.

24 Marmot M. Improvement of social environment to improve health. *Lancet* 1998; 351: 57–60. Note also that prior to the 1950s the social class gradient in coronary heart disease mortality in Britain tended in the opposite direction. The upper classes, with longer-standing exposure to affluent diets and low levels of physical activity, had slightly higher rates.

25 Krieger N. Theories for social epidemiology in the 21st century: an ecosocial perspective. *International Journal of Epidemiology*, 2001; 30 (August).

26 Sen A. *Poverty and Famines. An Essay on Entitlement and Deprivation*. Oxford: Oxford University Press, 1981.

27 Marmot MG, Shipley MJ, Rose G. Inequalities in death – specific explanations of a general pattern. *Lancet* 1984; 1: 1003–6.

28 Davey Smith G, Neaton JD, Wentworth D, et al. Socioeconomic differentials in mortality risk among men screened for the Multiple Risk Factor Intervention Trial: Part I, results for 300,685 white men. *American Journal of Public Health* 1996; 86: 486–96; Davey-Smith G, Neaton JD, Wentworth D, et al. Socioeconomic differentials in mortality risk among men

screened for the Multiple Risk Factor Intervention Trial: Part II, results for 20,224 black men. *American Journal of Public Health* 1996; 86: 497–504.

29 Leon, D. Common threads: underlying components of inequalities in mortality between and within countries. In: Leon D, and Walt G (eds.) *Poverty, Inequality and Health.* Oxford: Oxford University Press, 2001, pp. 58–87.

30 Leon DA, Davey Smith G. Infant mortality, stomach cancer, stroke, and coronary heart disease: ecological analysis. *British Medical Journal* 2000; 320: 1705–6.

31 Selye H. *The Stress of Life.* New York: McGraw Hill, 1956.

32 Sapolsky RM. Endocrinology alfresco: psychoendocrine studies of wild baboons. *Recent Progress in Hormone Research* 1993; 48: 437–68.

33 Shively CA, Laird KL, Anton RF. The behaviour and physiology of social stress and depression in female cynomolgus monkeys. *Biological Psychiatry* 1997; 41: 871–82.

34 Sapolsky RM. Hormonal correlates of personality and social contexts: from non-human to human primates. In: Panter-Brick C, Worthman CM (eds). *Hormones, Health and Behavior.* New York: Cambridge University Press, 1999, pp. 18–46.

35 Lynch JW, Davey Smith G, Kaplan GA, House JS. Income inequality and mortality: importance to health of individual income, psychosocial environment, or material conditions. *British Medical Journal* 2000; 320: 1200–4. In an earlier analysis this research group showed that inter-state differences in health care provision did not account for life expectancy differences between US states; see: Kaplan GA, Pamuk ER, Lynch JW, Cohen RD, Balfour JL. Inequality in income and mortality in the United States: analysis of mortality and potential pathways. *British Medical Journal* 1996; 312: 999–1003. This left open the question as to whether the differences were due to variations in social cohesion or material circumstances, or both.

36 Wilkinson RG. *Unhealthy Societies. The Afflictions of Inequality.* London: Routledge, 1996.

37 Kawachi I, Kennedy BP, Lochner K, Prothrow-Stith D. Social capital, income inequality and mortality. *American Journal of Public Health* 1997; 87: 1491–8.

38 Wolf S, Bruhn GH. *The Power of a Clan: A 25-year Prospective Study of Roseto, Pennsylvania.* New Brunswick, NJ: Transaction Publishers, 1993.

39 Feachem R. Health decline in Eastern Europe. *Nature* 1994; 367: 313–14; Bobak M, Marmot M. East–West mortality divide and its potential explanations: proposed research agenda. *British Medical Journal* 1996; 312: 421–5.

40 Watson P. Explaining rising mortality among men in Eastern Europe. *Social Science and Medicine* 1995; 41: 923–34; Kennedy B, Kawachi I, Brainerd E. The role of social capital: the Russian mortality crisis. *World Development* 1998; 26: 2029–43.

41 Leon D, Chenet L, Shkolnikov VM, et al. Huge variations in Russian mortality rates 1984–94: artefact, alcohol, or what? *Lancet* 1997; 350: 383–8. As was argued in chapter 1, the strong transient gain in life expectancy in Russia in the mid-1980s affords further evidence of the important influence of alcohol consumption patterns on Russian mortality.

42 Wadberg P, McKee M, Shkolnikov V, Chenet L, Leon DA. Economic change, crime, and mortality crisis in Russia: regional analysis. *British Medical Journal* 1998; 317: 312–18.

43 Kunitz SJ. *Disease and Social Diversity: The European Impact on the Health of Non-Europeans.* Oxford: Oxford University Press, 1994.

44 Keating D, Hertzman C. *Developmental Health and the Wealth of Nations.* London: Guilford, 1999.

10 Global environmental change: overstepping limits

1 Vitousek PM, Mooney HA, Lubchenco J, Melillo JM. Human domination of Earth's ecosystems. *Science* 1997; 277: 494–9.

2 Daily GC. *Nature's Services. Societal Dependence on Natural Ecosystems.* Washington, DC: Island Press, 1997.

3 Loh J, Randers J, MacGillivray A, et al. *Living Planet Report.* London: Earthscan, 1998.

4 Binswanger and Smith KR. Paracelsus and Goethe: founding fathers of environmental health. *Bulletin of the World Health Organization* 2000; 78: 1162–5.

5 Postel S, Daily G, Ehrlich PR. Human appropriation of renewable fresh water. *Science* 1996; 271: 785–8.

6 Postel S. *Pillar of Sand: Can the Irrigation Miracle Last?* New York: Norton, 1999.

7 Ehrlich P, Holdren J. Impact of population growth. *Science* 1971; 171: 1212–17. This paper proposed the well-known equation $I = PAT$, where I is the impact on the environment, P is the population size, A is the level of affluence and consumption and T is the type of technology used.

8 The calculations and their sources here have been described in: McMichael AJ, Powles JW. Human numbers, environment, sustainability and health. *British Medical Journal* 1999; 319: 977–80.

9 Rees W. Revisiting carrying capacity: area-based indicators of sustainability. *Population and Environment* 1996; 17: 195–215.

10 Ponting C. *A Green History of the World.* London: Penguin, 1991.

11 Xenophon, in the fifth century BC, argued that it was man's economic task to reorganize and manage nature according to the principle of 'harmonia'. His view that nature was the only true source of wealth promoted the economic primacy of agriculture in both Greek and Roman societies, and it anticipated the economic ideas of the Physiocrats in eighteenth-century Europe.

12 Hardin G. The tragedy of the commons. *Science* 1968 162:1243–8. Other prominent American commentators were Rachel Carson, Paul Ehrlich and Barry Commoner – see n. 4, ch. 1. See also n. 18, ch. 6: the provocative, though controversial, *The Limits to Growth*, based on computer modelling was published. British science, usually more cautious, produced in 1972 the influential *A Blueprint for Survival.*

13 Levins R. Preparing for uncertainty. *Ecosystem Health* 1995; 1: 47–57.

14 Intergovernmental Panel on Climate Change. *Special Report on Emission Scenarios.* Cambridge: Cambridge University Press, 2000.

15 Editorial. *The Guardian.* London, UK, 19 April 2000.

16 Hippocrates. Airs, waters and places. An essay on the influence of climate, water supply and situation on health. In: Lloyd GER (ed.) *Hippocratic Writings*. London: Penguin, 1978, p. 148.

17 Fagan B. *Floods, Famines and Emperors. El Niño and the Fate of Civilisations*. New York: Basic Books, 1999. See also: Diaz HF, Kovats RS, McMichael AJ, Nicholl N. Climate and human health linkages on multiple timescales. In: PD Jones, TD Davies, AEJ Ogilvie, et al. (eds.) *Climate and Climatic Impacts Through the Last 1000 Years*. Dordrecht: Kluwer Academic Press, 2000.

18 Intergovernmental Panel on Climate Change. *Third Assessment Report*, vol I. Cambridge: Cambridge University Press, 2001.

19 Duchin JS, Koster FT, Peters CJ, et al. Hantavirus pulmonary syndrome: a clinical description of 17 patients with a newly recognized disease. *New England Journal of Medicine* 1994; 330: 949–55.

20 Rapid regional cooling in Western Europe, via this mechanism, may have triggered the onset of previous ice-ages: ice-sheets over northern Europe would reflect away part of the incoming solar radiation. See, for example, Broecker WS. Thermohaline circulation, the achilles heel of our climate system: will man-made carbon dioxide upset the current balance? *Science* 1997; 278: 1582–8; Broecker WS. Was a change in thermohaline circulation responsible for the little ice age? *Proceedings of the National Academy of Science* 2000; 97: 1339–42.

21 Intergovernmental Panel on Climate Change. *Third Assessment Report*, vol II. Cambridge: Cambridge University Press, 2001.

22 Various studies associating the El Niño–Southern Oscillation with malaria oubtbreaks have been reported by Menno Bouma. See, for example, Bouma MJ, van der Kaay HJ. The El Niño Southern Oscillation and the historic malaria epidemics on the Indian subcontinent and Sri Lanka: an early warning system for future epidemics? *Tropical Medicine and International Health* 1996; 1: 86–96. The idea of such climatic warnings has a long history. Robert Plot, Secretary to the (UK) Royal Society, analysed weather observations in 1683–84 and concluded that if the same observations were made 'in many foreign and remote parts at the same time' we would 'probably in time thereby learn to be forewarned certainly of divers emergencies (such as heats, colds, dearths, plagues, and other epidemical distempers)'. For a general review, see Kovats, R.S. El Niño and human health. *Bulletin of the World Health Organization* 2000; 78: 1127–35.

23 Martens WJM, Kovats RS, Nijhof S, et al. Climate change and future populations at risk of malaria. *Global Environmental Change* 1999; 9 Supplement: S89–S107. An alternative approach to modelling eschews the use of widely accepted biological theory about the relationship of temperature and rainfall to malaria transmissibility, and relies on extrapolating the statistically observed relationship in today's world to a warmer and wetter future world. This approach makes some dubious assumptions that, for example, when northern China acquires the climatic conditions of Mediterranean Europe it will also acquire the same level of social/economic/technological modulation of malaria transmission.

24 Colwell R. Global climate and infectious disease: the cholera paradigm. *Science* 1996; 274: 2025–31.

25 Parry MC, Rosenzweig C, Iglesias A, et al. Climate change and global food security: a new assessment. *Global Environmental Change* 1999; 9 Supplement: S51–S67.

26 Dyson T. Prospects for feeding the world. *British Medical Journal* 1999; 319: 988–91.

27 de Gruijl F. Health effects from the sun's ultraviolet radiation, and ozone as a stratospheric sunscreen. *Global Change and Human Health* 2000; 1: 26–40.

28 Shindell DT, Rind D, Lonergan P. Increased polar stratospheric ozone losses and delayed eventual recovery owing to increasing greenhouse gas concentrations. *Nature* 1998; 392: 589–29. An additional worry is that, at warmer temperature, more water vapour will accumulate in the stratosphere and that this will form polar stratospheric clouds – the medium upon which the ozone-destroying reaction takes place and which can also remove the naturally present nitric acid molecules that scavenge the potentially ozone-destroying chlorine radicals.

29 UN Environment Programme. *Scientific Assessment of Ozone Depletion: 1998.* Nairobi: UNEP, 1998.

30 Slaper H, Velders GJM, Daniel JS, et al. Estimates of ozone depletion and skin cancer incidence to examine the Vienna Convention achievements. *Nature* 1998; 384: 256–8.

31 Watson RT, Dixon JA, Hamburg SP, et al. *Protecting Our Planet. Securing our Future. Linkages Among Global Environmental Issues and Human Needs.* UNEP, USNASA, World Bank, 1998; Crutzen PJ, Stoermer EF. The 'Anthropocene'. *IGBP Newsletter* 2000; 41: 17–18.

32 Everyone's favourite is the apparently spectacular, and most recent, event of 65 million years ago when the dinosaurs and many other species were wiped out – creating a moment of opportunity for the mammal survivors, including our wide-eyed ancestors, the primitive primates. That holocaust may well have been due to a large asteroid crashing into the Yucatan Peninsula, with or without accompanying massive vulcanic eruptions in the Deccan region of northern India. The earlier mass extinctions were apparently due to great changes in world climate caused by critical tectonic reconfigurations of continents. The extinction that ushered in the Age of Dinosaurs, for example, and brought the Permian Period to a close around 240 million years ago, occurred as the Pangean continental conglomerate drifted over the southern pole, acquired a huge mantle of glaciation, and world temperatures plunged.

33 McNeill J. *Something New Under the Sun. An Environmental History of the Twentieth Century.* London: Allen Lane, 2000.

34 Myers N. Biodiversity's genetic library. In: Daily G. *Nature's Services. Societal Dependence on on Natural Ecosystems.* Washington, DC: Island Press, 1997, pp. 255–73.

35 However, genetic resistance has already begun to emerge to this plant-manufactured environmentally friendly pesticide. Ominously, the resistance gene appears to be a dominant, not recessive, gene. This would mean that it cannot be deliberately diluted by swamping the resistant organisms with susceptible breeding mates.

36 In Britain, many species of wild bees are declining as natural habitat is eliminated. For example, as farmland, industry and paved roads extend, the red clover from which the bumble-bee derives its sustenance is becoming much more sparse. On an international scale,

the Varroa mite that naturally parasitises the Asian bees (*Apis cerano*) has now entered populations of European bees (*Apis mellifera*) and is decimating many of the hive populations.

37 Mooney H, Hobbs R. (eds.) *Invasive Species in a Changing World.* Washington, DC: Island Press, 2000.

38 Crosby A. *Ecological Imperialism. The Biological Expansion of Europe, 900–1900.* Cambridge: Cambridge University Press (Canto edn), 1986.

39 Meyer WB . *Human Impact on the Earth.* Cambridge: Cambridge University Press, 1996, pp. 76–7.

40 See also chapter 5. Most of the statistics are negative: for example, the catch from the north Atlantic and southeast Atlantic fisheries peaked three decades ago and has declined by over 60% since then.

41 A prion, as we saw in chapter 4, is a rogue molecule that can induce malformation in other normal molecules produced by the non-mutated version of the same gene. Thus, the prion 'replicates'. Hence, if an exogenous prion (from ingested meat) enters the cells of brain, it can subvert the normal prion protein molecules. Groups of affected brain cells then die. The irony is that the normal prion molecule is actually one of the brain's protective devices, acting to neutralise the damage of oxidative free radicals.

42 In 1997, for example, research in the Netherlands revealed that people living near turkey farms harboured drug-resistant enterococci, a diarrhoeal disease organism. Since vancomycin is one of the dwindling minority of antibiotics still useable against multi-drug-resistant bacteria, this finding has serious implications.

43 Lovelock J. *Gaia.* Oxford: Oxford University Press, 1989.

44 Margulis L. Quoted in Capra F. *The Web of Life.* New York: Anchor Books, 1996, p. 106.

45 UN Environment Programme. *Global Environment 2000.* London: Earthscan, 1999.

11 Health and disease: an ecological perspective

1 Turner J. Introduction. In: Shepard P. *Traces of an Omnivore.* Washington, DC: Island Press, 1996.

2 Loh J, Randers J, MacGillivray A, et al. *Living Planet Report.* London: Earthscan, 1998.

3 Corwin EHL (ed.) *Ecology of Health.* The New York Academy of Medicine Institute of Public Health. New York: Commonwealth Fund, 1949. The British epidemiologist Jerry Morris, in his seminal book *The Uses of Epidemiology.* Edinburgh and London: E&S Livingston, 1957, asks what social changes underlie the observable biological changes that are the manifestations of altered states of health.

4 Kreiger N. Theories for social epidemiology in the 21st century: an ecosocial perspective. *International Journal of Epidemiology,* 2001; 30 (August).

5 Lee K, Dodgson R. Globalisation and cholera: implications for global governance. *Global Governance* 2000; 6: 213–36.

6 Evans-Pritchard EE, Gillies E (eds.) *Witchcraft, Oracles and Magic Among the Azande.* Oxford: Oxford University Press, 1976.

7 Hippocrates. Airs, waters and places. An essay on the influence of climate, water supply and situation on health. In: Lloyd GER (ed.) *Hippocratic Writings.* London: Penguin, 1978, p. 148.

8 The historical roots of our ecological crisis. *Science* 1967; 155: 1203–7. See also n. 25 in ch. 1.

9 Moore SE, Cole TJ, Poskitt EM, et al. Season of birth predicts mortality in rural Gambia. *Nature* 1997; 388: 434–6.

10 McMichael AJ, Powles JW. Human numbers, environment, sustainability and health. *British Medical Journal* 1999; 319: 977–80.

11 Levins R. Dealing with uncertainty. *Ecosystem Health* 1995; 1: 47–57.

12 Wilson EO. *Consilience. The Unity of Knowledge.* New York: Alfred A Knopf, 1998.

13 Kaufman S. *At Home in the Universe. The Search for Laws of Complexity.* London: Viking, 1995.

14 Funtowicz SO, Ravetz JR. *Uncertainty and Quality in Science for Policy* Dordrecht: Kluwer, 1990.

15 Barbara Kingsolver. *The Poisonwood Bible.* London: Faber and Faber, 1999, pp. 524–5.

16 Dubos R. *Mirage of Health: Utopias, Progress, and Biological Change.* New York: Harper and Row, 1959.

17 Hughes CC, Hunter JM. Disease and 'development' in Africa. *Social Science and Medicine* 1970; 3: 443–93.

18 White GF, Bradley DJ, White AU. *Drawers of Water.* Chicago: University of Chicago Press, 1972.

19 Pépin J. Zaïre (Congo): resurgence of trypanosomiasis ('patients within borders'). *Lancet* 1997; 349: sIII 10–11.

20 Morse SS. Factors in the emergence of infectious diseases. *Emerging Infectious Diseases* 1995; 1: 7–15.

21 Harb M, Faris R, Gad AM, et al. The resurgence of lymphatic filariasis in the Nile delta. *Bulletin of the World Health* Organization 1993; 71: 49–54.

22 This proposition was the centrepiece of the 1998 annual World Health Report of WHO (Geneva: WHO, 1998). See also: Gwatkin DR. Health inequalities and the health of the poor. *Bulletin of the World Health Organization* 2000; 78: 3–17; Farmer P. Social inequalities and emerging infectious diseases. *Emerging Infectious Diseases* 1996; 2: 258–69.

23 The lines of argument are well presented in: Pearce N. Traditional epidemiology, modern epidemiology, and public health. *American Journal of Public Health* 1996; 86: 678–83; and Rothman KJ, Adami HO, Trichopoulos D. Should the mission of epidemiology include the eradication of poverty? *Lancet* 1998; 352: 810–13.

24 McMichael PD. *Development and Social Change: A Global Perspective.* Thousand Oaks, CA: Pine Forge, 2000; Saul JR. *The Unconscious Civilisation.* Concord, Ont.: Anansi, 1995.

25 McMichael AJ, Beaglehole R. The changing global context of public health. *Lancet* 2000; 356: 495–9.

26 Gray, J. *False Dawn. The Delusions of Global Capitalism.* London: Granta, 1998.

27 Wang J, et al. *Measuring Country Performance on Health: Selected Indicators for 115 Countries.*

Washington, DC: The World Bank, 1999. The estimates are based on an analysis of data from 115 low and middle-income countries.

12 Footprints to the future: treading less heavily

1 Natural selection has been largely eliminated in wealthy societies. The coevolution between humans and microbes presumably continues at low level everywhere, and at higher levels in poorer populations with high death rates in early life. Meanwhile, the fertility rate differences between major regions results in a change in the gene frequencies that determine humankind's more superficial biological features (facial form, skin pigmentation, etc.). However, since the difference in fertility rates between populations, and to a large extent within populations, is now primarily due to cultural and economic factors, it imparts no systematic 'fitness'-related selection in relation to biological attributes. It was ever thus.

2 Vitousek PM, Mooney HA, Lubchenco J, Melillo JM. Human domination of Earth's ecosystems. *Science* 1997; 277: 494–9.

3 Crutzen PJ, Stoermer E. The 'Anthropocene'. *IGBP Newsletter* 2000; 41: 17–18.

4 Crabbé P, Holland A, Ryszkowski L, Westra L (eds.) *Implementing Ecological Integrity. Restoring Regional and Global Environmental and Human Health.* Dordrecht: Kluwer, 1999.

5 Lander ES, Weinberg RA. Journey to the Center of Biology. *Science* 2000; 287: 1777–82.

6 And this in a twenty-first-century world in which Samuel Huntington foresees a 'clash of civilisations' arising from differing philosophical and religious value systems, not from competing political ideologies or imperial ambitions. See: Huntington S. *The Clash of Civilisations and the Remaking of World Order.* New York: Pocket Books, 1998.

7 Wilson EO. *Consilience. The Unity of Knowledge.* New York: Alfred A Knopf, 1998.

8 Caldwell LK. *Between Two Worlds. Science, the Environmental Movement and Policy Choice.* Cambridge: Cambridge University Press, 1990.

9 Costanza R, Daly H, Folke C, et al. *BioScience* 2000; 50: 149–55.

10 Wilson EO. *The Diversity of Life.* New York: Norton, 1992.

11 Hardin G. The tragedy of the commons. *Science* 1968; 162: 1243–8.

12 Dasgupta PS, Folke C, Maler K-G. The environmental resource base and human welfare. In: Lindahl-Kiessling K, Landberg H (eds.) *Population, Economic Development and the Environment.* Oxford: Oxford University Press, 1995, pp. 25–50.

13 Dasgupta PS. Population, poverty and the local environment. *Scientific American* 1995 (February): 40–5.

14 World Commission on Environment and Development. *Our Common Future.* Oxford: Oxford University Press, 1987.

15 Medawar P. Quoted in Dubos R. *Man Adapting.* New Haven, CT: Yale University Press, 1965, p. 433.

16 Cassen R, Visaria P. India: looking ahead to one and a half billion people. *British Medical Journal* 1999; 319: 995–7.

17 Cohen J. *How Many People Can the Earth Support.* New York: Norton, 1995.

18 Willey D. An optimum world population. *Medicine, Conflict and Survival* 2000; 16: 72–94.

19 Rees W. Revisiting carrying capacity: area-based indicators of sustainability. *Population and Environment* 1996; 17: 195–215.

20 Daily GC. *Nature's Services. Societal Dependence on Natural Ecosystems.* Washington, DC: Island Press, 1997.

21 Wackernagel M, Rees W. *Our Ecological Footprint. Reducing Human Impact on the Earth.* Gabriola Island, BC, Canada: New Society Publishers, 1996.

22 A figure of 3 hectares per person has been estimated by David Willey of the Optimum Population Trust (UK), on the basis of land needs for agriculture, pasture, forest, energy, urban development and a small 'screw-up' factor. See Willey (2000), n. 18.

23 Virchow R. Quoted in Dubos R. *Man Adapting.* New Haven, CT: Yale University Press, 1965, p. 393.

24 Vitousek PM, Ehrlich PR, Ehrlich AH, Matson PA. Human appropriation of the products of photosynthesis. *BioScience* 1986; 36: 368–73.

Index

Numbers in italics indicate *tables* or *figures*. Notes are shown by the page number followed by 'n' and the chapter and note numbers e.g. 370 (n2.11); 'p' refers to the preface.

CPSIA information can be obtained
at www.ICGtesting.com
Printed in the USA
LVHW08*2111221018
594409LV00010B/153/P